Sexually Transmitted Infections: Advances in Diagnosis and Management

Sexually Transmitted Infections: Advances in Diagnosis and Management

Edited by Cyrus Gibson

STATES
ACADEMIC PRESS
www.statesacademicpress.com

States Academic Press,
109 South 5th Street,
Brooklyn, NY 11249, USA

Visit us on the World Wide Web at:
www.statesacademicpress.com

ISBN: 978-1-63989-481-9

Cataloging-in-Publication Data

Sexually transmitted infections : advances in diagnosis and management / edited by Cyrus Gibson.
p. cm.
Includes bibliographical references and index.
ISBN 978-1-63989-481-9
1. Sexually transmitted diseases. 2. Sexually transmitted diseases--Diagnosis.
3. Sexually transmitted diseases--Treatment. I. Gibson, Cyrus.
RC200 .S49 2022
616.951--dc23

Table of Contents

Preface

Sexually Transmitted Infections (STIs) are the infections that commonly spread by sexual activity. There are no initial symptoms of sexually transmitted infections, which increase the risk of passing the infections to others. The signs and symptoms of these infections comprise of pelvic pain, ulcers around the genitals, and vaginal and penile discharge. Many different types of parasites, bacteria and viruses can be transmitted sexually. Trichomoniasis is an example of a parasitic STI. Bacterial sexually transmitted infections include gonorrhea, syphilis and chlamydia. HIV/AIDS, genital herpes and genital warts are viral STIs. Some sexually transmitted infections can spread by non-sexual contacts such as breastfeeding, during childbirth, and contact with the donor tissue and blood. The objective of this book is to give a general view of the sexually transmitted infections. It provides significant information on these infections to help develop a good understanding. This book is a vital tool for all researching and studying this field.

This book is a result of research of several months to collate the most relevant data in the field.

When I was approached with the idea of this book and the proposal to edit it, I was overwhelmed. It gave me an opportunity to reach out to all those who share a common interest with me in this field. I had 3 main parameters for editing this text:

1. Accuracy - The data and information provided in this book should be up-to-date and valuable to the readers.
2. Structure - The data must be presented in a structured format for easy understanding and better grasping of the readers.
3. Universal Approach - This book not only targets students but also experts and innovators in the field, thus my aim was to present topics which are of use to all.

Thus, it took me a couple of months to finish the editing of this book.

I would like to make a special mention of my publisher who considered me worthy of this opportunity and also supported me throughout the editing process. I would also like to thank the editing team at the back-end who extended their help whenever required.

Editor

1

Female Infertility Associated to *Chlamydia trachomatis* Infection

Agustín Luján, Silvina Fili and María Teresa Damiani

Abstract

Chlamydia trachomatis (CT) is the most common agent of bacterial sexually transmitted infections, both in developed and developing countries. It clearly constitutes a major burden on public health. Screening programs and current research are mainly focused on decreasing the high incidence of chlamydial infections as well as their associated morbidity.

The greater clinical impact of CT infections occurs in women of reproductive age. Acute CT infections are often associated to urethritis, mucopurulent cervicitis, endometritis, salpingitis, and pelvic inflammatory disease (PID). A vast proportion of CT infections are likely underestimated because of their asymptomatic clinical course. This leads to repeat and chronic infections, which have deleterious impact on the female reproductive health. Among the complications of the CT chronic infections are PID, ectopic pregnancy, preterm birth, tubal obstruction and female infertility, which are of great interest in the reproduction field.

Keywords: *Chlamydia trachomatis*, intracellular pathogens, bacterial sexually transmitted infections, tubal obstruction, female infertility

1. Introduction

Chlamydia trachomatis (CT) is the most frequent bacterial agent causing sexually transmitted infections (STIs) worldwide. According to the latest World Health Organization (WHO) report, approximately 100 million new infections occur annually [1]. According to the Centre for Disease Control (CDC), around 1.4 million new CT cases were reported in 2013, only in the United States [2].

In this chapter, we briefly present the current knowledge about the cell biology of the bacteria, reviewing the mechanisms of establishment of CT intracellular niche, the inducers of persistent infections, and the pathogen factors that may be involved in the damage of female reproductive tract. Then, we analyze the host factors that may contribute to the development of infertility, mainly immune response and genetic predisposition, hormonal status, and sexual behavior. Undiagnosed and untreated infections, repeat and persistent infections, and coinfections are likely responsible for the detrimental sequelae on woman fertility of CT pathogenesis.

This chapter specially focuses on the consequences of chronic diseases after CT infections, mainly pelvic inflammatory disease, tubal infertility, and adverse pregnancy outcome, which are of therapeutic interest in the reproduction field.

2. The bacteria: Intracellular life cycle, *Chlamydia trachomatis* serovars and virulence factors

2.1. Chlamydial developmental cycle and intracellular niche

CT is a highly evolved pathogen that has a reduced genome, first sequenced by Stephens and collaborators in 1998. Its chromosome consists of approximately one million base pairs and encodes for up to 600 proteins [3]. Analysis of chlamydial genes reveals that this bacterium heavily depends on host cell for nutrition and replication, indicating a complex evolution for adaptation to an obligate intracellular lifestyle.

CT has tropism for genital mucosal epithelium, which promotes its own uptake into non-phagocytic cells. Chlamydial infection and propagation rely upon a unique biphasic life cycle that begins by contact of infectious, environmentally resistant, elementary bodies (EBs) with the apical surface of the epithelial cell. Several mechanisms are involved in the invasion of host cell, likely parasite-specified phagocytosis and receptor-mediated endocytosis [4]. Multiple receptors have been proposed to mediate the interaction between the EB and the host cell, among them, the mannose receptor, the mannose 6-phosphate receptor, and the estrogen receptor [5]. Other host molecules such as heparan sulfate proteoglycans [6,7], and protein disulfide isomerase also participate in EB binding to the eukaryotic cells [8]. Concomitantly, multiple bacterial adhesins and ligands such as glycosaminoglycan [9], the major outer membrane protein (MOMP) [10], OmcB [11], and PmpD [12] facilitate EB attachment to host cells. Translocated actin-recruiting phosphoprotein (TARP) is a bacterial protein that nucleates actin and promotes host cell cytoskeleton remodeling to force bacterium uptake [13–15].

The infectious EBs enter the host cell in membrane-bound vesicles that travel toward the perinucleus and fuse to form a single vacuole termed the inclusion. Once inside this modified phagosome, EBs differentiate into metabolically active but non-infectious reticulate bodies (RBs) that are the replicative bacterial forms. RBs asynchronously multiply by binary fission within the confines of the growing inclusion. After numerous rounds of replication, RBs re-differentiate back into infectious EBs to be ready for spreading to adjacent cells [16,17]. The ability of CT to cycle between resting and replicating organisms accounts for a drawback in the eradication of this intracellular pathogen. Finally, the infectious bacteria are released by two independent mechanisms, the host cell lysis, or the extrusion of the inclusion [18]. A scheme of chlamydial developmental life cycle is shown in Figure 1.

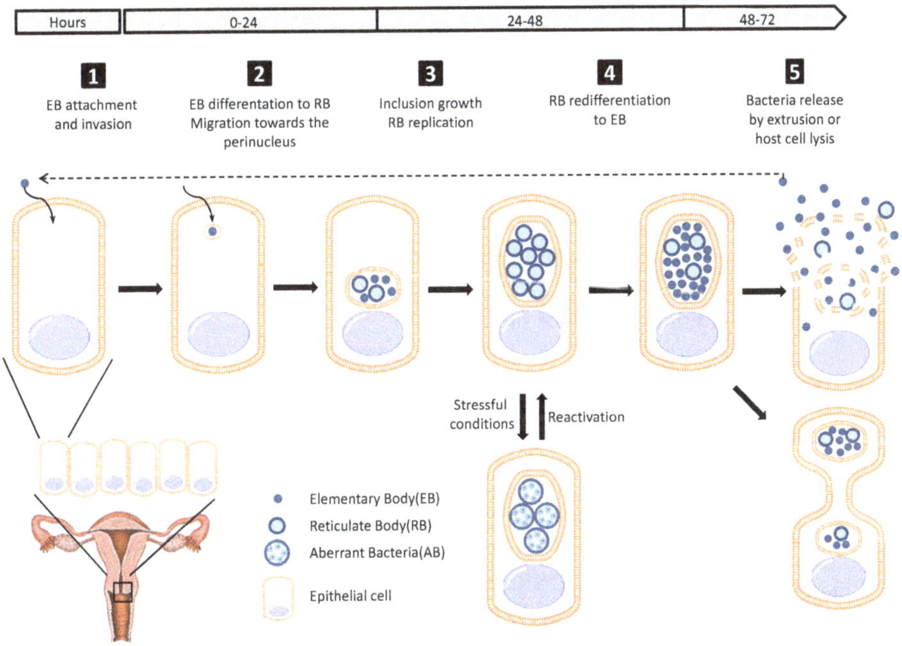

Figure 1. *Chlamydia trachomatis* developmental cycle. Chlamydial infection begins with attachment of the infectious bacterial form, the elementary body (EB) to uncharacterized host cell receptors. Signal transduction events are triggered, and EBs entry into the host cell in small vesicles. These CT-containing vesicles are actively modified by the bacteria; they travel toward the perinucleus and fuse to form a single vacuole named "the inclusion". Once internalized, EB differentiates into the replicative bacterial form, the reticulate body (RB), which multiplies by binary fission. At the end, RBs re-differentiate to EBs that are released by host cell lysis or extrusion of the inclusion. The whole cycle is completed in 40–72 hours. In a stressful environment, RBs enter a latent stage where it persists until more favorable growing conditions. These aberrant bacteria (AB) are present in persistent and chronic infections.

In response to stress, CT enters into a low replicative viable state that is termed "persistent or aberrant bacterial form", which is able to resume normal replication as soon as conditions are again favorable. Among the inducers of the persistent bacterial state stand the sphingolipid deprivation and tryptophan lack, the presence of interferon gamma (IFN-γ), or certain antibiotics such as penicillin. The evasion strategy has been linked to the capacity of these bacteria to cause latent and chronic infections. Thus, the onset of the infection is generally not detected and re-infection may occur, especially when infected couples are involved. Furthermore, the fact that CT clearance is rarely followed up, combined with the ability of this pathogen to persist, contributes to the occurrence of long-term infections [19].

Undoubtedly, an essential issue to chlamydial growth and development is the establishment of its intracellular niche. Early chlamydial gene expression is required to inclusion generation, to avoid immune system surveillance, and to hijack host cell functions [20]. These bacteria actively modify the inclusion membrane by exclusion or recruitment of selected host proteins, mainly Rab proteins, the master controllers of intracellular traffic [16,21]. Increasing evidence points out that the invading bacteria subvert trafficking not only to circumvent the lysosomal degradative route but also to facilitate the delivery of host nutrients to the growing inclusion [17,22]. As soon as the chlamydial inclusion is formed, it dissociates from the classical phagocytic pathway and barely interacts with endocytic vesicles [23]. Instead, chlamydial inclusion intersects Golgi-derived vesicles [24–27], multivesicular bodies [28], and lipid droplets [29,30]. By this strategy, these bacteria take over the infected cell for sphingomyelin, cholesterol, and neutral lipid acquisition like pirates [31–34]. In addition, CTs possess other mechanisms, such as transporter molecules, finely adapted to acquire amino acids, nucleotides, and energy from the host cell [22,35–38]. At present, the strategies developed by CTs to re-route intracellular trafficking and to co-opt host cell functions for their benefit are being actively studied.

2.2. Bacterial genotypes and virulence factors

Different strains of CT have been described based on genome sequencing and the antigenic properties of the major outer membrane protein (MOMP) [39]. There are more than 20 distinct serovars (serologically variant strains) of CT currently identified, on the basis of monoclonal antibody-based typing assays [40–42]. In general, CTs have been grouped into three main pathobiotypes: ocular infections (serovars A to C), sexually transmitted diseases (D to K), and lymphogranuloma venereum (L_1 to L_3). Serovars A, B, and C have tropism for the ocular epithelium, causing from acute conjunctivitis to trachoma, a serious eye disease endemic in Africa and Asia that is characterized by chronic conjunctivitis and can lead to infectious blindness. Serovars D through K have emerged as the major causing agents of sexually transmitted diseases. They preferentially infect squamocolumnar epithelial cells of female reproductive system and the male genitourinary tract. E and D serovars are isolated from genital tract infections with the most frequency worldwide. Occasionally, they cause conjunctivitis or pneumonia in newborns infected during labor. Serovars L1 to L3 are responsible for a systemic illness, the lymphogranuloma venereum that is associated with genital ulcer disease in tropical countries [43,44] (Table 1).

Chlamydia genotyping is useful to determine tissue tropism [45–47]. Several studies attempted to directly link disease severity with CT serovars; however, they often failed because of small number of samples and high variability in results [48]. Intensive research is conducted to confidently associate CT serotypes to higher pathogenic potential, clinical course, or disease outcome. Nevertheless, at present, bacterial ability to ascend and colonize female upper reproductive tract is not clearly associated to a particular CT serovar.

On the other hand, CT gene polymorphisms determine distinct antigenic challenge to the immune system [49]. Certain bacterial polymorphisms may induce an altered immune response [50]. In consequence, they are able to cause immunological disorders, especially in susceptible individuals. Chlamydial infections often precede the initiation of autoimmune diseases, and frequently, these bacteria are found within autoimmune lesions. Bacterial proteins similar to host self-proteins might be the underlying cause of diverse autoimmune diseases [51,52]. This molecular mimicry may elicit an immune response to both self and microbial proteins. Chlamydial heat shock protein 60, DNA primase, and OmcB proteins represent the strongest cases for molecular mimicry [53]. The most frequent autoimmune diseases connected to chlamydial infections are intestinal inflammatory pathologies and rheumatic or connective-tissue diseases [54,55]. Further research is required to unravel the molecular machinery involved in the complex pathogen-host cell interaction.

Chlamydial strains and clinical diseases			
Serovars	Host	Acute	Chronic
A–C	Newborns / Both sexes	Conjunctivitis	Trachoma
D–K	Newborn	Ophthalmia neonatorum	Neonatal pneumonia
	Men	Urethritis	Proctitis Epididymitis
	Women	Urethritis Cervicitis	Mucopurulent cervicitis Pelvic inflammatory disease Tubal infertility Ectopic pregnancy Premature rupture of membranes Chorioamnionitis Premature delivery Puerperal infection Cervical neoplasia
L_{1-3}	Both sexes		Lymphogranuloma venereum
Different serovars and bacterial polymorphism	Both sexes		Autoimmune diseases Reactive arthritis Collagenopathies Reiter´s syndrome Inflammatory bowel disease Crohn´s disease

Table 1. Chlamydial serovars, tissue tropism and clinical diseases. Acute and chronic pathologies occur in men, women and newborns following CT infections. Serovars A to C have tropism for ocular epithelium, causing from acute conjunctivitis to infectious blindness or trachoma. Serovars D to K infect epithelial cells of the genitourinary system, generating a broad range of acute and chronic pathologies that damage reproductive tissue and may infect newborns during labor. Serovars L_{1-3} cause lymphogranuloma venereum. Several autoimmune diseases are associated to diverse CT strains.

Several putative virulence factors have been postulated, including the polymorphic outer membrane autotransporter family of proteins (pmp), type III secretion system (TTSS) effectors, a large cytotoxin, and stress response proteins may contribute to increase the CT-associated pathogenicity. Pmp proteins are strongly immunogenic and trigger pro-inflammatory cytokine responses [56]. Chlamydial TTSS effectors mediate the interaction with the host as they are injected to the cytoplasm and alter host cell functioning [57–59]. Important TTSS effectors are the inclusion (Inc) proteins that are bacterial proteins present at the inclusion membrane. For instance, IncA promotes the fusion of individual CT-containing vesicles to form a single inclusion [60,61]. Natural IncA bacterial mutants are associated with reduced virulence [62]. Another TTSS effector is TARP, mentioned in the previous section, as a bacterial protein that favors CT internalization via an actin recruiting mechanism [34,63]. Additionally, a chlamydial cytotoxin glycosylates the eukaryotic protein Rac1, and thereby induces actin reorganization and promotes the invasion of host cell [64,65]. Chlamydial glycolipid exoantigens [66] and the lipopolysaccharide [67] may constitute additional virulence factors. Other proteins encoded by the cryptic plasmid or related to the ability of the bacteria to survive under stressful metabolic conditions such as iron or tryptophan deprivation are thought to increase virulence and pathogenicity [68,69]. Chlamydial stress proteins, GroEL and GroES, may activate toll-like receptors and trigger a potent inflammatory response, injuring host reproductive tissues [70–73].

In addition to CT serovars and virulence molecules, other bacterial factors may be involved in the pathogenicity and chlamydial infection outcome, such as the pathogen load, route of infection, bacterial ability to enter persistent state, ascension capacity and strength to colonize genital upper tract, resistance to antibiotic treatment, and so on. Further studies are needed to determine the contribution of each bacterial factor to the development of severe damage on the female reproductive system.

3. The host: Immunological and genetic factors, age and hormonal status, and sexual behavior

3.1. Immunological and genetic factors

An important issue that contributes to CT pathogenesis is its remarkable ability to avoid the host immune system. Several strategies are displayed by these bacteria to prevent immune degradation, such as its intracellular lifestyle, its ability to escape from phagolysosomal pathway, its resistance to interferon gamma (IFN-γ), among others lesser known bacterial molecules. Actually, host immune response has opposite results on chlamydial infection outcome. A low immune response generates a suitable environment for pathogen colonization, while a strong immune response could lead to excessive inflammation and tissue damage. Pathogens own characteristics in conjunction with host genetic susceptibility are important in determining the severity of the illness.

At the site of invasion, an intense inflammation occurs, attracting different types of cells, such as macrophages, neutrophils, T and B lymphocytes, natural killers, and dendritic cells. Locally, there is an increased production of reactive oxygen species (ROS) that produces oxidative DNA damage, lipid peroxidation, energy depletion, modulation of gene expression, and proteins synthesis. Oxidative stress provokes pathologic changes that harm reproductive tissues. In addition, a broad collection of pro- and anti-inflammatory cytokines are released including IFN-γ, tumor necrosis factor (TNF-α), interleukin (IL) IL-1β, IL-2, IL-3, IL-4, IL-5, IL-6, IL-8, IL-10, IL-12, IL-13, IL-17, IL-22, vascular endothelial growth factor (VEGF), granulocyte-macrophage colony-stimulating factor (GM-CSF), and lactoferrin. These mediators trigger cellular inflammatory responses that mediate direct damage to the tissues [74,75]. Most of them are involved in the pathophysiology of tubal infertility, birth defects, and miscarriage [76].

In addition to the inflammatory response, CT infection evokes vigorous local and systemic humoral and cell-mediated immune responses. Several CT-specific antibodies, IgG isotype rather than secretory IgA, are found in circulation and in the cervicovaginal fluid of the female genital tract. These antibodies can neutralize chlamydial antigens; nevertheless, they do not assure resolution of the infection. Antibodies toward the bacterial MOMP protein are prevalent in primary chlamydial infections, whereas antibodies against CT-hsp10 and hsp60 are present in recurrent or persistent infections and correlate with severe sequelae such as tubal infertility, ectopic pregnancy, and PID [77–79]. Regarding the cell-mediated immune response, the T-helper lymphocytes type 1 (Th1) secrete IFN-γ, IL-2, and IL-12 and play a role in the resolution of infection [80,81]. On the other hand, the T-helper lymphocytes type 2 (Th2), which support the humoral immune response, produces IL-4, IL-5, IL-6, and IL-10 and participates in the developing tubal scarring [82]. The inflammatory response occurs, at the same extent, in both initial and repeat infections, whereas T-cell responses are predominant in the latter ones [80,83].

Actually, host immune response is considered as one of the most important determinants in chlamydial infection outcome. A delicate balance between pro- and anti-inflammatory cytokines is needed to clear infection, avoiding tissue injuring. At this point, host genetic predisposition is a major player of pathology and CT-related infertility development [84].

Host genetic polymorphisms may encode aberrant or dysfunctional toll-like receptors (TLR) and nucleotide-binding oligomerization domain proteins (NOD) that do not appropriately recognize CT. These individuals have an impaired bacterial clearance and a high risk to develop an aberrant immune response, favoring CT persistence [85–88]. Identifying host genetic factors and bacterial virulence factors involved in immunoevasion and immunopathology remains a major priority in research for preventing chlamydial infection and its sequelae. Furthermore, the understanding of local innate and adaptive immune responses and their actors along the genital tract will be crucial for designing new therapeutic approaches and for developing a protective vaccine.

3.2. Age and hormonal status

CT preferentially targets young women at reproductive age. It has been reported that the highest incidence occurs in women between 16 to 24 years [89]. Therefore, the impact on female reproductive health is very important. Notwithstanding younger women are at higher risk of contracting a chlamydial infection, the rates of developing PID increase with age, being more frequent in the 30 to 40 decade [90]. After menopause, the frequency of chlamydial infections decreases substantially [91].

Accordingly, estrogen and progesterone are important for the establishment of chlamydial infection. Furthermore, estrogen receptors have been involved in the internalization of CT [92,93]. Sex hormones affect the clinical outcome of chlamydial infections; thus, follicle stimulating hormone (FSH), luteinizing hormone (LH), estradiol (E2), progesterone (P4), and prolactin (PRL) are involved not only in the establishment of chlamydial infection but also in the development of sequelae on reproductive tissue [94,95]. Additionally, oral contraceptive use was found to be a risk factor for CT infection. Several studies have attempted to elucidate the relation between the hormonal status at the time of infection and its contribution to tubal occlusion in genital chlamydial infection. Unfortunately, the role of sex steroids in infection outcome is far from being fully understood. Sex hormones have been shown to modulate immune responses and to have antioxidant effects in the female genital tract [96–98]. However, the mechanisms by which sex hormones may benefit or impair the colonization of genital tissues by pathogenic microorganisms should be further investigated.

3.3. Sexual behavior and other host factors

Sexual initiation at young age and a higher number of sexual partners are associated with increased risk of CT infection [99]. In a similar manner, having sex without protection favors CT contagion. This sexual behavior is also associated with higher incidence of sexually transmitted pathogens such as *Neisseria gonorrhoeae, Candida albicans, Human Immunodeficiency Virus,* among others [100–103]. Taken together, unsafe and high-risk sexual conduct is linked to impairment of women reproductive health, and particularly to tubal infertility. As it has been previously mentioned, some women have a genotypic predisposition to develop an abnormal immune response and severe inflammation following CT infection. In these women, there is a high rate of tubal obstruction and CT-related infertility, independent of sexual behavior [84].

In general, multiple sexual partners and unsafe intercourse increase the risk of CT recurrent infections and coinfection with other sexually transmitted pathogens. Thereby, the high chance to suffer repeat and chronic infections that target women reproductive tissue raises the infertility-associated pathologies.

4. Pathogen-host interplay: Establishment of latent, repeat, and persistent infections and coinfections

CT survival and replication heavily hinge on host cells. In fact, CT has evolved in relationship with human cells. However, little is known about the molecular basis of CT interaction with host epithelia and immune system. An increasing number of bacterial and host factors interplay for the establishment of chlamydial infection and determine the pathologic profile and clinical disease outcome. A simple scheme is shown in Figure 2 summarizing the main CT and host factors that jointly with environmental factors and the failure in diagnosis and treatment, lead to unsolved, latent, and long-term chlamydial infections.

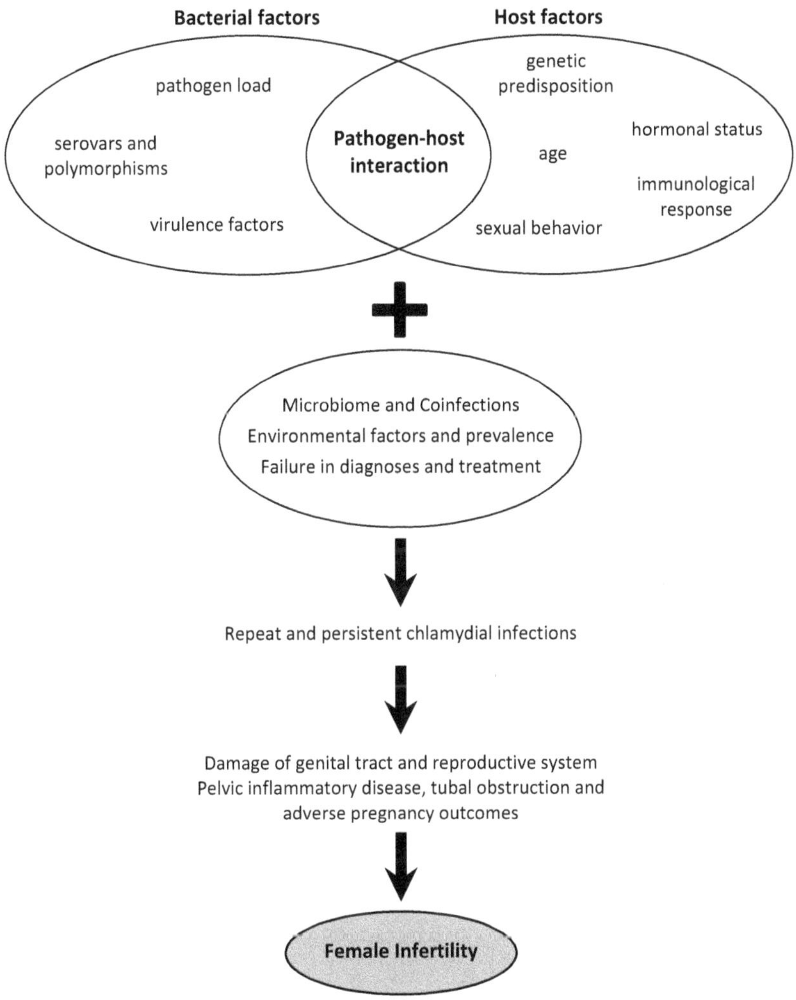

Figure 2. Bacterial and host factors involved in the development of female infertility. Bacterial factors such as CT genotypes and serovars, virulence factors, and pathogen burden, in conjunction with, host factors such as genetic predisposition and immune response, age and hormonal status, and sexual behavior participate in the establishment of the infection and pathology. Other elements that take part in the development of CT-related diseases are microbiome and coinfections with other sexually transmitted pathogens, environmental factors, and local prevalence, and most importantly, the failure in diagnosis and treatment of chlamydial infections. Taken together, these factors sustain repeat and persistent chlamydial infections that damage female reproductive health.

Microbiome (microbial flora present at the genital tract) and the presence of other sexually transmitted pathogens may be important for the colonization of reproductive tissue and the establishment of chlamydial infection. The presence of lactobacilli in the vagina confers protection against the acquisition of chlamydial infection [104]. In contrast, indole-generating bacteria present in the microbiome or bacterial vaginosis allow CT to synthesize tryptophan, and consequently, to avoid the anti-chlamydial activity of IFN-γ [45,65]. Coinfections are more frequent in vaginosis and women with high-risk sexual behavior [100]. Clearly, coinfections exacerbate host immune response and inflammation; therefore, they favor scarring and sequelae on female reproductive system and increase the likelihood of tubal infertility.

The worst scenarios involve silent and latent infections that underline chronic persistent chlamydial infection and frequent re-infections [1]. Chlamydial infections may persist in the female upper genital tract for months in the absence of treatment. They are often asymptomatic or alternate quiescent stages with periods of clinical manifestations [105]. Actually, chronic chlamydial infections may be because of the reactivation of asymptomatic latently infected deep-seated cells. The presence of aberrant bacterial forms responsible for chlamydial persistence constitutes a long-time challenge to the immune system. Host immunopathological response can damage the fallopian tube and generate female infertility [65,92].

Reinfections, persistent infections, and treatment failure account for repeat infections that represent a substantial proportion of the chlamydial infections detected annually [106]. Repeat infection is not the sole determinant of severe genital tract pathology and sequelae. However, repeat infection increases the risk of developing tubal obstruction and female infertility [76].

Increasing evidence indicates that long-term persistence of viable aberrant chlamydial organisms within host cells is associated with inflammatory and autoimmune diseases in extragenital tissues.

In definitive, the pathogen-host interplay and the concurrency of exogenous factors appear to be related to CT-induced immunopathology. In spite of the substantial worldwide impact of chlamydial disease, the bacterial and host factors that result in infertility are still not clear. Current efforts are focused on discovering what CT is doing to the host cells to prevent sequelae and undesired consequences of infection.

5. Mechanisms of pathogenicity and clinical course

CT infects both sexes; however, chlamydial infections constitute primarily a female health issue since the consequences are more damaging to the reproductive tissue in women than in men. In males, CT can infect urethra, epididymis, prostate, seminal vesicles, and testis. Usually, chlamydial infections are symptomatic, less frequent, and more easily eradicated in men than in women. Nevertheless, chlamydial infection in the male genitourinary tract might induce severe damage to seminiferous tubules, spermatogenesis, and sperm cells morphology that can result in impaired male fertility [107].

Here, we focus on chlamydial infections occurring in women. In first world countries, 3 to 5% of women younger than 30 years old will be infected by CT at any point in time [90,108]. And, in over 70% of the cases, CT infection of the female genitourinary tract is asymptomatic, spoiling the prevalence or incidence rates. Consequently, it is difficult to assess the incidence of sequelae, mainly PID, tubal obstruction, and female infertility, attributable to genital CT infection.

In women, CT is the major cause of mucopurulent cervicitis (MPC) and PID. Other manifestations of chlamydial infections are vaginitis, urethritis, salpingitis, endometritis, tubo-ovarian abscess, pelvic peritonitis, periappendicitis, and perihepatitis. The symptoms more frequently reported consist of abdominal pain, dysuria, vaginal itching, and abnormal vaginal discharge. However, the most important feature of chlamydial infection in the female genital tract is the occurrence of asymptomatic infection that remains subclinical for long periods in a high rate [109,110]. Asymptomatic ascending bacteria from the cervix may produce two groups of pathologies: (i) PID-associated complications such as chronic pelvic pain, tubal obstruction, and female infertility [111,112] and (ii) adverse pregnancy outcomes such as ectopic pregnancy, miscarriage, premature rupture of membranes, chrioamnionitis, preterm birth, stillbirths, and puerperal and neonatal infections [113–115].

General consensus in the medical community agrees that chlamydial PID is the most common preventable cause of tubal infertility and adverse pregnancy outcome [1]. However, the lack of systematic detection of the bacteria weakens these estimations, usually performed by analysis of a reduced number of cases. Approximately 20% of women with chlamydial lower genital tract infection will develop PID, 4% chronic pelvic pain, 3% tubal infertility, and 2% adverse pregnancy outcome [107]. In developing countries, the incidence and prevalence of CT infections and their harmful consequences on female reproductive tissue are not accurately known since CT infection is not routinely screened.

There is conclusive evidence that women who have suffered PID have higher risk to develop tubal infertility. A study demonstrated that 16.5% of women with abnormal laparoscopic findings likely resulting of acute PID failed to conceive, in comparison to 2.7% in control women; 10.8% developed tubal infertility, and 9.1% went through ectopic pregnancy. Therefore, PID increases the probability of permanent damage on female reproductive system. CT is the most common causing agent of PID; however, a drawback of this analysis is the lack of the identification of the infectious agent underlying the PID. Several randomized controlled trials to assess the value of CT screening found it helpful to reduce the incidence of PID among infected women [116–118]. The chance to develop tubal infertility after a single episode of PID is around 10% [112]. Furthermore, each episode of PID doubled the risk of tubal damage [119] independent of whether the infection was asymptomatic or not.

One of the most serious sequelae of PID and persistent chlamydial infections is the fibrosis and scarring obstruction of the fallopian tubes that leads to tubal infertility. However, the risk of tubal infertility due to CT infections is lower than PID incidence [76]. The proportion of tubal infertility among all causes of infertility varies from 40% in first-world countries to 85% in developing countries [1]. Undiagnosed and untreated chlamydial infections usually evolve to long-term persistent infections, in which chlamydial antigens chronically stimulate the host immune system. Abnormal humoral and cell-mediated immune responses and severe inflammation have been implicated in the development of immunopathological damage of fallopian tubes. Thus, the interaction between CT and the host becomes relevant for the illness outcome. However, the exact pathologic mechanism of CT-induced tubal damage and tubal infertility has not been elucidated yet.

In addition, acute and chronic maternal chlamydial infections constitute a significant risk factor for adverse pregnancy outcomes and newborns contagion. Untreated and persistent infections are strongly associated with ectopic pregnancy, which is the tubal development of the embryo and constitute the main cause of maternal mortality in the first trimester of pregnancy in developing countries. In addition, miscarriage, chrioamnionitis, low birth weight, stillbirth, premature rupture of membranes, and preterm birth are frequent pathological consequences of chlamydial infections [51,113,114]. Several mechanisms may contribute to the development of these pathologies, including direct fetal infection, placental damage, and severe puerperal maternal illness [120–124]. Nevertheless, the exact nature of chlamydial infection pathogenesis during pregnancy remains unexplained.

CT infections can also be vertically transmitted to newborns during labor, resulting in chlamydial conjunctivitis and/or pneumonia, which may possibly involve similar pathogenesis mechanisms to those occurring in the female genital tract.

Controversial reports point out CT as a risk factor for cervical carcinoma, independent of human papillomavirus [107]. It has been shown that CT interferes with multiple proapoptotic pathways to guarantee survival within host cells [125,126]. In addition, CT activates prosurvival signaling pathways for bacterial nutrient acquisition, expression of antiapoptotic factors, and synthesis of proinflammatory cytokines [127,128]. On the other hand, CT interferes with chromosome segregation and cytokinesis. In consequence, multinucleated cells and cells with aberrant number of chromosomes are often observed in cell cultures infected with CT [129]. Taken together, these findings suggest that persistent chlamydial infections might play a role in the development of cervical neoplasia. Further research is needed to shed light to this issue.

The high prevalence and incidence estimates worldwide, in conjunction to the diversity of clinical entities and long-term consequences of chlamydial infections, propel further research of the bacterial and host factors involved in the pathogenesis and damage to the reproductive system.

6. Important challenges: Prevention, diagnosis, and treatment of chlamydial infections

The widespread incidence and prevalence of sexually transmitted infections, especially among young population, made them a priority public-health concern worldwide. Screening, control programmes, and education in sexual behavioral aspects and contraception are fundamental for the prevention of chlamydial infections and their long-term sequelae, mainly PID and tubal infertility.

Routine screening allows the identification of asymptomatic carriers of CT and contributes to the early detection of chlamydial infections. Appropriated diagnostic services are required to obtain reliable results. The most confident tests for the detection of CT involve nucleid acid amplification techniques that are not available in all laboratories, especially in third-world countries. Nucleic acid amplification tests are more sensitive than culture or antigen tests.

Improvement in molecular diagnostics will lead to improvement in treatment and prevention of damage to reproductive tissues. It has been shown that screening is cost-effective even in low prevalence populations, due to the high costs of treatment of complications resulting from undiagnosed and untreated chlamydial infections [130]. The implement of additional targeted screening of women at risk will contribute to reduce the CT-associated infertility.

Additionally, clinicians should be aware about the latest therapeutic management of chlamydial cervicitis and PID. Different antibiotics such as azithromycin, doxycycline, ofloxacin, erythromycin, and amoxicillin may be useful for treating genital chlamydial infections [131]. The antibiotic selection depends on the characteristics of the drug itself like pharmacokinetics, half-life, and bioavailability, concentration in mucous membranes and genital tissues, development of gastrointestinal tract side effects, safe use in pregnancy, as well as, the characteristics of the host and the clinical course of chlamydial infection. The effectiveness of therapy relies on timely treating sex partners and to abstain from sexual intercourse until completing the whole antibiotic scheme.

Unceasing efforts are conducted for the development of a chlamydial vaccine. Nevertheless, until now, no effective chlamydial vaccines are available. The knowledge of bacterial factors involved in pathogenicity will help in addressing optimal vaccine design that prevents not only chlamydial infection but also progression to infertility.

Acknowledgements

The authors acknowledge CONICET (PIP), Foncyt (PICT 2116) and UNCuyo grants to M.T.D. for their support in research. They apologize to those investigators whose work could not be cited because of space constraints.

Author details

Agustín Luján, Silvina Fili and María Teresa Damiani*

*Address all correspondence to: meteresadamiani@gmail.com

Laboratory of Phagocytosis and Intracellular Transport, IHEM-CONICET, School of Medicine, University of Cuyo, Mendoza, Argentina

References

[1] World Health Organization. Prevalence and incidence of selected sexually transmitted infections, Chlamydia trachomatis, Neisseria gonorrhoeae, syphilis and Tricho-

monas vaginalis: Methods and results used by WHO to generate 2005 estimate. WHO. 2011;1–38.

[2] CDC. Incidence, Prevalence, and Cost of Sexually Transmitted Infections in the United States. CDC Fact Sheet. 2013;40(February):1–4.

[3] Stephens RS, Kalman S, Lammel C, Fan J, Marathe R, Aravind L, et al. Genome sequence of an obligate intracellular pathogen of humans: Chlamydia trachomatis. Science (Internet). 1998;282(5389):754–759.

[4] Hybiske K, Stephens RS. Mechanisms of Chlamydia trachomatis entry into nonphagocytic cells. Infect Immun. 2007;75(8):3925–3934.

[5] Cocchiaro JL, Valdivia RH. New insights into Chlamydia intracellular survival mechanisms. Cell Microbiol. 2009;11(11):1571–1878.

[6] Dautry-Varsat A, Subtil A, Hackstadt T. Recent insights into the mechanisms of Chlamydia entry. Cell Microbiol. 2005;7(12):1714–1722.

[7] Chen JC, Stephens RS. Chlamydia trachomatis glycosaminoglycan-dependent and independent attachment to eukaryotic cells. Microb Pathog. 1997;22(1):23–30.

[8] Abromaitis S, Stephens RS. Attachment and entry of chlamydia have distinct requirements for host protein disulfide isomerase. PLoS Pathog. 2009;5(4):1–12.

[9] Menozzi FD, Pethe K, Bifani P, Soncin F, Brennan MJ, Locht C. Enhanced bacterial virulence through exploitation of host glycosaminoglycans. Mol Microbiol. 2002;43(6):1379–1386.

[10] Su B, Karint M. Mitogen-activated gene expression protein kinase cascades and regulation of gene expression. Curr Opin Immunol. 1996;8(3):402–411.

[11] Fadel S, Eley A. Chlamydia trachomatis OmcB protein is a surface-exposed glycosaminoglycan-dependent adhesion. J Med Microbiol. 2007;56(1):15–22.

[12] Mölleken K, Schmidt E, Hegemann JH. Members of the Pmp protein family of Chlamydia pneumoniae mediate adhesion to human cells via short repetitive peptide motifs. Mol Microbiol. 2010;78(4):1004–1017.

[13] Engel J. Tarp and Arp: How Chlamydia induces its own entry. Proc Natl Acad Sci U S A. 2004;101(27):9947–9948.

[14] Lane BJ, Mutchler C, Al Khodor S, Grieshaber SS, Carabeo RA. Chlamydial entry involves TARP binding of guanine nucleotide exchange factors. PLoS Pathog. 2008;4(3):1–11.

[15] Jewett TJ, Miller NJ, Dooley CA, Hackstadt T. The conserved tarp actin binding domain is important for chlamydial invasion. PLoS Pathog. 2010;6(7):1–11.

[16] Damiani MT, Gambarte Tudela J, Capmany A. Targeting eukaryotic Rab proteins: A smart strategy for chlamydial survival and replication. Cell Microbiol. 2014;16(9): 1329–1338.

[17] Gambarte Tudela J, Capmany A, Romao M, Quintero C, Miserey-Lenkei S, Raposo G, Goud B, Damiani MT. The late endocytic Rab39a GTPase regulates the interaction between multivesicular bodies and chlamydial inclusions. J Cell Sci. 2015;128(16):3068–3081.

[18] Hybiske K, Stephens RS. Mechanisms of host cell exit by the intracellular bacterium Chlamydia. Proc Natl Acad Sci U S A. 2007;104(27):11430–11435.

[19] Beatty WL, Byrne GI, Morrison RP. Repeated and persistent infection with Chlamydia and the development of chronic inflammation and disease. Trends Microbiol. 1994;2(3):94–98.

[20] Bastidas RJ, Elwell CA, Engel JN, Valdivia RH. Chlamydial intracellular survival strategies. Cold Spring Harb Perspect Med. 2013;3(5): 1–20.

[21] Rzomp KA, Scholtes LD, Briggs BJ, Whittaker GR, Scidmore MA. Rab GTPases are recruited to chlamydial inclusions in both a species-dependent and species-independent manner. Infect Immun. 2003;71(10):5855–5870.

[22] Hackstadt T, Fischer ER, Scidmore MA, Rockey DD, Heinzen RA. Origins and functions of the chlamydial inclusion. Trends Microbiol. 1997;5(7):288–293.

[23] Fields KA, Hackstadt T. The chlamydial inclusion: Escape from the endocytic pathway. Annu Rev Cell Biol. 2002;18:221–245.

[24] Moore ER, Fischer ER, Mead DJ, Hackstadt T. The chlamydial inclusion preferentially intercepts basolaterally directed sphingomyelin-containing exocytic vacuoles. Traffic. 2008;9(12):2130–2140.

[25] Rejman Lipinski A, Heymann J, Meissner C, Karlas A, Brinkmann V, Meyer TF, et al. Rab6 and Rab11 regulate Chlamydia trachomatis development and golgin-84-dependent Golgi fragmentation. PLoS Pathog. 2009;5(10): 1–12.

[26] Capmany A, Damiani MT. Chlamydia trachomatis intercepts golgi-derived sphingolipids through a rab14-mediated transport required for bacterial development and replication. PLoS One. 2010;5(11): 1–17.

[27] Leiva N, Capmany A, Damiani MT. Rab11-Family of Interacting Protein 2 associates with chlamydial inclusions through its Rab-binding domain and promotes bacterial multiplication. Cell Microbiol. 2013;15(1):114–129.

[28] Beatty WL. Trafficking from CD63-positive late endocytic multivesicular bodies is essential for intracellular development of Chlamydia trachomatis. J Cell Sci. 2006;119(Pt 2):350–359.

[29] Cocchiaro J, Kumar Y, Fischer ER, Hackstadt T, Valdivia RH. Cytoplasmic lipid droplets are translocated into the lumen of the Chlamydia trachomatis parasitophorous vacuole. Proc Natl Acad Sci U S A. 2008;105(27):9379–9384.

[30] Saka HA, Valdivia R. Emerging roles for lipid droplets in immunity and host-pathogen interactions. Annu Rev Cell Dev Biol. 2012;28(1):411–437.

[31] Derré I, Swiss R, Agaisse H. The lipid transfer protein CERT interacts with the Chlamydia inclusion protein IncD and participates to ER-Chlamydia inclusion membrane contact sites. PLoS Pathog. 2011;7(6): 1–13.

[32] Elwell CA, Jiang S, Kim JH, Lee A, Wittmann T, Hanada K, et al. Chlamydia trachomatis co-opts gbf1 and cert to acquire host sphingomyelin for distinct roles during intracellular development. PLoS Pathog. 2011;7(9): 1–20.

[33] Robertson KD, Gu L, Rowe RK, Beatty WL. Inclusion biogenesis and reactivation of persistent Chlamydia trachomatis requires host cell sphingolipid biosynthesis. PLoS Pathog. 2009;5(11): 1–9.

[34] Clifton DR, Fields KA, Grieshaber SS, Dooley CA, Fischer ER, Mead DJ, et al. A chlamydial type III translocated protein is tyrosine-phosphorylated at the site of entry and associated with recruitment of actin. Proc Natl Acad Sci U S A. 2004;101(27): 10166–10171.

[35] Grieshaber S, Swanson JA, Hackstadt T. Determination of the physical environment within the Chlamydia trachomatis inclusion using ion-selective ratiometric probes. Cell Microbiol. 2002;4(5):273–283.

[36] Vandahl BBS, Stensballe A, Roepstorff P, Christiansen G, Birkelund S. Secretion of Cpn0796 from Chlamydia pneumoniae into the host cell cytoplasm by an autotransporter mechanism. Cell Microbiol. 2005;7(6):825–836.

[37] Trentmann O, Horn M, Van Scheltinga ACT, Neuhaus HE, Haferkamp I. Enlightening energy parasitism by analysis of an ATP/ADP transporter from chlamydiae. PLoS Biol. 2007;5(9):1938–1951.

[38] Derré I, Pypaert M, Dautry-Varsat A, Agaisse H. RNAi screen in Drosophila cells reveals the involvement of the tom complex in Chlamydia infection. PLoS Pathog. 2007;3(10):1446–1458.

[39] Mylonas I. Female genital Chlamydia trachomatis infection: Where are we heading? Arch Gynecol Obstet. 2012;285(5):1271–1285.

[40] Stephens RS, Sanchez-Pescador R, Wagar EA, Inouye C, Urdea MS. Diversity of Chlamydia trachomatis major outer membrane protein genes. J Bacteriol. 1987;169(9): 3879–3885.

[41] Baehr W, Zhang YX, Joseph T, Su H, Nano FE, Everett KD, et al. Mapping antigenic domains expressed by Chlamydia trachomatis major outer membrane protein genes. Proc Natl Acad Sci U S A. 1988;85(11):4000–4004.

[42] Millman K, Black CM, Johnson RE, Stamm E, Jones RB, Hook EW, et al. Population-based genetic and evolutionary analysis of Chlamydia trachomatis urogenital strain variation in the United States. J Bacteriol. 2004;186(8):2457–2465.

[43] Stothard DR, Boguslawski G, Jones RB. Phylogenetic analysis of the Chlamydia trachomatis major outer membrane protein and examination of potential pathogenic determinants. Infect Immun. 1998;66(8):3618–3625.

[44] Brown WJ, Rockey DD. Identification of an antigen localized to an apparent septum within dividing chlamydiae? Infect Immun. 2000;68(2):708–715.

[45] Nelson DE, Virok DP, Wood H, Roshick C, Johnson RM, Whitmire WM, et al. Chlamydial IFN-gamma immune evasion is linked to host infection tropism. Proc Natl Acad Sci U S A. 2005;102(30):10658–10663.

[46] Borges V, Nunes A, Ferreira R, Borrego MJ, Gomes JP. Directional evolution of chlamydia trachomatis towards niche-specific adaptation. J Bacteriol. 2012;194(22):6143–6153.

[47] Jeffrey BM, Suchland RJ, Quinn KL, Davidson JR, Stamm WE, Rockey DD. Genome sequencing of recent clinical Chlamydia trachomatis strains identifies loci associated with tissue tropism and regions of apparent recombination. Infect Immun. 2010;78(6):2544–2553.

[48] Dean D, Oudens E, Bolan G, Padian N, Schachter J. Major outer membrane protein variants of *Chlamydia trachomatis* are associated with severe upper genital tract infections and histopathology in San Francisco. J Infect Dis 1995;172(4):1013–1022.

[49] Brunham RC, Plummer FA, Stephens RS. Bacterial antigenic variation, host immune response, and pathogen-host coevolution. Infect Immun. 1993;61(6):2273–2276.

[50] Mascellino MT, Ciardi MR, Oliva A, Cecinato F, Hassemer MP, Borgese L. Chlamydia trachomatis detection in a population of asymptomatic and symptomatic women: Correlation with the presence of serological markers for this infection. New Microbiol. 2008;31(2):249–256.

[51] Domeika M, Domeika K, Paavonen J, Mårdh PA, Witkin SS. Humoral immune response to conserved epitopes of Chlamydia trachomatis and human 60-kDa heat-shock protein in women with pelvic inflammatory disease. J Infect Dis. 1998;177(3): 714–719.

[52] Swanborg RH, Boros DL, Whittum-Hudson JA, Hudson AP. Molecular mimicry and horror autotoxicus: Do chlamydial infections elicit autoimmunity? Expert Rev Mol Med. 2006;8(29):1–23.

[53] Linhares IM, Witkin SS. Immunopathogenic consequences of Chlamydia trachomatis 60 kDa heat shock protein expression in the female reproductive tract. Cell Stress Chaperones. 2010;15(5):467–473.

[54] Peña AS, Karimi O, Crusius JBA. A new avenue to investigate: The autophagic process. From Crohn's disease to Chlamydia. Drugs Today. 2009;45(Suppl. B):113–117.

[55] Carter JD, Inman RD, Whittum-Hudson J, Hudson AP. Chlamydia and chronic arthritis. Ann Med. 2011;44(8):1–9.

[56] Henderson IR, Nataro JP. Virulence functions of autotransporter proteins. Infect Immun. 2001;69(3):1231–1243.

[57] Subtil A, Blocker A, Dautry-Varsat A. Type III secretion system in Chlamydia species: Identified members and candidates. Microbes Infect. 2000;2(4):367–369.

[58] Betts HJ, Wolf K, Fields KA. Effector protein modulation of host cells: Examples in the Chlamydia spp. arsenal. Curr Opin Microbiol. 2009;12(1):81–87.

[59] Beeckman DSA, Vanrompay DCG. Zoonotic *Chlamydophila psittaci* infections from a clinical perspective. Clin Microbiol Infect. 2009;15(1):11–17.

[60] Hackstadt T, Scidmore MA, Shaw EI, Fischer ER. The Chlamydia trachomatis IncA protein is required for homotypic vesicle fusion. Cell Microbiol. 1999;1(2):119–130.

[61] Delevoye C, Nilges M, Dehoux P, Paumet F, Perrinet S, Dautry-Varsat A, et al. SNARE protein mimicry by an intracellular bacterium. PLoS Pathog. 2008;4(3): 1–14.

[62] Geisler WM, Suchland RJ, Whittington WL, Stamm WE. Quantitative culture of Chlamydia trachomatis: relationship of inclusion-forming units produced in culture to clinical manifestations and acute inflammation in urogenital disease. J Infect Dis. 2001;184(10):1350–1354.

[63] Jewett TJ, Fischer ER, Mead DJ, Hackstadt T. Chlamydial TARP is a bacterial nucleator of actin. Proc Natl Acad Sci U S A. 2006;103(42):15599–15604.

[64] Belland RJ, Scidmore MA, Dean D, Hogan D, Whitmire WM, McClarty G, et al. Chlamydia trachomatis cytotoxicity associated with complete and partial cytotoxin genes. Proc Natl Acad Sci U S A. 2001;98(24):13984–13989.

[65] Carlson JH, Hughes S, Hogan D, Cieplak G, Sturdevant DE, McClarty G, et al. Polymorphisms in the Chlamydia trachomatis cytotoxin locus associated with ocular and genital isolates. Infect Immun. 2004;72(12):7063–7072.

[66] Vora GJ, Stuart ES. A role for the glycolipid exoantigen (GLXA) in chlamydial infectivity. Curr Microbiol. 2003;46(3):217–223.

[67] Brade L, Nurminen M, Makela PH, Brade H. Antigenic properties of *Chlamydia trachomatis* lipopolysaccharide. Infect Immun. 1985;48(2):569–572.

[68] Omsland A, Sixt BS, Horn M, Hackstadt T. Chlamydial metabolism revisited: Interspecies metabolic variability and developmental stage-specific physiologic activities. FEMS Microbiol Rev. 2014;38(4):779–801.

[69] Wood H, Fehlner-Gardner C, Berry J, Fischer E, Graham B, Hackstadt T, et al. Regulation of tryptophan synthase gene expression in Chlamydia trachomatis. Mol Microbiol. 2003;49(5):1347–1359.

[70] Witkin SS, Jeremias J, Toth M, Ledger WJ. Cell-mediated immune response to the recombinant 57-kDa heat-shock protein of Chlamydia trachomatis in women with salpingitis. J Infect Dis. 1993;167(6):1379–1383.

[71] Kol A, Lichtman AH, Finberg RW, Libby P, Kurt-Jones EA. Cutting edge: Heat shock protein (HSP) 60 activates the innate immune response: CD14 is an essential receptor for HSP60 activation of mononuclear cells. J Immunol. 2000;164(1):13–17.

[72] LaVerda D, Albanese LN, Ruther PE, Morrison SG, Morrison RP, Ault KA, et al. Seroreactivity to Chlamydia trachomatis Hsp10 correlates with severity of human genital tract disease. Infect Immun. 2000;68(1):303–309.

[73] Kinnunen A, Molander P, Morrison R, Lehtinen M, Karttunen R, Tiitinen A, et al. Chlamydial heat shock protein 60-specific T cells in inflamed salpingeal tissue. Fertil Steril. 2002;77(1):162–166.

[74] Jha R, Srivastava P, Salhan S, Finckh A, Gabay C, Mittal A, et al. Spontaneous secretion of interleukin-17 and -22 by human cervical cells in Chlamydia trachomatis infection. Microbes Infect. Elsevier Masson SAS; 2011;13(2):167–178.

[75] Spear GT, Kendrick SR, Chen HY, Thomas TT, Bahk M, Balderas R, et al. Multiplex immunoassay of lower genital tract mucosal fluid from women attending an urban STD clinic shows broadly increased IL1ß and lactoferrin. PLoS One. 2011;6(5):1–7.

[76] Low N, Egger M, Sterne JAC, Harbord RM, Ibrahim F, Lindblom B, et al. Incidence of severe reproductive tract complications associated with diagnosed genital chlamydial infection: The Uppsala Women's Cohort Study. Sex Transm Infect. 2006;82(3): 212–218.

[77] Agrawal T, Vats V, Salhan S, Mittal A. Mucosal and peripheral immune responses to chlamydial heat shock proteins in women infected with Chlamydia trachomatis. Clin Exp Immunol. 2007;148(3):461–468.

[78] Srivastava P, Jha R, Bas S, Salhan S, Mittal A. In infertile women, cells from Chlamydia trachomatis infected sites release higher levels of interferon-gamma, interleukin-10 and tumor necrosis factor-alpha upon heat-shock-protein stimulation than fertile women. Reprod Biol Endocrinol. 2008;6:20.

[79] Mascellino MT, Margani M, Oliva A. Helicobacter pylori: Determinant and markers of virulence. Dis Markers. 2009;27(3-4):137–156.

[80] Darville T, Hiltke TJ. Pathogenesis of genital tract disease due to Chlamydia trachomatis. J Infect Dis. 2010;201(S2):114–125.

[81] Morrison SG, Su H, Caldwell HD, Morrison RP. Immunity to murine Chlamydia trachomatis genital tract reinfection involves B cells and CD4+ T cells but not CD8+ T cells. Infect Immun. 2000;68(12):6979–6987.

[82] Holland MJ, Bailey RL, Conway DJ, Culley F, Miranpuri G, Byrne GI, et al. T helper type-1 (Th1)/Th2 profiles of peripheral blood mononuclear cells (PBMC); responses to antigens of Chlamydia trachomatis in subjects with severe trachomatous scarring. Clin Exp Immunol. 1996;105(3):429–435.

[83] Horne AW, Stock SJ, King AE. Innate immunity and disorders of the female reproductive tract. Reproduction. 2008;135(6):739–749.

[84] Lal JA, Malogajski J, Verweij SP, De Boer P, Ambrosino E, Brand A, et al. Chlamydia trachomatis infections and subfertility: Opportunities to translate host pathogen genomic data into public health. Public Health Genomics. 2013;16(1-2):50–61.

[85] Ingalls RR, Rice PA, Qureshi N, Takayama K, Juey Shin Lin, Golenbock DT. The inflammatory cytokine response to Chlamydia trachomatis infection is endotoxin mediated. Infect Immun. 1995;63(8):3125–3130.

[86] Prebeck S, Kirschning C, Dürr S, da Costa C, Donath B, Brand K, et al. Predominant role of toll-like receptor 2 versus 4 in Chlamydia pneumoniae-induced activation of dendritic cells. J Immunol. 2001;167(6):3316–3323.

[87] Heine H, Müller-Loennies S, Brade L, Lindner B, Brade H. Endotoxic activity and chemical structure of lipopolysaccharides from Chlamydia trachomatis serotypes E and L2 and Chlamydophila psittaci 6BC. Eur J Biochem. 2003;270(3):440–450.

[88] Welter-Stahl L, Ojcius DM, Viala J, Girardin S, Liu W, Delarbre C, et al. Stimulation of the cytosolic receptor for peptidoglycan, Nod1, by infection with Chlamydia trachomatis or Chlamydia muridarum. Cell Microbiol. 2006;8(6):1047–1057.

[89] Walker J, Tabrizi SN, Fairley CK, Chen MY, Bradshaw CS, Twin J, et al. Chlamydia trachomatis incidence and re-infection among young women – Behavioural and microbiological characteristics. PLoS One. 2012;7(5):1–9.

[90] Price MJ, Ades AE, de Angelis D, Welton NJ, Macleod J, Turner K, et al. Incidence of Chlamydia trachomatis infection in women in England: Two methods of estimation. Epidemiol Infect. 2014;142(3):562–576.

[91] Bender N, Herrmann B, Andersen B, Hocking JS, van Bergen J, Morgan J, et al. Chlamydia infection, pelvic inflammatory disease, ectopic pregnancy and infertility: Cross-national study. Sex Transm Infect. 2011;87(7):601–608.

[92] Hall JV, Schell M, Dessus-Babus S, Moore CG, Whittimore JD, Sal M, et al. The multi-faceted role of oestrogen in enhancing Chlamydia trachomatis infection in polarized human endometrial epithelial cells. Cell Microbiol. 2011;13(8):1183–1199.

[93] Borth N, Massier J, Franke C, Sachse K, Saluz HP, Hänel F. Chlamydial protease CT441 interacts with SRAP1 co-activator of estrogen receptor and partially alleviates its co-activation activity. J Steroid Biochem Mol Biol. 2010;119(1–2):89–95.

[94] Sonnex C. Influence of ovarian hormones on urogenital infection. Sex Transm Infect. 1998;74(1):11–19.

[95] Agrawal T, Vats V, Wallace PK, Salhan S, Mittal A. Role of cervical dendritic cell subsets, co-stimulatory molecules, cytokine secretion profile and beta-estradiol in development of sequalae to Chlamydia trachomatis infection. Reprod Biol Endocrinol. 2008;6:46.

[96] Wan C, Latter JL, Amirshahi A, Symonds I, Finnie J, Bowden N, et al. Progesterone Activates Multiple Innate Immune Pathways in Chlamydia trachomatis-Infected Endocervical Cells. Am J Reprod Immunol. 2014;71(2):165–177.

[97] Beagley KW, Gockel CM. Regulation of innate and adaptive immunity by the female sex hormones oestradiol and progesterone. FEMS Immunol Med Microbiol. 2003;38(1):13–22.

[98] Kaushic C, Zhou F, Murdin AD, Charles R, Zhou FAN. Effects of estradiol and progesterone on susceptibility and early immune responses to Chlamydia trachomatis infection in the female reproductive tract. Infect Immun.2000 Jul;68(7):4207–4216.

[99] Macleod J, Salisbury C, Low N, McCarthy A, Sterne JAC, Holloway A, et al. Coverage and uptake of systematic postal screening for genital Chlamydia trachomatis and prevalence of infection in the United Kingdom general population: Cross sectional study. BMJ. 2005;330(7497):940.

[100] Wiesenfeld HC, Hillier SL, Krohn MA, Landers DV, Sweet RL. Bacterial vaginosis is a strong predictor of Neisseria gonorrhoeae and Chlamydia trachomatis infection. Clin Infect Dis. 2003;36(5):663–668.

[101] Korn AP, Hessol NA, Padian NS, Bolan GA, Donegan E, Landers DV, et al. Risk factors for plasma cell endometritis among women with cervical Neisseria gonorrhoeae, cervical Chlamydia trachomatis, or bacterial vaginosis. Am J Obstet Gynecol. 1998;178(5):987–990.

[102] Da Silva CS, Adad SJ, De Souza MAH, Barcelos ACM, Terra APS, Murta EFC. Increased frequency of bacterial vaginosis and Chlamydia trachomatis in pregnant women with human papillomavirus infection. Gynecol Obstet Invest. 2004;58(4):189–193.

[103] Quintero CA, Tudela JG, Damiani MT. Rho GTPases as pathogen targets: Focus on curable sexually transmitted infections. Small GTPases. 2015;(May):1–11.

[104] Gong Z, Luna Y, Yu P, Fan H. Lactobacilli inactivate Chlamydia trachomatis through lactic acid but not H2O2. PLoS One. 2014;9(9):e107758.

[105] Richmond SJ, Sparling PF. Genital chlamydial infections. Am J Epidemiol. 1976;103(5):428–435.

[106] Batteiger BE, Tu W, Ofner S, Pol B Van Der, Diane R, Orr DP, et al. Repeated Chlamydia trachomatis genital infections in adolescent women. J Infect Dis. 2011;201(1): 42–51.

[107] Paavonen J, Eggert-Kruse W. Chlamydia trachomatis: Impact on human reproduction. Hum Reprod Update. 1999;5(5):433–447.

[108] Lewis D, Newton DC, Guy RJ, Ali H, Chen MY, Fairley CK, et al. The prevalence of Chlamydia trachomatis infection in Australia: A systematic review and meta-analysis. BMC Infect Dis. 2012;12(1):113.

[109] Bé Bé Ar C, De Barbeyrac B. Genital Chlamydia trachomatis infections. Clin Microbiol Infect. 2009;15:4–10.

[110] Haggerty CL, Gottlieb SL, Taylor BD, Low N, Xu F, Ness RB. Risk of sequelae after Chlamydia trachomatis genital infection in women. J Infect Dis. 2010;(2):S134–S155.

[111] Chernesky MA, Lee H, Schachter J, Burczak JD, Stamm WE, McCormack WM, et al. Diagnosis of Chlamydia trachomatis urethral infection in symptomatic and asymptomatic men by testing first-void urine in a ligase chain reaction assay. J Infect Dis. 1994;170(5):1308–1311.

[112] Hillis SD, Joesoef R, Marchbanks PA, Wasserheit JN, Cates W, Westrom L. Delayed care of pelvic inflammatory disease as a risk factor for impaired fertility. Am J Obstet Gynecol. Mosby; 1993;168(5):1503–1509.

[113] Martin DH, Koutsky L, Eschenbach DA, Daling JR, Alexander ER, Benedetti JK, et al. Prematurity and perinatal mortality in pregnancies complicated by maternal Chlamydia trachomatis infections. JAMA. 1982;247(11):1585–1588.

[114] Gravett MG. Independent associations of bacterial vaginosis and Chlamydia trachomatis infection with adverse pregnancy outcome. JAMA. 1986;256(14):1899.

[115] Gencay M, Koskiniemi M, Saikku P, Puolakkainen M, Raivio K, Koskela P, et al. Chlamydia trachomatis seropositivity during pregnancy is associated with perinatal complications. Clin Infect Dis. 1995;21:424–426.

[116] Oakeshott P, Kerry S, Aghaizu A, Atherton H, Hay S, Taylor-Robinson D, et al. Randomised controlled trial of screening for Chlamydia trachomatis to prevent pelvic inflammatory disease: The POPI (prevention of pelvic infection) trial. BMJ. 2010;340:c1642.

[117] Herzog SA, Althaus CL, Heijne JC, Oakeshott P, Kerry S, Hay P, et al. Timing of progression from Chlamydia trachomatis infection to pelvic inflammatory disease: A mathematical modelling study. BMC Infect Dis. 2012;12(1):187.

[118] Price MJ, Ades AE, De Angelis D, Welton NJ, MacLeod J, Soldan K, et al. Risk of pelvic inflammatory disease following Chlamydia trachomatis infection: Analysis of prospective studies with a multistate model. Am J Epidemiol. 2013;178(3):484–492.

[119] Paavonen J, Lehtinen M. Immunopathogenesis of chlamydial pelvic inflammatory disease: The role of heat-shock proteins. Infect Dis Obs Gynecol. 1994;2(3):105–110.

[120] Khader SA, Gopal R. IL-17 in protective immunity to intracellular pathogens. Virulence. 2010;1(5):423–427.

[121] Agrawal T, Bhengraj AR, Vats V, Salhan S, Mittal A. Expression of TLR 2, TLR 4 and iNOS in cervical monocytes of Chlamydia trachomatis-infected women and their role in host immune response. Am J Reprod Immunol. 2011;66(6):534–543.

[122] Gupta R, Vardhan H, Srivastava P, Salhan S, Mittal A. Modulation of cytokines and transcription factors (T-Bet and GATA3) in CD4 enriched cervical cells of Chlamydia trachomatis infected fertile and infertile women upon stimulation with chlamydial inclusion membrane proteins B and C. Reprod Biol Endocrinol. 2009;7:84.

[123] Balasubramaniam ES, Van Noorden S, El-Bahrawy M. The expression of interleukin (IL)-6, IL-8, and their receptors in fallopian tubes with ectopic tubal gestation. Fertil Steril. 2012;98(4):898–904.

[124] Lewis ME, Belland RJ, Abdel Rahman YM, Beatty WL, Aiyar AA, Zea AH, et al. Morphologic and molecular evaluation of Chlamydia trachomatis growth in human endocervix reveals distinct growth patterns. Front Cell Infect Microbiol. 2014;4:71.

[125] Fan T, Lu H, Hu H, Shi L, McClarty GA, Nance DM, et al. Inhibition of apoptosis in chlamydia-infected cells: Blockade of mitochondrial cytochrome c release and caspase activation. J Exp Med. 1998;187(4):487–496.

[126] Rajalingam K, Al-younes H, Müller A, Meyer TF, Szczepek AJ, Rudel T, et al. Epithelial cells infected with Chlamydophila pneumoniae are resistant to apoptosis. Infect Immun. 2001 Dec;69(12):7880–7888.

[127] Buchholz KR, Stephens RS. The extracellular signal-regulated kinase/mitogen-activated protein kinase pathway induces the inflammatory factor interleukin-8 following Chlamydia trachomatis infection. Infect Immun. 2007;75(12):5924–5929.

[128] Rajalingam K, Sharma M, Lohmann C, Oswald M, Thieck O, Froelich CJ, et al. Mcl-1 is a key regulator of apoptosis resistance in Chlamydia trachomatis-infected cells. PLoS One. 2008;3(9) :1–11.

[129] Grieshaber SS, Grieshaber NA, Miller N, Hackstadt T. Chlamydia trachomatis causes centrosomal defects resulting in chromosomal segregation abnormalities. Traffic. 2006;7(8):940–949.

[130] Puolakkainen M, Hiltunen-Back E, Reunala T, Suhonen S, Lähteenmäki P, Lehtinen M, et al. Comparison of performances of two commercially available tests, a PCR assay and a ligase chain reaction test, in detection of urogenital Chlamydia trachomatis infection. J Clin Microbiol. 1998;36(6):1489–1493.

[131] Horner PJ. Azithromycin antimicrobial resistance and genital Chlamydia trachomatis infection: Duration of therapy may be the key to improving efficacy. Sex Transm Infect. 2012;88(3):154–156.

2

Genital Herpes

Selma Emre and Ayse Akkus

Abstract

Genital herpes simplex virus (HSV) infections are among the most commonly seen sexually transmitted infections in the world. Genital herpes is a serious health problem because the infection continues through life with remissions and relapses, it causes recurring painful ulcers, and there is no known cure for it. The real prevalence of the genital herpes infection is unknown due to asymptomatic cases. The majority of infected individuals are not aware of the infection due to short duration of symptoms and signs or its asymptomatic nature. The clinical presentation of genital herpes shows certain differences in terms of the primary attack following the first encounter with the virus and recurrent attacks. There is a strong relationship between HSV-2 positivity and human immunodeficiency virus (HIV). A serious complication of genital herpes in the mother during pregnancy, neonatal herpes, has a mortality risk of 60% if not treated. Antiviral therapy is safe and effective, for both episodic treatment and chronic suppression of HSV. Epidemiology, clinical presentation, laboratory, and treatment options of genital herpes are summarized in this chapter.

Keywords: genital herpes, herpes simplex viruses, sexually transmitted diseases

1. Introduction

Genital herpes is a sexually transmitted infection which is seen throughout the world and continues through life. It is the most common cause of diseases accompanied by genital ulceration. Genital herpes is a serious health problem because the infection continues through life with remissions and relapses, it causes recurring painful ulcers, the virus transmitted from mother to infant causes serious neonatal infections, and there is no known cure for it [1, 2].

Herpes simplex viruses (HSV) are the most common human pathogens causing infections in orofacial and genital regions. Genital herpes infection is caused by herpes simplex virus 1 (HSV-1) and herpes simplex virus 2 (HSV-2). HSV-1 mainly causes infection in oral, facial, and ocular regions and in the central nervous system (CNS) and is transmitted during childhood. While in the past genital herpes infections were mostly caused by HSV-2 and orofacial infections were mostly caused by HSV-1, HSV-1 is reported to cause genital herpes at an increasing rate today, particularly in developed countries [3, 4]. One of the important reasons behind the increase in HSV-1-induced genital herpes cases in developed countries is decreased seroprevalence of HSV-1 and the fact that the host has not encountered with the virus prior to the onset of sexual activity. Another important reason is suggested to be changing sexual behaviors among the youth such as oral sex. HSV-2 is usually transmitted through sexual contact and causes genital infection. HSV-2 may cause orofacial infections as well, which cannot be clinically distinguished from HSV-1-induced infections. However, HSV-2-induced orofacial infections are very rare [5, 6].

Herpes simplex viruses stay with infected individuals latently for lifetime. Their presentation is quite variable depending on the immune condition of the host, site of entry of the virus, and whether the disease is primary or secondary [7]. Genital herpes infection has some serious results. First of all, HSVs transmitted from the mother to the neonatal cause serious mortality and morbidity. The second serious risk is the fact that genital herpes infections facilitate human immunodeficiency virus (HIV) and play a role in the spread of HIV [8].

2. Epidemiology

Genital HSV infections are among the most commonly seen sexually transmitted infections in the world. The real prevalence of the genital herpes infection is unknown due to asymptomatic cases. The most common cause of the genital herpes infection is HSV-2, but the number of primary genital herpes cases induced by HSV-1 is on the rise. The prevalence of infections induced by HSV-1 and HSV-2 varies between countries. While HSV-1 prevalence is about 60–80% worldwide, its prevalence in developing countries varies between 70 and 100%. HSV-2 prevalence is reported to vary between 7 and 80% depending on the country, age group, and sexual life characteristics. More than 500 million people are estimated to be infected with HSV-2 worldwide, which corresponds to 16% of the world population in between the ages of 15–49. It is also estimated that 20 million new cases occur every year [5, 6, 9].

HSV-1 seroprevalence is associated with age, race, geographical location, and socioeconomic status. HSV-2 is associated with age, race, geographical location, socioeconomic status, sexually transmitted disease history, onset of sexual activity, and number of the sexual partner. The most significant determining factor in genital HSV infections is lifetime sexual partner count. It was found in a study conducted in the United States that HSV-2 infection and HSV1/HSV2 co-infection are closely associated with lifetime sexual activity, smoking status, and recreational drug use [1, 10].

HSV-1 is typically transmitted during childhood and with non-sexual contact. While HSV-1-induced genital herpes prevalence varies between geographical regions, almost half of all new genital herpes cases are caused by HSV-1 in European countries [12]. HSV-1 seropositivity is estimated to be 40–63% in the United States, while HSV-2 seropositivity is estimated to be

16–18% [10]. While HSV-1 prevalence was 62% in the United States between 1988 and 1994, it dropped to 57.7% between 1999 and 2004. However, HSV-1 seroprevalence was found to increase in those who were diagnosed with genital herpes only [3]. Having orofacial HSV-1 infection during childhood may protect against genital HSV-1 infection in later years and silent HSV-2 seroconversion occurs more frequently in individuals with HSV-1 immunity. In other words, the transmission rate, duration of disease, and severity of disease are decreased in those who have immunity against a HSV type due to cross-immunity. The presence of HSV-1 antibodies does not prevent HSV-2 transmission. However, HSV-2 infection may be milder or asymptomatic in those with positive HSV-1 antibodies [7, 10, 11].

HSV-2 positivity occurs in adolescence when sexual activity begins and prevalence rate consistently increases toward adult ages. HSV-2 seroprevalence during pregnancy is reported to be 7–40% in different parts of the world. It is reported in rates varying between 60 and 95% in those infected with HIV and female sex workers [5]. The region with the highest HSV-2 prevalence and incidence is sub-Saharan Africa. Prevalence goes as high as 80% for men and over the age of 35 for women. HSV-2 seroprevalence is lower in European countries and reports vary greatly between countries. In cross-sectional studies for Europe between 1989 and 2000, HSV-2 seroprevalence was found to be 4% in Great Britain and Wales, whereas it was found to be 24% in Bulgaria. While it was 20–30% in Germany and Switzerland, it went as high as 40% in Turkey. The lowest prevalence is reported in Asian countries with 10–30% [12–14].

HSV-2 seroprevalence was found to be 17.2% in the United States in 1999–2000 and 14% between 2005 and 2010. It is believed that behaviors reducing sexual risk factors improved hygiene and life conditions, improved socioeconomic conditions, and shrinking families might have had effective in the decrease in HSV-1 and HSV-2 prevalence [3, 10].

3. Structure of herpes simplex viruses

More than 80 virus types were identified in the herpesvirus family. However, only eight herpesviruses cause diseases in humans. Herpesviruses, which are human pathogens, are HSV-1 (HHV-1), HSV-2 (HHV-2), varicella zoster virus (VZV, HHV-3), Epstein-Barr virus (EBV, HHV-4), cytomegalovirus (CMV, HHV-5), human herpesvirus 6 (HHV-6), human herpesvirus 7 (HHV-7), and human herpesvirus 8 (HHV-8). Herpesviruses, which are the first two types of HHVs and responsible for genital herpes infections, are referred to as herpes simplex viruses [15].

HSVs are members of the alpha herpesviridea subfamily of the herpesvirus family and have a large double-stranded DNA genome. The diameter of the viral nucleocapsid is approximately 100 nm and the diameter of the virus is approximately 250 nm. The structure of the virus consists of a nucleus containing the DNA in the center, an icosahedral capsid surrounding the nucleus, a tegument consisting of an amorphous protein layer surrounding the capsid, and an envelope surrounding all of these [7, 12]. The envelope is a glycoprotein outer cover and is typically derived from the host cell membrane while the DNA-containing capsid passes through the nuclear membrane of the host cell. These glycoproteins play an important role during entry into the host cell. Even though DNA sequences of HSV-1 and HSV-2 are very similar, they have different antigenic structures due to differences in envelope proteins [16].

HSVs are required to attach to at least three different cell surface receptors to start the infection. As a result of this attachment, the plasma membrane and the virus envelope join and the virus enters into the cell as a result. The viral envelope contains at least 12 different glycoproteins involved in the virus' entry into and exit from the cell (gB, gC, gD, gE, gH, gI, gK, gL, and gM) [17]. Five different envelope proteins are involved in the virus entry process. Surface glycoproteins of HSVs mediate attachment to and entry into host cell surface and also stimulate the host's immune system [12]. Heparan sulfate proteoglycans (HSPGs) on the cell surface are attachment regions for HSVs. gB and gC bind HSPGs and are necessary for attachment. Fırst, gD binds cell surface receptor and starts changes which allow for membrane fusion of other glycoproteins. Nectin-1 is a cell adhesion molecule, which gD binds and also the main HSV receptor found in epithelial cells and neurons [12, 17, 18].

The viral genome is required to pass through the cell surface and cytoplasm and reach the nucleus for the replication of the virus. Entry of the virus into nucleus occurs in three stages. The first stage is the absorption of the virion to the cell surface, the second stage is passing through nuclear pores after passing through the plasma membrane, and the third stage is the introduction of the viral DNA from the capsid [16]. HSVs mostly use their own DNA synthesis mechanisms for genome replication; however, they are dependent on the host's RNA polymerase II for transcription of viral genes. Viral DNA synthesize requires at least seven viral proteins. At least six viral proteins allow for robust expression of viral genes and mobilize cellular proteins for effective synthesis of the viral DNA and proteins. Other viral proteins, mainly thymidine kinase (TK), ribonucleotide reductase, dUTPase, and uracyl DNA glycosylase, control viral nucleic acid metabolism. These proteins are potential targets of antiviral treatment [12].

4. Pathophysiology

Host's immune system is the most important factor which determines the transmission, severity, and frequency of recurrence of the infection. Humoral and cellular immune systems limit the spread of the virus in immune-competent individuals. In experiments with both humans and rats, CD4+ and CD8+ T lymphocytes, macrophages, natural killer cells, and inflammatory cytokines such as interferon-γ were shown to be involved in protection against HSVs [5, 19]. While individuals with mild cellular immune deficiency experience frequent recurrences and slower resolution, individuals with severe immune deficiency are at a higher risk of disseminated, treatment-resistant, and chronic disease. More frequent and severe recurrent herpes infections in acquired immunodeficiency syndrome (AIDS) patients indicate the importance of cellular immunity, CD4+ T cells in particular [9]. Humoral immune system, on the other hand, does not affect disease severity. However, it is involved in reduction of virus titer in inoculation region and neural tissues during primary infection [5, 19]. Another cell that is primarily affected in genital herpes and involved in immune response against HSV-2 is keratinocytes. Keratinocytes infected with HSV-2 show up-regulation of antiviral cytokines such as interferon alpha, beta, tumor necrosis factor-alpha (TNF-α), colony-stimulating factors, growth factors, defensins, selectins, lymphocyte function-associated antigens, and Toll-like receptors [20].

Genital HSV infections are more common in women compared to men. Studies show that women are more vulnerable to transmission than men. This vulnerability is believed to arise from anatomic characteristics of women, the structure of the genital epithelium, longer exposure to inoculum, and a higher rate of viral reactivation among men than women. When it comes to sexual transmission, the risk of transmission from man to woman is higher than the risk of transmission from woman to man. The virus is easily deactivated with water, soap, and drying and transmission through objects is not likely [21].

The virus, which enters into the body through skin or mucosa, starts the cytolytic replication within epithelial cells. In this period, virions within epithelial cells are observed histologically as intranuclear inclusions. Cells turn into multinucleated giant cells due to cytolytic properties of HSVs. Epithelial cells break up due to cell damage, and the space between separated cells is filled with liquid. Resulting blisters contain cellular debris, inflammatory cells, and virion products [5].

HSVs are neurotropic human pathogens. Following the replication in epithelial cells, the virus is absorbed by sensory neurons that innervate these tissues. The virus travels through neuron body and to neural ganglia via retrograde microtubule-associated transport and remains latently in neural ganglia without leading to cell death in neurons. It is unknown why and how HSVs remain latently. However, after a single lytic infection, the virus gains ability to protect against host's defense system. The latent virus genome is kept within sensory neurons in a balanced manner and all viral lytic genes are suppressed. The virus may reactivate to continue its replication due to various triggering factors and reaches epithelial cells via anterograde transport. Infected cells do not spread virus for the duration of latent infection and disease symptoms are not observed in the host. Trigeminal and sacral ganglia are the regions where HSV-1 and HSV-2 viruses most frequently remain latent. Recurrent genital herpes infection usually occurs as a result of reactivation of the virus remaining latent in sacral root ganglia [9, 17, 22]. Many factors such as traumas, inflammatory diseases, ultraviolet, menstruation, immune suppression, fatigue, and psychological stress may lead to reactivation of the latent virus. Following the virus reactivation, the virus reaches mucosa and skin once more from dorsal root ganglia through peripheral nerves. The infection maybe symptomatic or asymptomatic and seroconversion of type-specific antibodies takes 4–6 weeks [11].

4.1. HSV/HIV relationship

There is a strong relationship between HSV-2 positivity and HIV. The risk of HIV transmission is three times higher in women and men infected with HSV-2 [23, 24]. Among HIV-positive patients in UK, HSV-1 seroprevalence was found to be 90%, HSV-2 seroprevalence was found to be 67%, and HSV-1 and HSV-2 co-incidence was found to be 64% [25]. Worldwide, more than half of individuals infected with HIV have HSV-2 infection. Genital herpes lesions are suggested to facilitate HIV acquisition due to disruptions in physical barriers of skin and mucosa. Another facilitating factor may be HIVs reaching a high number of CD4+ cells due to increased cellular inflammatory response. HSV-2 infection is believed to have played a facilitating role in HIV endemic in sub-Saharan Africa. HSV suppression treatment has not been shown to prevent HIV transmission [13, 20, 26]. In addition, HSV-2 infection is suggested to accelerate HIV disease and increase viral load. HSV treatment with acyclovir has been shown to slow down HIV progression in individuals co-infected with HIV and HSV-2. Some authors recommend that HIV-infected patients are checked for HSV-2 and co-infected individuals receive suppression treatment for HSV-2. However, this subject has not been fully illuminated. Although it is known that HSV-2 positivity facilitates HIV transmission, there is no evidence showing that it accelerates AIDS progression. On the other hand, HIV viral load has been reported to increase HSV-2 activity [26].

5. Clinic

Genital herpes lesions are formed by both HSV-1 and HSV-2 viruses. Severity of clinical signs varies significantly. Since the majority of individuals infected with HSV do not realize a clinical symptom, they are not diagnosed with genital herpes. Therefore, they continue to spread the virus without knowing that they are infected. While mild and moderate symptoms and signs are observed in some patients, the first attack may be as severe as to require hospitalization in others. HSV-1-induced genital herpes may be milder and recur less frequently than the infection induced by HSV-2. The incubation period after the transmission of the virus is not known with certainty. The primary infection occurs 2–12 days (4 days on average) after sexual contact. In one study, based on the data obtained from patients who were aware of having the primary attack, the time between the sexual contact and the primary attack may vary from 1 to 49 days and thus it is suggested that the incubation period may be longer than expected [27].

The majority of infected individuals are not aware of the infection due to short duration of symptoms and signs or its asymptomatic nature. For this reason, genital herpes should be considered in patients with nonspecific genital symptoms. The clinical presentation of genital herpes shows certain differences in terms of the primary attack following the first encounter with the virus and recurrent attacks [28].

5.1. Primary genital herpes

Although episodes in most primary genital herpes cases are asymptomatic or atypical, clinical signs are similar for both HSV-1 and HSV-2 in terms of the classical symptomatic first episode. In the prodromal period, patients may have headache, fever, anorexia, malaise, and painful inguinal and femoral lymphadenopathy. Following the prodromal period which lasts for 2–24 h, patients experience localized or regional pain and tingling and burning sensations. Constitutional symptoms are present in 80% of patients [11, 27]. Primary lesions begin about 4–7 days after sexual contact on labia minora, introitus, and urethral meatus in women and on penis shaft and glans in men as painful, erythematous, clustering vesicles, and papules in varying sizes. Painful and inflammatory vulvar edema is present in women. Other than the genital region, lesions may be seen on perineum and hips. Proctitis is one of the important initial symptoms in homosexual men. Irregular erosions and ulcers are formed due to ruptured vesicles. Since circulating antibodies are not on a sufficient level, autoinoculation may occur in other anatomical regions during or after the primary genital infection in particular. Lesions are crusted and heal without scarring after 2–3 weeks. In this period, patients may spread the virus for approximately 12 days. Atypical course may be present in women with cervical lesions, which are usually overlooked, and it is more difficult to make a diagnosis. The moist property of the genital region in women may lead to more severe clinical signs. Dysuria is also more common in women. Autonomic dysfunction and aseptic meningitis, which lead to urinary retention, are complications seen in this period. These lesions may sometimes occur without said complications. In primary genital herpes infections, aseptic meningitis is seen in 30% of women and 10% of men [7, 11]. The most common and unsettling symptom during the first episode is reported to be pain in women. In men, on the other hand, lesions are reported to be the most common and unsettling symptom. Surveys made with patients show that female patients experience more work force loss during the first genital herpes attack compared to male patients [29].

5.2. Recurrent genital herpes

The virus remaining latent in sensory neural ganglia following the primary genital herpes reactivates and causes recurrent infections. Recurrent lesions occur more commonly in men. Recurrence is observed in 70–90% of HSV-2-positive individuals and in 20–50% of HSV-1-positive individuals who have had a symptomatic primary genital infection [5]. Recurrences are six times more frequent in HSV-2 infections compared to HSV-1 infections [1]. One to two days prior to recurrent lesions, prodromal signs such as itching, tingling, paresthesia, and pain in lumbosacral dermatomes are observed. Recurrent genital herpes lesions involve less grouped lesions compared to primary genital herpes and tend to be unilateral (**Figure 1**). It

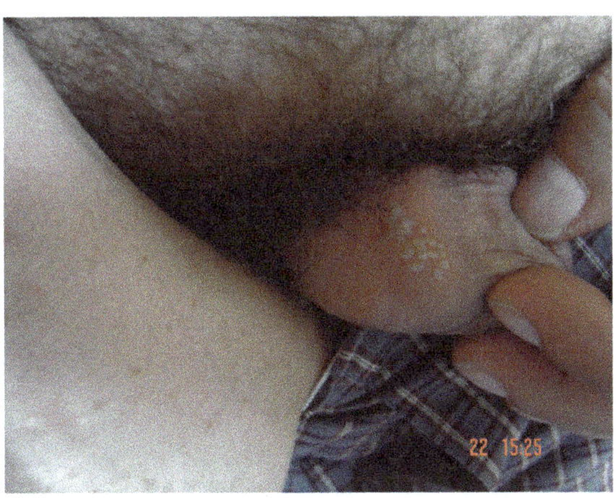

Figure 1. Painful grouped vesicles are seen. By the courtesy of Dr. Zekayi Kutlubay.

is usually not accompanied by systemic symptoms. Lesions are painful; however, the pain is milder compared to primary infection. Lesions usually heal within 7–8 days and viral spread lasts shorter and its concentration is lower. Recurrences may occur on thighs, lower abdomen, hips, and genital organs. Fissures, erythematous patches, excoriations, and linear ulcerations may be seen as atypical lesions [1, 11, 30]. Recurrent infections become sparse in time. That being said, recurrences have been reported in 25% of patients in the fourth year of infection [5].

5.3. Asymptomatic genital viral shedding

Genital herpes infections are characterized by lifelong viral shedding after the first genital herpes attack. Viral shedding in individuals infected with genital herpes continues with both lesional and asymptomatic periods. Fifty to ninety percent of transmissions occur from infected individuals who are not aware of their infections during the asymptomatic viral shedding period. Only 25% of HSV-2-seropositive individuals have genital herpes history. The majority of infected individuals either carries the infection asymptomatically or is not aware of symptoms [1, 2]. The period with the highest risk of transmission is the active disease period which involves visible lesions. Shedding continues for 1 week after symptomatic attacks. However, viral reactivation is characterized by asymptomatic viral shedding in most patients. The asymptomatic shedding property of the virus is the most significant reason behind its spread. Viral shedding is very common in HSV-2-seropositive patients, whereas it is less common in asymptomatic HSV-1 patients. The cell shredding rate is 3–5% in cell cultures obtained from women infected with genital HSV-2 in asymptomatic period; however, this rate goes up to 28% when wipe samples are examined using the polymerase chain reaction (PCR) method.

Studies show that the highest shedding rates are seen within the first year following the onset of the infection. In a study involving 377 adults with genital herpes, viral shedding was examined by applying the PCR method to anogenital swab and found to be 33.6% within the first year after the first attack, 20.6% between 1 and 9 years, and 16.7% over 10 years. Subclinical viral shedding was shown to be similar in both men and women.

5.4. Neonatal herpes

A rare yet serious complication of genital herpes in the mother during pregnancy, neonatal herpes, has a mortality risk of 60% if not treated. It may lead to mortality and permanent sequels in 30% of cases in spite of antiviral treatment. Neonatal herpes is estimated to be about 10 in 100,000 live births worldwide. This corresponds to approximately 14,000 neonatal herpes (4000 HSV-1 and 10,000 HSV-2) cases every year. The highest number of neonatal herpes cases belongs to Africa due to high HSV-2 positivity rate among women and high birth rate. HSV-1 infections cause more neonatal herpes cases than HSV-2 infections in the United States, Europe, and the West of the Pacific [31].

Transmission from the mother to the infant mostly (85%) occurs during vaginal birth due to viral shedding. Intrauterine (5%) and postnatal (10%) transmission cases are less common [2, 8]. Its clinical manifestation involves eye, mouth, and skin infection, central nervous system disease, or disseminated disease which starts within the first 28 days of life. Eye, mouth, and skin infection is present in 45% of cases and characterized by vesicular lesions without CNS involvement or disseminated disease. CNS disease is observed in about 30% of cases and characterized by lethargy, feeding difficulty, and seizures. CNS disease may be accompanied by skin lesions. The mortality is 6% and permanent moderate and severe neurological damage is 50% with intravenous (IV) acyclovir treatment. Disseminated disease consists of the remaining 25% of cases and presents multiple organ involvement with clinical sepsis. The mortality is 30% in spite of acyclovir treatment [20].

6. Laboratory

Although genital herpes can be diagnosed via patient history and examination, herpes diagnosis may not always be easy. There may be atypical localizations such as hip and thigh or atypical presentations such as vulvar/penile/perianal fissures, recurrent erythema, recurrent pain, cystitis, urethritis, and genital discharge without lesions. On the other hand, various diseases causing ulcers in the genital region such as Behcet's disease, Crohn's disease, other sexually transmitted diseases, and fixed drug eruption may mimic herpes. In such cases, the patient may be subjected to unnecessary antiviral treatments and experience negative social and psychosocial effects due to the diagnosis. For a thorough infection management, the clinical diagnosis must be supported with laboratory confirmation. Supporting the diagnosis is also important for detection of possible cases, further consulting services, and prevention of serious complications such as neonatal herpes [32–34].

6.1. Virus detection and typing

It refers to displaying the viral genome on the skin or mucosal membrane. The best test sample is vesicle content. Samples must be sent to the laboratory in saline or virus transport medium [30]. Virus detection methods are mainly divided into four groups: cell culture, molecular methods (nucleic acid amplification tests (NAATs)), direct viral antigen detection, and cytological examinations [34]. The most commonly preferred methods are cell culture and PCR, which is a NAAT method. It is possible to distinguish between HSV-1 and HSV-2 using these two methods. It is absolutely necessary to distinguish between HSV-1 and HSV-2 in newly diagnosed genital herpes cases [35]. Because viral shedding is intermittent, the fact that no infected cell is detected does not mean that the HSV infection is not present [36].

Cell culture has lost its previous significance since it has low sensitivity in cases of healing lesions and ulcerative lesions and requires more time compared to PCR. NAAT methods such as PCR are accepted as the reference test by many centers due to their high sensitivity [30, 34, 36, 37]. Other advantages of NAAT methods include reproducibility, speed, and labor efficiency [38]. Direct viral antigen detection is a good alternative since it results in a matter of hours and is a commercially accessible method. However, it has certain disadvantages such as low specificity and sensitivity values and inability to distinguish types. Cytological methods based on detection of cellular changes such as Tzanck are not recommended due to lack of specificity and sensitivity. Similarly, these methods do not allow for distinguishing types as well [34].

6.2. Serology

Immunoglobulin M (IgM) antibodies can be detected in blood 7–10 days after encountering the infectious agent. They remain detectable for about 1–2 weeks, while they remain positive for about 6 weeks in some individuals. They become positive again within a short time frame in recurrent infections [39]. Detection of IgG antibodies may require 2 weeks to 3 months following the transmission of the virus and they remain positive for lifetime [5]. Although IgM detection in IgG negativity during the window period in the first infection in particular may be important for primary infection diagnosis, it is not recommended for routine practice [34, 40].

HSV-1 IgG antibodies do not allow for distinguishing between genital and oropharyngeal infections, HSV-2 IgG antibodies can be used to confirm genital herpes infection diagnosis. For this reason, detection of type-specific HSV IgG antibodies, especially HSV-2, is very important to use type-specific serological tests for an accurate and effective genital herpes management [6, 34].

Detection of type-specific HSV IgG antibodies is a rapid, effective, and reliable method in infection diagnosis. Although it does not provide information related to infection time, it is possible to support primary infection diagnosis in individuals who are believed to have *the first genital herpes attack*. When used together with direct virus detection methods, primary infection diagnosis is possible with observing the initially negative IgG value, which is specific to HSV type, becoming positive in repeated PCR tests. Serology is also effective in detection of asymptomatic HSV-2 carries and possible viral shedders [30]. Especially *patients with negative direct virus detection tests, yet recurrent or atypical genital symptoms and partners of individuals diagnosed with genital herpes* are suitable indications. If the partner is HSV-2-negative, it is important to detect the infection to take protective measures. It is also important to know the HSV serology in case of pregnancy to protect against neonatal herpes, which is a serious condition, and take necessary measures. Moreover, HSV-2 infection increases the risk of HIV transmission independently and leads to disease progression in HIV-seropositive patients. Therefore, HSV serology should be explored especially for *individuals with multiple partners and/or HIV-seropositive individuals* to control sexually transmitted diseases and manage HIV. HSV serology has no indication in general population [34]. **Table 1** shows how to interpret laboratory findings in detail.

Type-specific serological tests are commercially available and the enzyme-linked immunosorbent assay (ELISA) method is widely used. They depend on detection of HSV-specific glycoprotein G1 or C1 (HSV-1) and glycoprotein G2 (HSV-2) as antigen [36]. These tests have a sensitivity of 97–100% and a specificity of 94–98% [5, 41]. Although there are multiple tests used for confirmation, the Western Blot test is accepted as the gold standard and can be found in only a number of reference centers [34].

	HSV-1 detection by direct method	HSV-2 detection by direct method	HSV-1-specific IgG	HSV-2-specific IgG	Interpretation
First assessment of genital lesions	Positive	Negative	Negative	Positive or negative	Acute HSV-1 infection. Repeat HSV-1-specific serology within 15–30 days
	Negative	Positive	Positive or negative	Negative	Acute HSV-2 infection. Repeat HSV-2-specific serology within 15–30 days
Recurrent genital lesions	Positive	Negative	Positive	Positive or negative	Recurrent HSV-1 infection
	Negative	Positive	Positive or negative	Positive	Recurrent HSV-2 infection
	Negative	Negative	Negative	Positive	Possible recurrent HSV-2 infection. Other potential causes of genital ulcerative disease should be considered
	Negative	Negative	Positive	Negative	Possible recurrent HSV-1 infection. Other potential causes of genital ulcerative disease should be considered

Table 1. Virological and serological approach to genital HSV infection.

7. Treatment

Systemic antiviral use is the essential point of genital herpes treatment. Studies have shown that systemic antiviral treatment limits the severity and duration of the genital herpes attack [42, 43]. The important point to keep in mind is that antiviral treatment does not eliminate latent infection and does not affect posttreatment recurrence risk and severity [36].

In treatment of HSV-1- and HSV-2-induced genital herpes, it is recommended to use acyclovir, valacyclovir, and famciclovir as the standard primary care [30, 36]. These are nucleoside analogs which inhibit herpesvirus DNA polymerase specifically. While acyclovir is available in IV and oral forms, valacyclovir and famciclovir are available in oral form only. These three agents have similar activities in terms of reducing disease severity, duration, and recurrence [44]. Acyclovir is the prototype drug since it is the first molecule used. It is safe and has high tolerability. Gastrointestinal system complaints, eruption, and temporary neurotoxic effects are possible. Nephrotoxicity may develop in insufficiently hydrated cases. Concurrent nephrotoxic drug use should be avoided, liver and kidney functions should be followed closely, and the dose should be adjusted in case of renal failure [45]. Valacyclovir is the prodrug form of acyclovir. Valacyclovir is converted to acyclovir by hepatic valacyclovir hydrolase. It has higher oral bioavailability. Its use is not licensed for children, adolescents, and pregnant women. Its side effect profile is similar to that of acyclovir. Famciclovir is the prodrug form of penciclovir, which is only available in topical form. It has a quite high oral bioavailability. Similar to valacyclovir, its use is not licensed for children, adolescents, and pregnant women. Possible side effects include headache, nausea, and diarrhea [30].

The effect of topical agents is weaker than systemic agents and they do not contribute to combined treatment. They are not recommended for use in case of genital herpes since they lead to an increase in resistance. Intravenous treatment should be considered only when oral agents cannot be tolerated and in complicated cases [35]. Washing with serum physiologic and using analgesic and topical anesthetic agents are additional approaches which may be beneficial.

7.1. Primary genital herpes

Primary infections are usually more severe and longer compared to recurrent attacks. Therefore, guides recommend systemic antiviral use in all primary genital herpes cases. It is recommended that treatment is started within the first 5 days. If new lesion formation continues, treatment should be started in cases older than 5 days as well. The patient should be followed up closely in terms of systemic symptoms, complications, and new lesion formation. In such cases, it may be necessary to prolong the standard treatment [35, 36, 46]. **Table 2** shows recommended doses in detail.

7.2. Recurrent genital herpes

Recurrent genital herpes attacks are usually self-limiting and not so irritating compared to the first attack. However, attacks may sometimes be very frequent (four to six times a year or more) and severe and reduced the individual's life quality. In such cases, two different regimens are used: the suppressive treatment and the intermittent treatment. Patient compliance and cost should be considered when choosing a treatment regimen. **Table 2** shows recommended doses in detail. Acyclovir is low in cost compared to the other two agents. Intermittent treatment seems to be more advantageous than suppressive treatment in terms of both patient compliance and cost. Although studies show that both treatment regimens are effective and safe, suppressive treatment is more effective [47]. Thus, the World Health Organization (WHO) recommends suppressive treatment at first and to stop the treatment after 1 year to reassess recurrence frequency [46]. Since the patient usually experiences an attack after stopping the treatment, it is recommended to wait at least for the second attack. The treatment may be restarted after reassessment for patients who have unacceptable attack frequency and symptoms [35].

First episode for genital herpes (adult, pregnant, immunosuppressive patients)	Oral doses[a]
Acyclovir[b]	400 mg three times a day for 5–10 days or 200 mg five times a day for 5–10 days
Valacyclovir	500–1000 mg twice a day for 5–10 days
Famciclovir	250 mg three times a day for 5–10 days
Suppressive therapy for recurrent genital herpes	
Acyclovir[b]	400 mg twice a day[d] 200 mg four times daily[c]
Valacyclovir	500 mg once a day or 1 g once a day[d]
Famciclovir	250 mg twice a day 500 mg twice a day[d]
Episodic therapy for recurrent genital herpes	
Acyclovir[b]	400 mg three times a day for 5 days[d] or 800 mg twice a day for 5 days or 800 mg three times a day for 2 days
Valacyclovir	500 mg twice a day for 3 days or 1 g once a day for 5 days[d]
Famciclovir	125–250 mg twice a day for 5 days or 1 g twice a day for 1 day or 500 mg for 1 dose followed by 250 mg twice a day for 2 days 500 mg twice a day for 5 days[d]

[a]First episode oral doses vary according to guidelines.

[b]Recommended as the first choice in the WHO STI guideline.

[c]Has a usage difficulty although it is found more efficient than the usage of 400 mg twice a day.

[d]The recommended dose for the people HIV+ and have more than 10 episodes a year.

Table 2. Treatment of genital herpes.

7.3. Management of complications

Complications such as urinary retention, meningoencephalitis, disseminated disease, pneumonia, and hepatitis, which are usually observed during the first attack and in immunosuppressive individuals, should be treated by hospitalizing the patient. The patient should be administered acyclovir 5–10 mg/kg IV every 8 h for 2–7 days or until clinical recovery is observed. The initial intervention should be followed up with oral antiviral treatment and the process should be completed in a total of 10 days. The treatment should be 21 days in case of HSV encephalitis [36].

7.4. Special cases

7.4.1. HSV management in pregnancy

Neonatal herpes during pregnancy is a serious health problem with high mortality and morbidity. Herpes must be managed carefully during pregnancy to minimize the risk of transmission to fetus. Primary/recurrent character of the maternal infection, presence of transplacental neutralizing antibodies, presence of premature rupture of membranes, fetal scalp electrode use, and labor method are factors which affect transmission [48]. Maximum risk occurs with the primary infection acquired during the third trimester.

7.4.1.1. Primary attack management

Treatment should not be delayed in case of primary attack. Oral acyclovir administration in standard dose (400 mg/three times/day) is recommended as primary care. If the maternal infection is disseminated, IV use should be considered [49]. Although all three agents are accepted to be safe, valacyclovir and famciclovir are not recommended for primary care due to insufficient data [49–51]. If the attack occurs during the first or the second trimester, suppressive treatment with acyclovir may be started again from the 36th week until labor [52, 53]. If the attack occurs during the third trimester, acyclovir administration should be continued until labor. Detection of type-specific HSV antibodies is recommended for pregnant women who apply due to primary attack during the third trimester. Detection of the same antibody type with the type isolated on genital swab usually indicates recurrent attack rather than primary attack. There is no elective C-section indication in such cases. Otherwise, if there is also any doubt, attacks in the third trimester should be treated as primary attack and elective C-section should be used [49].

7.4.1.2. Recurrent attack management

Existing protective antibodies of the pregnant woman with recurrent attack protect the fetus against transplacental transmission. Thus, neonatal herpes is not common in recurrent herpes cases. While antiviral treatment is not recommended for recurrent attacks before the 36th week, standard treatment may be considered in severe cases [54, 55]. It has been shown that suppressive treatment with acyclovir from the 36th week until labor reduces viral shedding, clinical herpes lesions, and requirement for C-section [56]. Vaginal birth should be preferred if there is no other obstetric contraindication. Even though vaginal birth is recommended in case of lesion presence during birth, the final decision should be made by the mother due to low neonatal herpes risk [49].

7.4.2. HSV management in HIV-positive patients

HSV is a condition that requires careful assessment in HIV+ patients. Similar to immunocompetent individuals, reactivation is subclinical in most cases [57]. However, the form of reactivation is closely related with the rate of immunosuppression and ulcerate, necrotic, painful, massive, multiple, and atypical lesions may be observed especially in patients with low CD4+ cell count [58]. Resistance is a high possibility in HIV+ patients. Antiviral treatment has been shown to be effective in HIV+ patients as well [59, 60]. However, antiviral treatment has not been found to be effective in preventing the transmission of HIV or HSV to the possible partner [61, 62]. **Table 2** shows doses for HIV+ patients.

7.5. Cases of resistance

Drug resistance should always be considered in cases where lesions become chronic or new attacks occur under antiviral treatment. Development of drug resistance against acyclovir and derivatives has been increasing due to high prevalence of herpes and frequent and prolonged use of accessible agents. There is a vast difference between immunocompetent and immunosuppressive cases in terms of drug resistance. Immunocompetent individuals rarely develop drug resistance, while drug resistance rates up to 36% have been reported for immunosuppressive cases in the literature. In a clinical study on patients with genital herpes, the acyclovir resistance rate has been found to be 0.18% for HIV-negative cases and 5.3% for HIV-positive cases [63–65].

Acyclovir resistance occurs through HSV thymidine kinase gene mutations. Phenotypically, it is observed as loss in TK activity, reduced TK production, or reduced affinity for substrate [66]. Acyclovir resistance is accompanied by cross-resistance against other nucleoside analogs such as valacyclovir, famciclovir, ganciclovir, and penciclovir since they share the same mechanism. While treatment with high doses of acyclovir and analogs is possible in cases of partial resistance, other treatment methods, which do not depend on TK, should be considered in cases of complete resistance [35, 67]. An oral agent other than acyclovir and analogs is not available. Foscarnet (40–80 mg/kg IV every 8 h) administration is the first choice after high doses of acyclovir in case of non-response to nucleoside analogs. Non-response to foscarnet is also possible, albeit rare. In such cases, IV cidofovir administration (5 mg/kg/week) may be considered [68]. Topical imiquimod is a good alternative in cases where IV treatment is not possible [69–71]. Although it is effective in resistant cases, topical cidofovir is disadvantaged due to lack of a commercially available preparation [72].

8. Protection from transmission

The first and most important approach is to inform asymptomatic partners and detection of possible asymptomatic carriers by assessing type-specific HSV-2 antibodies. Although it is not possible to fully protect HSV-2-seronegative partners from transmission, it is possible to minimize the risk. The primary reason behind sexual transmission is asymptomatic viral shedding. Both HSV-1- and HSV-2-induced genital herpes cases may involve asymptomatic viral shedding. Viral shedding is more common in individuals with frequent and severe attacks in particular. The first step to protection is to encourage condom use. It has been shown to have quite high effectiveness in regular use and higher effectiveness in transmission from man to woman [73]. Sexual intercourse should be avoided during active attack periods. Asymptomatic viral shedding responsible for transmission can be suppressed with all systemic antiviral treatments [74, 75]. A reverse transcriptase inhibitor analog also approved for HIV, gel form of tenofovir, has been shown to protect HSV-seronegative women against transmission when used 12 h prior to intercourse [76]. SPL7013 gel (VivaGel®) is a microbicide developed to protect against HIV and HSV. It has been found to have strong antiviral activity when used 3 h before intercourse [77].

Efforts to develop a vaccine for HSV-1 and HSV-2 are among the priorities of WHO. Although there is no licensed HSV vaccine available as of now, there are numerous vaccines at clinical and preclinical study stages. Studies have gained pace, thanks to a better understanding of immune response against HSV [78]. Vaccines generally have two different purposes: reduction of disease activity and viral shedding (therapeutic) and prevention of infection occurrence (prophylactic). The most common HSV vaccines used in human clinical studies are glycoprotein subunit (gp D2) vaccines. A HSV subunit vaccine, HerpeVac, is a prophylactic vaccine and has the most intensive clinical study. In a study on HSV-1- and HSV-2-seronegative women, it has been found that the vaccine provides 58% protection against HSV-1; however, it has no protective effect against HSV-2 [79]. Clinical phase II studies of four prospective vaccines with therapeutic indications still continue today. First results of studies on GEN-003, a gD2/ICP4 protein subunit vaccine with Matrix M adjuvant, indicate that the vaccine reduces viral shedding by about 50% [80]. HerpV, a peptide vaccine with 32 peptides complexed with heat shock proteins and Q-21 adjuvant, is another therapeutic vaccine and reduces viral shedding by 15%. The other two vaccines (codon-optimized polynucleotide vaccine and VCL-HB01/HM01) are DNA vaccines and research results are awaited for these vaccines. Phase I studies for HSV529, a replication-defective HSV-2 vaccine, have started with both therapeutic and prophylactic indications [81].

9. Consultancy

It is very important to inform herpes-seropositive individuals and their partners accurately and completely and eliminate their concerns. Because it is possible to improve their life quality through the right consultancy, transmission can be minimized and cases such as neonatal herpes may be prevented. It is not an accurate and complete approach to provide medical services only. Patients should be provided consultancy in the first visit. A healthy consultancy and information should involve the following:

- ***General***: HSV is not a race- or gender-specific infection. While having multiple partners increases the risk, it may be seen in monogamous individuals as well. Transmission is possible without clinical lesions and symptoms (asymptomatic viral shedding). Recurrences are likely to happen.
- ***Treatment***: It is possible to reduce lesion duration and severity, attack frequency, asymptomatic viral shedding, and negative psychological effects on the patient using antiviral systemic treatment [44, 82].

- ***Protection***: It is important that current and future partners are informed by the HSV-positive individual. Partner status should be determined by serology and HSV-negative partners should be informed about possible measures. Intercourse should be avoided during active lesion presence and transmission risk should be minimized by condom use. HSV+ women should be informed about the neonatal herpes risk, and obstetricians and gynecologists should be urged to inform patients during pregnancy. In addition, it should be mentioned that HIV transmission risk is increased in HSV-2-positive individuals.
- ***Psychology***: Mental health of individuals may be negatively affected upon diagnosis due to shame, guilt, fear, and despair. Words such as "chronic, incurable, attack" should be avoided during the visit to prevent increased concern. The patient may not understand what is told during the first visit due to the shock caused by the diagnosis. For this reason, the patient should be followed up in future visits. The individual may overcome the difficulty by sharing experiences with or learning from others with the same infection. There are various support platforms which can be used for this purpose and the individual may be referred to such platforms [35, 36, 83].

Author details

Selma Emre[1]* and Ayse Akkus[2]

*Address all correspondence to: dr_semre@yahoo.com

1 Department of Dermatology, Medical School, Yildirim Beyazit University, Ankara, Turkey

2 Dermatology Clinic, Tunceli State Hospital, Tunceli, Turkey

References

[1] Beauman JG. Genital herpes: A review. American Family Physician. 2005;**72**(8):1527-1534

[2] Brugha R, Keersmaekers K, Renton A, Meheus A. Genital herpes infection: A review. International Journal of Epidemiology. 1997;**26**(4):698-709

[3] Xu F, Sternberg MR, Kottiri BJ, McQuillan G, Lee FK, Nahmias AJ, Berman SM, Markowitz LE. Trends in herpes simplex virus type 1 and type 2 seroprevalence in the United States. Journal of American Medical Association. 2006;**296**(8):964-973. DOI: 10.1001/jama.296.8.964

[4] Kortekangas-Savolainen O, Orhanen E, Puodinketo T, Vuorinen T. Epidemiology of genital herpes simplex virus type 1 and 2 infections in southwestern Finland during a 10-year period (2003-2012). Sexually Transmitted Diseases. 2014;**41**(4):268-271. DOI: 10.1097/OLQ.0000000000000101

[5] Gupta R, Warren T, Wald A. Genital herpes. Lancet. 2007;**370**:2127-2137. DOI: 10.1016/S0140-6736(07)61908-4

[6] Wald A, Ericsson M, Krantz E, Selke S, Corey L. Oral shedding of herpes simplex virus type 2. Sexually Transmitted Infections. 2004;**80**(4):272-276. DOI: 10.1136/sti.2003.007823

[7] Fatahzadeh M, Schwartz RA. Human herpes simplex virus infections: Epidemiology, pathogenesis, symptomatology, diagnosis, and management. Journal of the American Academy of Dermatology. 2007;**57**(5):737-763. DOI: 10.1016/j.jaad.2007.06.027

[8] Cunningham AL, Taylor R, Taylor J, Marks C, Shaw J, Mindel A. Prevalence of infection with herpes simplex virus types 1 and 2 in Australia: A nationwide population based survey. Sexually Transmitted Infections. 2006;**82**:164-168. DOI: 10.1136/sti.2005.016899

[9] Cunningham AL, Diefenbach RJ, Miranda-Saksena M, Bosnjak L, Kim M, Jones C, Douglas MW. The cycle of human herpes simplex virus infection: Virus transport and immune control. The Journal of Infectious Diseases. 2006;**194**:S11-S18. DOI: 10.1086/505359

[10] Beydoun HA, Dail J, Ugwu B, Boueiz A, Beydoun MA. Socio-demographic and behavioral correlates of herpes simplex virus type 1 and 2 infections and co-infections among adults in the USA. International Journal of Infectious Diseases. 2010;**14**(Suppl 3):e154-e160. DOI: 10.1016/j.ijid.2009.12.007

[11] Koren M, Decker CF. Genital herpes. Disease-a-Month. 2016;**62**(8):287-293. DOI: 10.1016/j.disamonth.2016.03.013

[12] Whitley RJ, Roizman B. Herpes simplex virus infections. Lancet. 2001;**357**(9367):1513-1518. DOI: 10.1016/S0140-6736(00)04638-9

[13] Rajagopal S, Magaret A, Mugo N, Wald A. Incidence of herpes simplex virus type 2 infections in Africa: A systematic review. Open Forum Infectious Diseases. 2014;**1**(2):e2014. DOI: 10.1093/ofid/ofu043

[14] Paz-Bailey G, Ramaswamy M, Hawkes SJ, Geretti. Herpes virus type 2: Epidemiology and management options in developing countries. Sexually Transmitted Infections. 2007;**83**:16-22. DOI: 10.1136/sti.2006.020966

[15] Suazo PA, Ibanez FJ, Retamel-Diaz AR, Pas-Fiblaz MV, Bueno SM, Kalergis AM, Gonzalez PA. Evasion of early antiviral responses by herpes simplex viruses. Mediators of Inflammation. 2015;**2015**:593757. DOI: 10.1155/2015/593757

[16] Mindel A. Herpes Simplex Virus. Berlin Heidelberg: Springer-Verlag; 1989. pp. 1-14. DOI: 10.1007/978-1-4471-1683-7

[17] Jaishankar D, Shukla D. Genital herpes: Insights into sexually transmitted infectious disease. Microbial Cell. 2016;**3**(9):438-450. DOI: 10.15698/mic2016.09.528

[18] Di Giovine P, Settembre EC, Bhargava AK, Luftig MA, Lou H, Cohen GH, Eisenberg RJ, Krummenacher C, Carfi A. Structure of herpes simplex virus glycoprotein D bound to the human receptor nectin-1. PLoS Pathogens. 2011;**7**(9):e1002277. DOI: 10.1371/journal.ppat.1002277

[19] Marques AR, Straus SE. Herpes simplex. In: Wolf K, Goldsmith LA, Katz SI, Gilchrest BA, Paller AS, Leffell DJ, editors. Fitzpatrick's Dermatology in General Medicine. 8th ed. McGraw Hill; eBook. 2008. pp. 1873-1885. DOI: 10.1036/0071466908

[20] Gardella C. Herpes simplex virus genital infections: Current concepts. Current Infectious Disease Reports. 2011;**13**:588-594. DOI: 10.1007/s11908-011-0209-5

[21] Wald A, Zeh J, Selke S, Warren T, Ashley R, Corey L. Genital shedding of herpes simplex virus among men. The Journal of Infectious Diseases. 2002;**186**(Suppl 1):S34–S39

[22] Nicoll MP, Proença JT, Efstathiou S. The molecular basis of herpes simplex virus latency. FEMS Microbiology Reviews. 2012;**36**:684-705. DOI: 10.1111/j.1574-6976.2011.00320.x

[23] Weiss HA, Buve A, Robinson NJ, Dyck EV, Kahindo M, Anagonou S, Musonda R, Zekeng L, Morison L, Carael M, Laga M, Hayes RJ. The epidemiology of HSV-2 infection and its association with HIV infection in four urban African populations. AIDS. 2001;**15**(Suppl 4):S97-S108

[24] Freeman EE, Weiss HA, Glynn JR, Cross PL, Whitworth JA, Hayes RJ. Herpes simplex virus 2 infection increases HIV acquisition in men and women: Systematic review and meta-analysis of longitudinal studies. AIDS. 2006;**20**:73-83

[25] Allan P, Das S. Prevalence of HSV-1/HSV-2 antibodies in HIV seropositive patients in Coventry, United Kingdom. Sexually Transmitted Infections. 2004;**80**(1):77. DOI:10.1136/sti.2002.003343

[26] Tan DH, Murphy K, Shah P, Walmsley SL. Herpes simplex virus type 2 and HIV disease progression: A systematic review of observational studies. BMC Infectious Diseases. 2013;**13**:502. DOI:10.1186/1471-2334-13-502

[27] Thin RN. Does first episode genital herpes have an incubation period? A clinical study. International Journal of STD & AIDS. 1991;**2**(4):285-286. DOI:10.1177/095646249100200412

[28] Auslander BA, Biro FM, Rosenthal SL. Genital herpes in adolescents. Seminars in Pediatric Infectious Diseases. 2005;**16**:24-30. DOI:10.1053/j.spid.2004.09.008

[29] Richards J, Krantz E, Selke S, Wald A. Healthcare seeking and sexual behavior among patients with symptomatic newly acquired genital herpes. Sexually Transmitted Diseases. 2008;**35**(12):1015-1021. DOI: 10.1097/OLQ.0b013e318182a596

[30] Sauerbrei A. Herpes genitalis: Diagnosis, treatment and prevention. Geburtsh Frauenheilk. 2016;**76**:1310-1317. DOI: 10.1055/s-0042-116494

[31] Looker KJ, Magaret AS, May MT, Turner KM, Vickerman P, Newman LM, Gottlieb SL. First estimates of the global and regional incidence of neonatal herpes infection. The Lancet Global Health. 2017;**5**(3):e300–e309. DOI: 10.1016/S2214-109X(16)30362-X

[32] Steben M. Genital herpes simplex virus infection. Clinical Obstetrics & Gynecology. 2005;**48**(4):838-844

[33] Gnann JW, Whitley RJ. Genital herpes. New England Journal of Medicine. 2016;**375**(7):666-674. DOI: 10.1056/NEJMcp1603178

[34] Legoff J, Péré H, Bélec L. Diagnosis of genital herpes simplex virus infection in the clinical laboratory. Virology Journal. 2014 May;**11**:83. DOI: 10.1186/1743-422X-11-83

[35] Patel R, Green J, Clarke E, Seneviratne K, Abbt N, Evans C, et al. 2014 UK national guideline for the management of anogenital herpes. International Journal of STD & AIDS. 2015;**26**(11):763-776. DOI: 10.1177/0956462415580512

[36] Workowski KA, Bolan GA. Sexually Transmitted Diseases Treatment Guidelines, 2015. MMWR Recommendations and Reports. 2015;**64**(RR-03):1-137

[37] Strick LB, Wald A. Diagnostics for herpes simplex virus: Is PCR the new gold standard? Molecular Diagnosis & Therapy. 2006;**10**(1):17-28

[38] Ramaswamy M. Diagnosis of genital herpes by real time PCR in routine clinical practice. Sexually Transmitted Infections. 2004;**80**(5):406-410. DOI: 10.1136/sti.2003.008201

[39] Amudha VP, Rashetha, Sucilathangam G, Cinthujah B, Revathy C. Serological profile of HSV-2 in STD patients: Evaluation of diagnostic utility of HSV-2 IgM and IgG detection. Journal of Clinical and Diagnostic Research. 2014 Dec;**8**(12):DC16-9. DOI: 10.7860/JCDR/2014/10586.5314

[40] Morrow R, Friedrich D. Performance of a novel test for IgM and IgG antibodies in subjects with culture-documented genital herpes simplex virus-1 or -2-infection. Clinical Microbiology and Infection. 2006;**12**(5):463-439. DOI: 10.1111/j.1469-0691.2006.01370.x

[41] Ashley RL. Performance and use of HSV type-specific serology test kits. Herpes. 2002;**9** (2):38-45

[42] Fife KH, Barbarash RA, Rudolph T, Degregorio B, Roth R. Valaciclovir versus acyclovir in the treatment of first-episode genital herpes infection. Results of an international, multicenter, double-blind, randomized clinical trial. The Valaciclovir International Herpes Simplex Virus Study Group. Sexually Transmitted Diseases. 1997;**24**(8):481-486

[43] Chosidow O, Drouault Y, Leconte-Veyriac F, Aymard M, Ortonne JP, Pouget F, et al. Famciclovir vs. aciclovir in immunocompetent patients with recurrent genital herpes infections: A parallel-groups, randomized, double-blind clinical trial. British Journal of Dermatology. 2001;**144**(4):818-824. DOI: 10.1046/j.1365-2133.2001.04139.x

[44] Lebrun-Vignes B, Bouzamondo A, Dupuy A, Guillaume J-C, Lechat P, Chosidow O. A meta-analysis to assess the efficacy of oral antiviral treatment to prevent genital herpes outbreaks. Journal of the American Academy of Dermatology. 2007;**57**(2):238-246. DOI: 10.1016/j.jaad.2007.02.008

[45] Kimberlin DW, Whitley RJ. Antiviral therapy of HSV-1 and HSV-2. In: Arvin A, Campadelli-Fiume G, Mocarski E, et al., editors. Human Herpesviruses: Biology, Therapy, and Immunoprophylaxis. Cambridge: Cambridge University Press; 2007. Contributors. Available from: https://www.ncbi.nlm.nih.gov/books/NBK47387/

[46] WHO Guidelines for the Treatment of Genital Herpes Simplex Virus. Geneva: World Health Organization; 2016. Available from: https://www.ncbi.nlm.nih.gov/books/NBK396232/

[47] Fife KH, Almekinder J, Ofner S. A comparison of one year of episodic or suppressive treatment of recurrent genital herpes with valacyclovir. Sexually Transmitted Diseases. 2006;**34**(5):297-301. DOI: 10.1097/01.olq.0000237853.69443.71

[48] Brown ZA, Wald A, Morrow RA, Selke S, Zeh J, Corey L. Effect of serologic status and cesarean delivery on transmission rates of herpes simplex virus from mother to infant. Journal of American Medical Association. 2003;**289**(2):203-209

[49] Foley E, Clarke E, Beckett VA, Harrison S, Pillai A, FitzGerald M, Owen P, Low-Beer N, Patel R. Management of Genital Herpes in Pregnancy Management of Genital Herpes in Pregnancy Guideline Development Group. 2014. Available from: https://www.rcog.org.uk/globalassets/documents/guidelines/management-genital-herpes.pdf

[50] Kang S-H, Chua-Gocheco A, Bozzo P, Einarson A. Safety of antiviral medication for the treatment of herpes during pregnancy. Canadian Family Physician. 2011;**57**(4):427-428

[51] Pasternak B, Hviid A. Use of acyclovir, valacyclovir, and famciclovir in the first trimester of pregnancy and the risk of birth defects. Journal of American Medical Association. 2010;**304**(8):859-866. DOI: 10.1001/jama.2010.1206

[52] Scott LL, Hollier LM, McIntire D, Sanchez PJ, Jackson GL, Wendel GD. Acyclovir suppression to prevent clinical recurrences at delivery after first episode genital herpes in pregnancy: An open-label trial. Infectious Diseases in Obstetrics and Gynecology. 2001;**9**(2):75-80. DOI: 10.1155/S106474490100014X

[53] Sheffield JS, Hollier LM, Hill JB, Stuart GS, Wendel GD. Acyclovir prophylaxis to prevent herpes simplex virus recurrence at delivery: A systematic review. Obstetrics & Gynecology. 2003;**102**(6):1396-1403

[54] Money D, Steben M. Guidelines for the management of herpes simplex virus in pregnancy. Journal of Obstetrics and Gynaecology Canada. 2008;**30**(208):514-526

[55] Westhoff GL, Little SE, Caughey AB. Herpes simplex virus and pregnancy: A review of the management of antenatal and peripartum herpes infections. Obstetrical & Gynecological Survey. 2011;**66**(10):629-638. DOI: 10.1097/OGX.0b013e31823983ec

[56] Hollier LM, Wendel GD. Third trimester antiviral prophylaxis for preventing maternal genital herpes simplex virus (HSV) recurrences and neonatal infection. Hollier LM, Wendel GD. Cochrane Database of Systematic Reviews. 2008;**23**(1):CD004946. DOI: 10.1002/14651858.CD004946.pub2

[57] Schacker T, Zeh J, Hu HL, Hill E, Corey L. Frequency of symptomatic and asymptomatic herpes simplex virus type 2 reactivations among human immunodeficiency virus-infected men. Journal of Infectious Diseases. 1998;**178**(6):1616-1622

[58] Strick LB, Wald A, Celum C. HIV/AIDS: Management of herpes simplex virus Type 2 infection in HIV type 1-infected persons. Clinical and Infectious Diseases. 2006;**43**(3):347-356. DOI: 10.1086/505496

[59] Romanowski B, Aoki FY, Martel AY, Lavender EA, Parsons JE, Saltzman RL. Efficacy and safety of famciclovir for treating mucocutaneous herpes simplex infection in HIV-infected individuals. Collaborative Famciclovir HIV Study Group. AIDS. 2000;**14**(9):1211-1217

[60] Conant MA, Schacker TW, Murphy RL, Gold J, Crutchfield LT, Crooks RJ, et al. Valaciclovir versus aciclovir for herpes simplex virus infection in HIV-infected individuals: two randomized trials. International Journal of STD & AIDS. 2002;**13**(1):12-21. DOI: 10.1258/0956462021924550

[61] Mujugira A, Magaret AS, Celum C, Baeten JM, Lingappa JR, Morrow RA, et al. Daily acyclovir to decrease herpes simplex virus type 2 (HSV-2) transmission from HSV-2/HIV-1 coinfected persons: A randomized controlled trial. Journal of Infectious Diseases. 2013;**208**(9):1366-1374. DOİ: 10.1093/infdis/jit333

[62] Celum C, Wald A, Lingappa JR, Magaret AS, Wang RS, Mugo N, et al. Acyclovir and transmission of HIV-1 from persons infected with HIV-1 and HSV-2. New England Journal of Medicine. 2010;**362**(5):427-439. DOİ: 10.1056/NEJMoa0904849.

[63] Jiang Y-C, Feng H, Lin Y-C, Guo X-R. New strategies against drug resistance to herpes simplex virus. International Journal of Oral Science. 2016;**8**(1):1-6. DOI: 10.1038/ijos.2016.3

[64] Langston AA, Redei I, Caliendo AM, Somani J, Hutcherson D, Lonial S, et al. Development of drug-resistant herpes simplex virus infection after haploidentical hematopoietic progenitor cell transplantation. Blood. 2002;**99**(3):1085-1088

[65] Reyes M. Acyclovir-resistant genital herpes among persons attending sexually transmitted disease and human immunodeficiency virus clinics. Archives of Internal Medicine. 2003;**163**(1):76. DOI: 10.1001/archinte.163.1.76

[66] Gilbert C, Bestman-Smith J, Boivin G. Resistance of herpesviruses to antiviral drugs: Clinical impacts and molecular mechanisms. Drug Resistance Updates. 2002;**5**(2):88-114

[67] Engel JP, Englund JA, Fletcher CV, Hill EL. Treatment of resistant herpes simplex virus with continuous-infusion acyclovir. Journal of American Medical Association. 1990;**263**(12):1662. DOI: 10.1001/jama.1990.03440120084042

[68] Piret J, Boivin G. Resistance of herpes simplex viruses to nucleoside analogues: Mechanisms, prevalence, and management. Antimicrobial Agents and Chemotherapy. 2011;**55**(2):459-472. DOİ: 10.1128/AAC.00615-10

[69] Brummitt CF. Imiquimod 5% cream for the treatment of recurrent, acyclovir-resistant genital herpes. Clinical and Infectious Diseases. 2006;**42**(4):575. DOI: 10.1086/499529

[70] Perkins N, Nisbet M, Thomas M. Topical imiquimod treatment of aciclovir-resistant herpes simplex disease: Case series and literature review. Sexually Transmitted Infections. 2011;**87**(4):292-295. DOI: 10.1136/sti.2010.047431

[71] Hirokawa D, Woldow A, Lee SN, Samie F. Treatment of recalcitrant herpes simplex virus with topical imiquimod. Cutis. 2011;**88**(6):276-277

[72] Lalezari J, Schacker T, Feinberg J, Gathe J, Lee S, Cheung T, et al. A randomized, double-blind, placebo-controlled trial of cidofovir gel for the treatment of acyclovir-unresponsive mucocutaneous herpes simplex virus infection in patients with AIDS. Journal of Infectious Diseases. 1997;**176**(4):892-898

[73] Magaret AS, Mujugira A, Hughes JP, Lingappa J, Bukusi EA, DeBruyn G, et al. Effect of condom use on per-act HSV-2 transmission risk in HIV-1, HSV-2-discordant Couples. Clinical and Infectious Diseases. 2015;**62**(4):456-461. DOI: 10.1093/cid/civ908

[74] Wald A, Selke S, Warren T, Aoki FY, Sacks S, Diaz-Mitoma F, et al. Comparative efficacy of famciclovir and valacyclovir for suppression of recurrent genital herpes and viral shedding. Sexually Transmitted Diseases. 2006;**33**(9):529-533. DOI: 10.1097/01.olq.0000204723.15765.91

[75] Gupta R, Wald A, Krantz E, Selke S, Warren T, Vargas-Cortes M, et al. Valacyclovir and acyclovir for suppression of shedding of herpes simplex virus in the genital tract. Journal of Infectious Diseases. 2004;**190**(8):1374-1381. DOI: 10.1086/424519

[76] Abdool Karim SS, Abdool Karim Q, Kharsany ABM, Baxter C, Grobler AC, Werner L, et al. Tenofovir gel for the prevention of herpes simplex virus type 2 infection. New England Journal of Medicine. 2015;**373**(6):530-539. DOI: 10.1056/NEJMoa1410649

[77] Price CF, Tyssen D, Sonza S, Davie A, Evans S, Lewis GR, et al. SPL7013 gel (VivaGel®) retains potent HIV-1 and HSV-2 inhibitory activity following vaginal administration in humans. Goepfert PA, editor. PLoS One. 2011;**6**(9):e24095. DOI: 10.1371/journal.pone.0024095

[78] Sandgren KJ, Bertram K, Cunningham AL. Understanding natural herpes simplex virus immunity to inform next-generation vaccine design. Clinical & Translational Immunology. 2016;**5**(7):e94. DOI: 10.1038/cti.2016.44

[79] Belshe RB, Leone PA, Bernstein DI, Wald A, Levin MJ, Stapleton JT, et al. Efficacy results of a trial of a herpes simplex vaccine. New England Journal of Medicine. 2012;**366**(1):34-43. DOI: 10.1056/NEJMoa1103151

[80] Wald A. Therapeutic HSV-2 vaccine (GEN-003) results in durable reduction in genital lesions at 1 year phase 1/2aclinical trial: GEN-003-001. 2014. Available from: https://www.genocea.com/assets/Wald-IDSA-2014-10-oct.pdf

[81] Johnston C, Gottlieb SL, Wald A. Status of vaccine research and development of vaccines for herpes simplex virus. Vaccine. 2016;**34**(26):2948-2952. DOI: 10.1016/j.vaccine.2015.12.076

[82] Apoola A, Radcliffe K. Antiviral treatment of genital herpes. International Journal of STD & AIDS. 2004;**15**(7):429-433. DOI: 10.1258/0956462041211153

[83] Warren T, Ebel C. Counseling the patient who has genital herpes or genital human papillomavirus infection. Infectious Disease Clinics of North America. 2005;**19**(2):459-476. DOI: 10.1016/j.idc.2005.03.011

3

Infection by Human Papillomavirus (HPV), *Chlamydia trachomatis* and *Ureaplasma urealyticum*, in Relation with Reproductive Failure

Adriana Ancer-Arellano, Jesus Ancer-Rodríguez, David Hardisson, Alberto Niderhauser-Garcia, Jose Sanchez-Hernández, Alvarez-Cuevas Salomón and Guadalupe Gallegos-Avila

Abstract

Recent studies suggest that besides oncogenic capacity, HPV could have etiological role on infertility, but more evidence is necessary to confirm these results. We present in this chapter the microbiological and clinical outcome of 104 infertile women aleatory selected, from northeast of Mexico: 84.6%, with genital infection (GI) by multiple germs: *Chlamydia trachomatis* (*Ct*) [86.5%], HPV [49%], *Ureaplasma urealyticum* (*Uu*) [47.11%] and *Mycoplasma hominis* [35.57%]. Significant association ($P \leq 0, 05$) was observed between the HPV presence and *Uu* diagnosis, assisted-reproduction unsuccessful like previous treatment, cervical cytology with inflammatory process, multiple sexual partners, white-dense-mucous, secretion into the vagina, and HPV diagnosed in early years. The more frequent genotypes of HPV present in the infertile women studied were 6/18/16/58/11 and 68. In 60% of them, more than two genotypes were founded. The most frequent associations of high-risk HPV (HPVhr) were 16/18, 16/58, 16/33, 16/52 and 18/58. Considering the isolate or combined presentation of HPVhr, 79.5% of these women would have a potential to develop cervix carcinoma. GI by HPV/*Uu*/*Ct* affects the fertility. Infertile women with GI that include these microorganisms with probed (HPV/*Ct*) or suspicious carcinogenic effect (*Uu*) would be considered a group of high risk for cervical cancer.

Keywords: genital infection, HPV, *Chlamydia trachomatis*, *Ureaplasma urealyticum*, Infertility, risk for cervical cancer

1. Introduction

At present, reproductive failure affects to a great population. Human infertility is defined by World Health Organization, like the absent of conception and outcome of healthy baby borne, after 1 year of unprotected intercourse. Infertility is a health complex problem with low quality life for the couples. Estimations on 2010 referred 1.9 and 10.5% of primary and secondary infertility, respectively, on women at reproductive age (20–40 years old). A high prevalence of fertility health is documented in South of Asia, Medium East, Central Europe, East Europe, and Central Asia [1].

Genitourinary unspecific infection is associated with unexplained infertility, subfertility, obstetric and gynecologic complications that not have known clear etiology for several decades like recurrent abortion, premature delivery, placenta dysfunction and preeclampsia [2, 3]. As well, assisted reproduction treatment for infertility had been associated with genital infection [4–7]. Specific treatment for genital infection is recommended to improve the successful of *in vitro* fertilization an embryo implantation [8, 9]. The low age of sexual activity initiation and with multiple sexual partners is a recognized risk factor for sexually transmitted genitourinary infection, but the absent or subtle clinical manifestations prevent the opportune treatment and persisting infection for long time and thus may exert detriment on the reproductive function [10].

Besides the still controversial participation of HPV on fertility and obstetric complications, the major bacteria implicated for a long time are *C. trachomatis,* and other atypical bacteria treated in next section: *U. urealyticum, M. hominis,* that were considered for a long time an improbable cause of female internal genital infection, were isolated from endometrial tissue and material obtained by hysteroscopy and laparoscopy procedures, in women with tubary obstruction, hidrosalpinx, and adherence syndrome [11–15]. In recent years, another species of Mycoplasmataceae, *M. genitalium,* has been considered an emerging sexually transmitted infection that exerts damage in female genital tract and is implicated in fertility problems [16–18].

2. Human papillomavirus

2.1. Classification

HPV belongs to *Papoviridae* family microorganism and comprises a group of approximately 200 small DNA viruses. According to its tissue tropism, HPV has been classified like *Alpha* HPV that affects epithelial mucosae and is subclassified into high risk and low risk of carcinogenic potential *Beta, gamma, nu* and *mu.* HPV has more potential to affect cutaneous epithelia and more associated with papilloma and external warts and had been associated with no melanocytic skin carcinoma [19, 20].

2.2. Epidemiology

The HPV infection has an epidemiologic importance. Registered prevalence is influenced by diagnostic test applied, the number and age of individuals of studied population, the geographic region studied [21]. Nevertheless, actually are considered the most common sexually transmitted viral infection worldwide, present in 11–12% of population and are 14 million people infected by first time each year. The incidence of HPV infection in the United States is one of higher, as 44.8%, and is present principally in women 20–24 years old [22]. In Mexico from 2005 to 2010, urogenital candidiasis and HPV infection present an incidence of 12.3/100,000 habitant between 15 and 24 years old and were higher between 20 and 24 years old. In this country had been estimated that toward 2050, there are not a clear tendency to diminish of the HPV infection. This situation is very worrying due to the potential malignancy of the lesions [23]. On the records of National Institute of Statistic and Geography of Mexico, were informed that 4417 women died by cervical cancer, in 2013 [24].

2.3. Biomedical importance

HPV infect principally undifferentiated keratinocytes into de basal level of stratified squamous epithelia, from mucous genital and oropharyngeal epithelia cutaneous and, as well as glandular cells of endocérvix [25–27]. HPV had been recognized as definitive anogenital carcinogen for male and female, mainly in uterine cervix cancer [28], alone or in combination with other germs [29]. Some estimations show that the presence of HPV represents 12 more opportunities to develop cervical cancer than general population [30] and the HPV infection the most important between the factor risk for cervical cancer [21]. Recently, HPV was associated, lung cancer [31–34] to larynx and pharynx carcinoma that their incidence are increasing in the last years [35, 36]. The global incidence of head and neck squamous cells and cervical cancer is similar; infection at both sites is strongly associated with sexual behavior: similarities in chromosomal aberrations, gene expression, and methylation and micro RNA profiles between Positive HPV head and neck squamous cells and cervical cancer. All of these observations were referred as argue to carry out comparative epidemiologic study of HPV infection and associated with carcinoma of head and neck and cervical cancer [37].

2.4. Their role in reproductive failure

Although is well known than many authors are interested to search carcinogenic roll of HPV, there are only a few studies about the effect of HPV infection on human reproduction [38–41]. There is evidence showing the adherence of HPV to the equatorial segment of sperm cell [42]. Epidemiologic data about the infection by HPV in infertile men associated high levels of seminal leukocytes, with altered movement and morphology of head sperm, with the HPV infection [43–45]. Previously, experimental studies had been demonstrated chromosomic damage in HPV infected sperm, depending of genotypes 16 and 3 [46, 47]. An association has been found between cervical HPV of high risk and premature membrane rupture and preterm new borne [48–50]. The genital infection by more than one genotype of HPV was higher in recurrent early lost pregnancy, and HPV was identified in placenta tissue of preterm delivery by preeclampsia [41]. The frequency of cervical HPV infection and high-grade lesion was higher in women that have indicated assisted reproduction than general population [6] and successful of assisted reproduction were affected by the presence of HPV [5, 7]. The HPV transmission from mother to child *in utero* was informed in several investigations [51–54]. These authors remark the risk to appear papillary lesions in oropharynx and larynx of new born from mothers infected by HPV.

3. Chlamydia trachomatis

3.1. Biology and classification

The family Chlamydiaceae consists of two clinically important genera, *Chlamydia* and *Chlamydophila*, with three species responsible for human disease: *Chlamydia trachomatis*, *Chlamydophila psittaci*, and *Chlamydophila pneumoniae* [55]. *C. trachomatis*, as all the members of the family Chlamydiaceae, is an obligate intracellular parasite whose developmental cycle occurs within a eukaryotic host. Infection of eukaryotic host cells is initiated by the metabolically inactive and the infectious elementary bodies (EBs). Through largely unknown mechanisms, EBs attach to and induce their internalization by host cells. Within the first few hours post infection, EBs differentiate to the larger and more pleomorphic reticulate bodies (RBs), which are metabolically active, noninfectious, and replicative. At the end of a successful developmental cycle, the cell lyses, releasing the EBs [56, 57].

3.2. Medical relevance

Chlamydia trachomatis is the most prevalent sexually transmitted bacterial infection, recognized worldwide, which causes a wide spectrum of diseases, including salpingitis, endometritis, and uterine, cervical lesions with scarring process, which often causes infertility in women [58]. Serotypes D-K of *C. trachomatis* has an etiologic relation to pelvic inflammatory disease; it has been isolated from superior genital tract in a quarter of women with pelvic inflammation and is possible that chronic process would be in relation to ovarian cancer [59]. The role of *C. trachomatis* with regard to inducing male factor infertility is a matter of debate. Chlamydial infection could potentially exert a strong influence on male infertility, as it is the main cause of urethritis and accessory gland inflammation in men. Sequelae of ascending infections might be occlusions in the canaliculi system of the genital tract, damage of the epithelial cells involved in spermatogenesis, and immunoreaction with the production of antisperm antibodies [60, 11]. Also, the relationship of *C. trachomatis* infection with semen quality and sperm morphology is still controversial [61, 62]. In men, are documented that *Chlamydia trachomatis* is responsible of epididymitis, orchitis, prostatitis and urethritis [63–66]. Then more, there are many evidence of that this infection cause sperm damage with low motility, altered morphology, and diminish of sperm concentration, with detriment of male fertility [67–71]. Sexually transmitted infections are hypothesized to play a role in the development of prostate cancer, perhaps due to inflammation-induced oncogenesis [71]. Eventually, more evidence supports this affirmation. An investigation to evaluate the possible role of *Chlamydia trachomatis* in the pathogenesis of prostate cancer assessed the presence of this bacterium in prostate biopsies of patients with prostate cancer, patients with benign prostatic hyperplasia

(BPH) and control subjects. Tissue sections were analyzed using a direct fluorescent-antibody (DFA) assay. When proliferative areas were compared, *C. trachomatis* was most frequently detected in prostate cancer group that in BPH patients ($p = 0.006$). In inflammation areas, *C. trachomatis* was most frequently detected in prostate cancer patients that in control subjects ($p = 0.008$). These data suggest an association between the presence of *C. trachomatis* and prostate cancer [72].

4. Mycoplasmataceae Genus

4.1. Biology and classification

Mycoplasma are microorganisms derived from Gram-positive bacteria characterized by: streamlined and very small genome, the absence of a cell wall, requiring cholesterol for membrane function and growth, and displaying genetic economy that determine a strict dependence of the host for nutrients and refuge [73, 74]. They have a parasitic lifestyle, invading target cells and existing and replicating for extended periods intracellularly [75]. From 200 species established into class Mollicutes, six of them: *Ureaplasma urealyticum, Mycoplasma hominis, Mycoplasma genitalium, Mycoplasma primatum, Mycoplasma spermatophilum* and *Mycoplasma penetrans* have like their main site of colonization, the genital tract [76]. These microorganisms can be commensal in low genitourinary tract of sexually active men and women and can live in close relationship to mammalian cells. Nevertheless, they may cause disorders and pathologies associated with infertility: non-gonococcal and non-chlamydial, epididymitis, urolitiasis, as well with reproductive problems and infertility [77–84].

4.2. Medical relevance

Gnarpe and Friberg in early seventies informed for the first time a high percentage (85%) of infertile patients with *Ureaplasma urealyticum* isolated from semen by specific culture, compared to low percentage (22%) in fertile men. Then, these authors showed by scanning electron microscopy, Mycoplasma adhered to sperm tail [85]. Similar observation was done in the following years by different authors [86–90]. The use of PCR techniques confirmed the presence of *Ureaplasma urealyticum* in seminal samples of subfertile men with sperm alterations [62, 91, 92]. Since two before decade, had been affirm that Mycoplasma have carcinogenic potential due to the long latency an infection chronicity that may induce malignant cellular transformation [93]. Recently, experimental studies demonstrated induction of genic expression altered in prostatic and cervical cells and progression to malignant transformation [94, 95]. *Mycoplasma hominis* and *Mycoplasma hyorhinis*, a mycoplasma frequently present in patients with AIDS, induce malignant transformation with increased karyotypic entropy, chromosomal aberrations and polysomy, in BPH-1 cells, after 9 months that were infected with these germs [96]. These observation had been supported a relationship between prostatitis and cancer, in etiologic association referred in 2002 [97].

5. Mechanism of genital coinfection by HPV, *chlamydia trachomatis* and *mycoplasmas*

The cervical overlaying columnar epithelia can be invaded by *Ureaplasma urealyticum* and *Chlamydia trachomatis* that produce severe inflammatory response, with discharge of exudative secretions and clinical signs and symptoms [98, 99]. Nevertheless, usually the appropriated diagnostic test will not be applied, and the treatment generally is unspecific. The presence of inflammatory cells in the genital ducts enhances the adherence of virus [100, 101], and *Chlamydia trachomatis* has been considered an enhancer to the entry of human immunodeficiency virus and HPV, the only one germ directly associated with the etiology of cervical cancer [101–104]. Several studies have demonstrated an association between *Chlamydia trachomatis* and a high risk HPV persistence [105, 106]. A study realized by Paba et al., (2008), in patients with intraepithelial neoplasia or cervical cancer, confirmed the association of *Chlamydia trachomatis* and multiple high risk HPV persistence, and like a consequence of viral integration, inhibition of cell apoptosis, overexpression of E6/E7 oncogenes and cellular transformation [107].

6. Our experience

6.1. Studies on male infectious factor of infertility

Our group has reported different studies in couples with infertility of unknown etiology, from northeast Mexico. In that patients with spontaneous and recurrent abortion and failure in assisted reproduction treatments, was frequently detected the presence in seminal fluid, urethral swab and cervix and vagina secretions, of *Chlamydia trachomatis* and *Ureaplasma urealyticum,* and *Mycoplasma hominis*. The diagnosis of *Chlamydia trachomatis* was made by direct immunofluorescence, the gold standard for this microorganism for a long of time. For detection of *Ureaplasma urealyticum* and *Mycoplasma sp.,* we practiced specific media culture, considered too, the gold standard. In morphologic seminal analysis, we described the presence of elementary bodies and inclusion vacuoles of Chlamydia and bacterial particles similar to Mycoplasmas, inside the cytoplasm, adhered to the principal piece and into the middle piece of the sperm [108].

A pattern of structural sperm alteration and inflammatory reaction with sperm phagocytosis, by leucocytes and macrophages, were described by semi thin section at light microscopy and thin section by transmission electron microscopy [109–113]. Beside this the infectious process result a diminish motility, vitality, linear movement and sperm concentration. These seminal parameters were associated with high levels of sperm chromatin fragmentation (SCD test), and high levels of reactive oxygen species (ROS) detected by NBT test. The antibiotic, antioxidant and drugs against the inflammation treatment determine the reduction of bacteriospermia, increase percentage of normal sperm, especially from acrosome damage, middle piece flagellum and nuclear defects. After 6 weeks of treatment, the probability of outcome of pregnancy with healthy newborn increased, and seminal parameters of predictive value were chromatin fragmentation, bacteriospermia and head sperm anomalies [114–117].

6.2. Studies on female infectious factor of infertility

After confirming that a very high percentage of couples in northern Mexico with incapacity to procreate, have *Chlamydia trachomatis* and *Ureaplasma urealyticum* infections in the ducts and organs of the seminal tract, associated with detrimental damage of fertilization capacity of the sperm, we studied the endometrium histopathology and *endometrialis bacteria.* Although endometritis is included into the internal genital infection, present in a high percentage of infertile couples, the study of endometrial biopsy is out of the diagnostic routine evaluation of infertility female factor. Microscopic analysis was performed on paraffin embedded and H&E stained tissue sections, observed at 1000X. In all the cases, it was possible to recognize, the presence of bacterial particles, identified according to their morphology, such as Chlamydia or Ureaplasma, which were previously diagnosed in genital secretions. The most frequent histopathologic findings at the endometrial tissue were interstitial edema (93%), lymphocytic and polymorphonuclear subepithelial infiltrate (72%) and in 48%, plasmocytic subepithelial infiltrate. The cell denudation of the lining epithelia was observed in 69% of biopsies, and in 62% of them, intracytoplasmic vacuole of epithelial cells, known as spongiosis, was observed. In a low percentage of cases, intraepithelial inflammatory cells (lymphocytes and polymorphonuclears) were found at the endometrium, both lining and glandular epithelia. Germinal center of inflammatory cells in the connective stroma also was observed. The concluding results of this study showed the invading endometrium with *Chlamydia trachomatis* and *Ureaplasma urealyticum* that were present too, into the mucus of uterine cavity and cervical duct. In view of glandular and stromal changes, inflammatory reaction and presence of bacteria into the stromal tissue and glandular and lining epithelia, endometritis due to *Chlamydia trachomatis* and *Ureaplasma urealyticum*, should be considered like an adverse condition to the female fertility as well implantation and normal embryo development. The clinician must consider the study of endometrial biopsy in all patients that need evaluation for infertility, even more if signs and symptoms of internal genital infection or chronic inflammatory process are present. Early diagnosis of genital infection and laboratory test performance looking for *Chlamydia trachomatis* and *Ureaplasma urealyticum* and its corresponding treatment could be prevent reproductive failure and scarring injuries and maybe can improve the results of reproduction treatments [118, 119]. While male genital infection by *Chlamydia trachomatis and Ureaplasma urealyticum* is generally asymptomatic, the women have a variable signs and symptoms of the sick, and clinical improvement is easier to appreciate; in male, their low and subtle clinical signs of infection and the treatment results can be see only by the study of seminal parameters in relation to the infection. For some years, we have focused on the investigation of the clinical and pathogenic aspects of the internal genital infections as well as the integral therapeutic management of male and female reproductive pathologies named as treatment of "binomials gineco-andrologic" of the infectious factor of Infertility [120, 121].

6.3. Study of HPV in infertile couples

In addition of sexually transmission of *Chlamydia trachomatis and Ureaplasma urealyticum*, along the clinical evaluation, is necessary to be in alert to another sexually transmitted germ. This chapter focuses on the results of the first work that we carried out about the importance of the presence of HPV in the population with infectious factor of infertility. The aim of this analysis was to establish the HPV and genotype prevalence, the relationship of HPV presence with other microorganism, and to describe clinical findings of the studied group of patients.

6.3.1. *Patients, material and methods*

6.3.1.1. *Study population*

For the present analysis, samples of mucous secretion from cervix and vagina and endocervical scrapes of 104 women randomly selected women, from patients attended at private clinic in Monterrey, México, for infertility and genitourinary infection since 2003–2014. Patients were recruited by verbal invitation at the time of consultation. They gave voluntary authorization, by Informed consent, to use the clinical data and results of the laboratory test for statistical analysis. Ethical issues were in accordance with the Helsinki Declaration and endorsed by the Ethics Committee of our institution (PA15-001). All selected patients had polymerase chain reaction (PCR) test for HPV in genital secretions and were tested by direct specimen test Kit for *Chlamydia trachomatis* detection (MicroTrak; Trinity Biotech, Wicklow, Ireland); the isolation of *Ureaplasma urealyticum* and *Mycoplasma hominis* was done using the Mycoplasma IST kit (BioMerieux, Marcy L' Etoile, France). For any other microorganism, we applied general culture.

6.3.1.2. *Clinical assessment*

An infertility medical history was taken and recorded on a standardized form by a single experienced clinician, who also performed external genital, vaginal exploration, pelvic examinations and realized the sampling of genital secretions. The data obtained from medical file were: demographic parameters, history of fertility and infertility, gestational losses and obstetric complications, treatment of infertility problems, history of cervical lesions, and surgical procedures, result of previous cervical-vaginal cytology Pap smears, signs and symptoms of genitourinary infections and pathological data of the cervix and vagina examination. At subjective appreciation, the clinical parameters were considered for semiquantitative record: low, medium, and high or abundant.

6.3.1.3. *HPV DNA extraction and genotyping*

For the extraction and purification of DNA from cervical samples, 100 μL of the cell suspension previously prepared was used. Silica extraction columns (Nucleospin® Blood, Machery-Nagel GmBH & Co., Germany) were used under the manufacturer's instructions. During the 12 years covered by this study, the technology for HPV diagnosis was changing. For this reason, different techniques were applied depending on the time when the patient arrives for medical treatment. In 34 patients, molecular detection of HPV-AND was carried out by PCR-Multiplex that detect 4–12 genotypes; for 36 patients, secretions from the cervix and vagina were tested for HPV capillary electrophoresis using "Applied Biosystems 3130 series genetic analyzer systems" and the software GeneMapper, which diagnostic 14–19 genotypes high and low risk. Molecular detection of ADN from HPV was done in the 36 patients by

Dual Priming Oligonucleotide, more specific and that detect 14–19 genotypes of HPV and in the 34 last patients *in situ* Hybridization with oligo specific probes to identified 20–28 HPV genotypes.

6.3.1.4. Statistical analysis

Absolute frequency of qualitative parameters is expressed in percentages. For quantitative variable was calculated media and, or median as well standard deviation. Sensitivity, specificity, positive and negative predictive values were calculated using (2 × 2) contingency tables. The association between clinical results and HPV and the association between other microorganisms present were calculated with Fisher's exact test. For all tests, the significance level was $P \leq 0.05$ and power of $(1-\beta) = 80\%$ for two-tail. The statistical software used was SPSS version 17 for Windows (SPSS Inc.)

6.3.2. Results

From 690 infertile couples attended from 2003 to 2012, the aleatory selected sample of 104 female partners was representative, according to medium probability ponderation of 48% for the different genotypess, that was estimated based in some reports [122]. A total of 104 female partners from couples with genitourinary infection were included in this study. Primary infertility was present in 65 couples and secondary infertility in 13 couples. The median age of the patients was 34 years (range, 22–55 years). The microorganisms identified on the group studied are *C. trachomatis* (86.5%), HPV (49%), *U. urealyticum* (47.11%), *M. Hominis* (35.57%), *E. coli* (20.2%), *C. Albicans* (17.3%) and *S. faecalis* (10.6%). In a high proportion of the vaginal samples, microbiota vaginal was reduced or absent in a (76.9%) and 86% have more than one pathogen germs. *C albicans* was present like solitary microorganism in 17.3% as well HPV was the only identified germ in one patient. Statistical analysis established positive correlation between HPV and *U. urealyticum* ($p = 0.05$) and decreased microbiota ($p = 0.001$).

The distribution of *C. trachomatis* was similar in the positive and negative to HPV group (**Figure 1**).

Between the clinical parameters taken into account for this investigation, some of them presented statistics correlation to the presence of HPV: the presence of more than one sexual partner ($p = 0.05$), genitourinary infection symptoms ($p = 0.01$), white mucous vaginal secretion fluxing from the uterine duct ($p = 0.05$), failure in assisted reproduction previously carried out ($p \leq 0.0001$), and previous HPV infection diagnosed by suspicious lesion or cytological exam ($p \leq 0.0001$) was in association to HPV (**Table 1**). For *Microbiota vaginalis*, the relationship to the presence of HPV was proportionally inversed.

Prevalent genotypes of HPV detected in the infertile patients studied group were; HPVar 6 (19.2%), HPVhr 18 (12.5%), HPVhr 16 (11.6%), HPVhr 58 (11.1%), HPVhr 52 (7.1%), HPVlr 11 (6.7%) and HPVhr 68 (7.5%). Thirteen different genotypes of PVH were detected in low frequency. These data are concentrated on **Table 2**. To consider the percentage of this frequency, it is necessary to remember that the results depend on the number of HPV search in each one of the three different tests applied that was not equal for all patients.

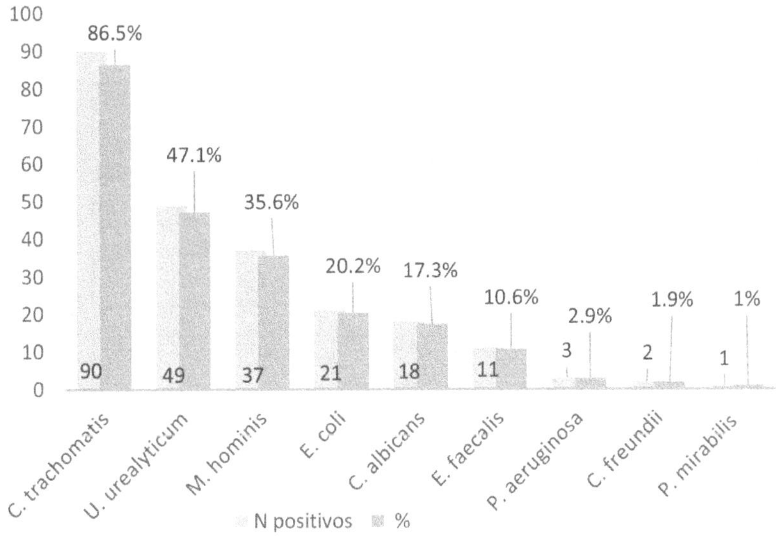

Figure 1. Microorganism identified into the cervix and vagina secretions of 104 female partners from couples with genitourinary infection. The most frequent bacteria in the genital sample of infertile women studied were *Chlamydia trachomatis*. However, if we considered that *Ureaplasma urealyticum* and *Mycoplasma hominis* belong to the same genus: Mycoplasmataceae, the presence of these bacteria, result of major importance in this group.

Combinations of more than one HPV genotypes were detected in 60% on the studied samples. From them 46.3% were the following associations between high risk for cancer HPV: 16/18, 18/58, 16/33, 16/52 and 18/52. In a similar percentage (44.8%) of women, low risk for cancer, principally HPV 6, was detected in combination with high risk HPV: 18, 52, 16 and 39. As well, we observed that three to five different HPV genotypes were present in 23.5% of the positive group infertile patients (**Figure 2**).

According to the results of this study, a total of 79.5% of positive HPV group of patients, presented one or more high-risk genotypes, and considering the statistical association between the positivity to HPV and the clinical history of previous HPV infections, this condition may represent a persistent infection or a reinfection. Consequently, we consider convenient a recommendation to take in account women with reproductive failure, like a group of risk of cervical cancer. There was statistical association between the positivity to HPV to clinical history of previous HPV infections. Would be very important, the simultaneously presence with *Ureaplasma urealyticum*, and *Chlamydia trachomatis*, sexually transmitted germs with suspicious carcinogenic potential, in a population in reproductive age, as we observed in this study.

With the results obtained from this study, it was not possible to establish an association between the abortions presented in 28 of the studied women, and the positivity to HPV. Nevertheless for future studies that include a high number of patients, is may be important to observe that low risk to cancer genotypes 6 and 11, were present in a high prevalence in this investigation, and their importance on the results of inseminations, in vitro fertilization and gestational loss, and are not defined now a days. Finally, our data confirm the recommendation to investigate HPV before to carry out *in vitro* fertilization, in view of the high frequency of failure of this treatment of infertility, when HPV is present.

	Total of cases		HPV positive		HPV negative		P
	N	%	N	%	N	%	
HPV previous diagnosis	46	44.2	33	64.7	13	24.5	0.0001
Pap. report: inflammation low/ moderate	33	32.0	21	41.2	12	23.1	0.05
Active genitourinary infection	67	64.4	39	76.5	28	52.8	0.01
Only one partner	67	64.4	28	54.9	39	73.6	0.05
≥2 sexual partner	37	35.6	23	45.1	14	26.4	0.05
Unsuccessfully FIV/ ICSI	15	100	11	73.3	4	26.7	0.002
White, dense mucus secretion	78	85.7	42	85.7	36	69.2	0.05
Ureaplasma urealyticum in vaginal secretion	49	47.1	29	56.9	20	37.7	0.05
Absence of vaginal microbiota	55	52.9	24	47.1	31	58.5	0.03
Diminished vaginal microbiota	25	24.0	17	33.3	8	15.1	0.03

The most frequent bacteria in the genital sample of infertile women studied were *Chlamydia trachomatis*. However, if we considered that *Ureaplasma urealyticum* and *Mycoplasma hominis* belong to the same genus: Mycoplasmataceae, the presence of these bacteria, result of major importance in this group.

Table 1. Microbiological and clinical data associated with HPV.

HPV genotype identified	Risk for cancer	Patients studied for genotype		Positive result	
		N	%	N	%
6	Low	104	100	20	19.2
16	Alto	103	99	12	11.6
18	High	104	100	13	12.5
58	High	72	69.2	8	11.1
52	High	98	94.2	7	7.1
11	Low	104	100	7	6.7
31	High	87	83.7	5	5.7
33	High	72	69.2	5	6.9
68	High	67	64.4	5	7.5
66	High	67	64.4	3	4.5
51	High	98	94.2	3	3.1

HPV genotype identified	Risk for cancer	Patients studied for genotype		Positive result	
		N	%	N	%
42	Low	66	63.5	2	3
39	High	69	66.3	3	4.3
59	High	69	66.3	1	1.4
45	High	73	69.2	1	1.4
35	High	73	69.2	1	1.4
71	Low	70	67.3	1	1.4
61	Low	69	66.3	1	1.4
55	Low	63	60.6	1	1.6
81	Low	1	1	1	–

Table 2. Prevalent genotypes of HPV detected by PCR in secretions of cervix and vagina of infertile women studied group.

The following description will give an illustration of some of cases included in this study resume of microbiologic and gineco obstetric data are included at the **Figures 3–5**.

Case 2. Women 34 years, previously treated with five intrauterine inseminations and three *in vitro* fertilization (IVF) with intracytoplasmic sperm injection (ICSI). This patient had been treated repeatedly too, for genitourinary infection, unsuccessfully. After abnormal findings in a colposcopy, and histopathologic diagnosis of koilocyte in a cervix biopsy the clinician decide to practice hysterectomy, principally to solve the recurrent infections. One year later, these women required medical assistance due to severe signs and symptoms of genitourinary infection. In the vaginal sample were presented HPV 18, 35, 39, 51, 56, 66 y 74 (**Figure 3**). **Case 3.** Woman of 29 years old attended by primary infertility of unknown etiology and had been treated two times by assisted reproduction, with negative results. At the time of her arrive to the specially clinic, she referred previous result of ASCUS in PAP and signs and symptoms of genitourinary infection: dysuria, pelvic pain, abnormal menstrual bleeding, and a fluxing of white secretion from the vagina. At genital exploration, hypertrophy and erythema of cervix and papillary lesion at vaginal wall were found. The secretion of cervix and vagina was positive to *C. trachomatis, U. urealyticum* and *C. albicans*. PCR detected genotypes 16, 31, 33, 52, and 54 (**Figure 4**).

Case 3. Female 31 years, with two pregnancy loss of the first trimester, in both were diagnosed by ultrasound a chorionic vesicle without embryo. This patient did not have any fertility treatment previously. She had some PAP inform with inflammation but in one of them was diagnosed metaplastic changes. Genital infection was clinically diagnosed, and multi-microbial infection was detected in samples of secretions. (**Figure 4**). **Case 4.** A 37-year-old woman, who had a child without fertility treatment and did not have a second pregnancy, despite having no contraceptive treatment. This patient required medical assistance for chronic infection that was resistant to many treatments implemented previously. In this case were found HPV 44

	16	18	26	31	33	35	39	45	51	52	53	56	58	59	66	68	73	82	6	11	40	42	43	44	54	55	61	70	71	81
16																														
18	4																													
26																														
31		1																												
33	2	1		1																										
35																														
39	1	1						1																						
45	1	1																												
51				1																										
52	2	2			1																									
53																														
56																														
58	4		1	1												1														
59																														
66	1																													
68	1	1																												
73																														
82																														
6	3	8		1	1	1	2			4		1	3	1	1															
11	2	1			1														3											
40																														
42																														
43																														
44																														
54																														
55																														
61																			1											
70																			1											
71																														
81																			1											
	16	18	26	31	33	35	39	45	51	52	53	56	58	59	66	68	73	82	6	11	40	42	43	44	54	55	61	70	71	81

Figure 2. HPV genotyping results: Combinations of HPV. The number inside the square represents the patients with at least two different genotypes HPV detected in cervical and vaginal secretions of the women studied. Inside the square is the number of cases identified with the combined presence in the sample of cervical secretion of different Genotype HPV. For example: 4 cases have a combination of 16 and 18 genotypes of HPVhr; another 4 cases have simultaneously HPVhr 16 and 58.

and HPV 52 in association to *C. trachomatis, U. urealyticum* that eventually may be an etiologic association to secondary infertility of this case. Then more, *S. faecalis* and *E.coli* were present as part of the microorganism found in genital secretions. *Lactobacillus acidophilus* was absent (**Figure 5**). **Case 5**. Another patient that not received infertility treatment, but do not have a baby, even to be active sexually and do not have protection contraceptive. This woman suffers urinary symptoms since 2 years ago, and clinical signs and symptoms of vaginal recurrent infection, resistant to previous treatments. The diagnostic test applied to vaginal and cervical fluids was positive to one of the most common HPV associations: 16 and 18, but HPV 39, *C. trachomatis, U. urealyticum* and *C. albicans* were part of the multiple germs infection (**Figure 5**).

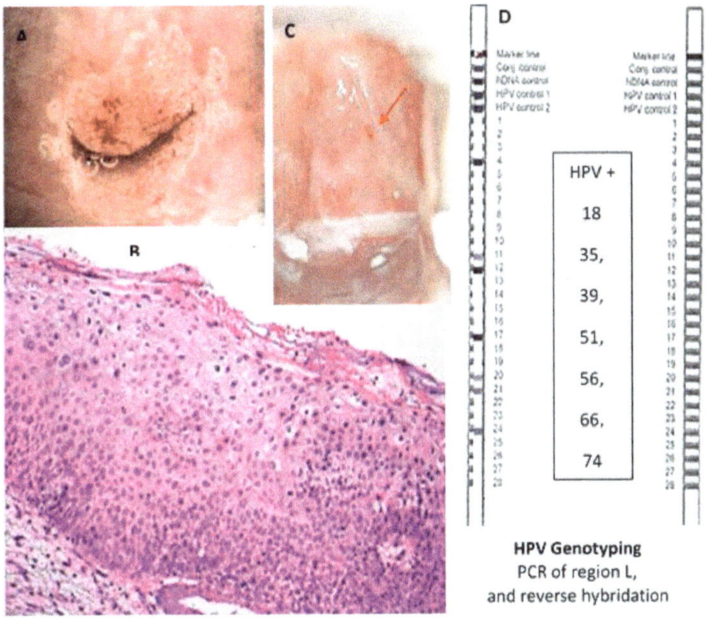

Figure 3. Infertile women with chronic genitourinary infection, and failure in assisted reproduction. Case 1. The patient was treated by hysterectomy due to persistent infection, after several fruitless treatment of assisted reproduction for primary infertility. The images illustrate clinical, histopathological and HPV test in vaginal secretions. (A) Abnormal colposcopy; (B) koilocyte was found in the cervix biopsy; (C) arrow shows lesion on vaginal fundus; (D) results of PCR and HPV genotyping of vaginal secretions. Multiple HPV were present, except the 74 of unknown significance, all correspond a high risk for cancer genotype.

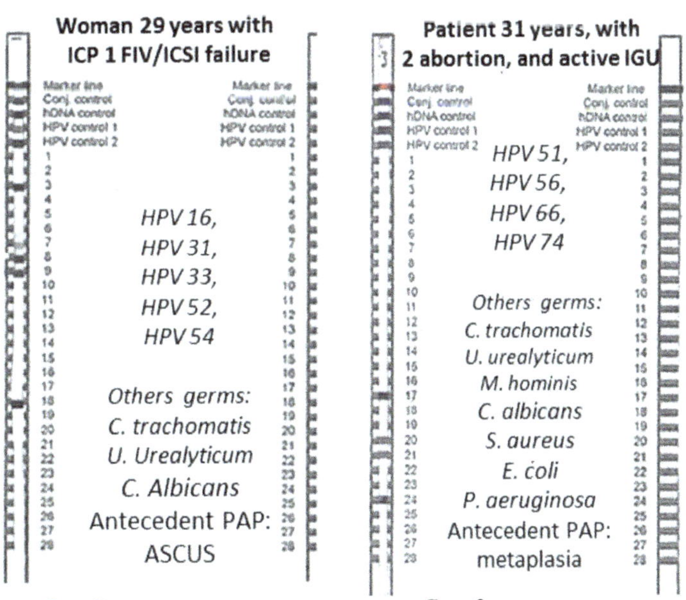

Case 2 Case 3

Figure 4. HPV genotypes combinations associated with genitourinary infection by multiple microorganisms.

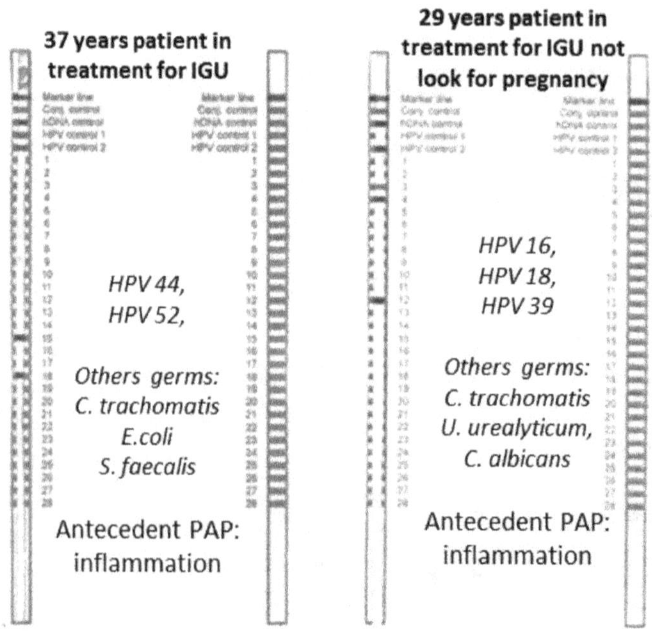

Case 4 Case 5

Figure 5. HPV genotypes combinations associated with genitourinary infection by multiple microorganisms in infertile patients.

7. Concluding remarks

This is a study carried out by aleatory selection of 104 infertile women attended by reproductive failure and genital infection; the main objective was to establish the relationship of HPV presence, with other microorganism and the genotype of HPV detected in this group of infertile women. All patients authorized the use of clinic and laboratory analysis data from her cervical and vaginal samples, to realize statistical analysis and sign an informed consent. The clinical parameters considered were: signs and symptoms of infection disease, results of previous assisted reproduction treatments, and the presence of previous abortions. These data were compared to genotype HPV present, and the diagnosis of others germs by laboratory test included direct investigation with immunofluorescence monoclonal antibodies to *Chlamydia trachomatis,* and bacterial cultures, included selective media to *U. urealyticum, M. hominis*. The microorganisms identified on the group studied are *C. trachomatis* (86.5%), HPV (49%), *U. urealyticum* (47.11%), *M. Hominis* (35.57%), *E. coli* (20.2%), *C. Albicans* (17.3%) and *S. faecalis* (10.6%). In a high proportion of the vaginal samples, microbiota vaginal was reduced or absent in a (76.9%) and 86% have more than one pathogen germs. *C albicans* was present like solitary microorganism in 17.3% as well HPV was the only identified germ in one patient. Statistical analysis established positive correlation between HPV and *U. urealyticum* ($p = 0.05$), and decreased microbiota ($p = 0.001$). The distribution of *C. trachomatis* was similar in the positive and negative to HPV group.

In this study, more than one sexual partner ($p = 0.05$), genitourinary infection symptoms ($p = 0.01$), white mucous vaginal secretion fluxing from the uterine duct ($p = 0.05$), failure in assisted reproduction before carry out, and previous HPV infection diagnosed by suspicious lesion or cytological exam ($p \leq 0.0001$) were in association to HPV. Prevalent genotypes of HPV detected in the infertile patients studied group were HPV six (19.2%), HPV 18 (12.5%), HPV 16 (11.5%), HPV 58 (7.2%), HPV 52 (6.7%), HPV 11 (6.7%) and HPV 68 (7.5%). Combinations of more than one HPV genotypes were detected in 60% on the studied samples. From them, 46.3% were the following associations between high risk for cancer HPV: 16/18, 18/58, 16/33, 16/52 and 18/52. In a similar percentage (44.8%) of women, low risk for cancer, principally HPV 6, was detected in combination with high risk HPV: 18, 52, 16 and 39. As well, we observed that three to five different HPV genotypes were present in 23.5% of the positive group infertile patients. According to the results of this study, a total of 79.5% of positive HPV group of patients, presented one or more high risk genotypes, and considering the statistical association between the positivity to HPV and the clinical history of previous HPV infections, this condition may represent a persistent infection or a reinfection. Consequently, we consider convenient a recommendation to take in account women with reproductive failure, like a group of risk of cervical cancer. With the results obtained from this study, was not possible to establish an association between the abortions presented on 28 of the studied women, and the positivity to HPV. Nevertheless for future studies that include a high number of patients, is may be important to observe that low risk to cancer genotypes 6 and 11, were present in a high prevalence in this investigation, and their importance on the results of inseminations, *in vitro* fertilization and gestational loss, still not defined now a days.

Acknowledgements

Authors acknowledge to"Center for Research and Development in Health Sciences (CIDICS) of Autonomous University of Nuevo León", for their assessment in molecular test for HPV, C. trachomatis and U. urealyticum, and for the financial support to this publication.

Author details

Adriana Ancer-Arellano[1], Jesus Ancer-Rodríguez[1], David Hardisson[2], Alberto Niderhauser-Garcia[1], Jose Sanchez-Hernández[3], Alvarez-Cuevas Salomón[1] and Guadalupe Gallegos-Avila[3]*

*Address all correspondence to: Guadalupe.gallegos@gmail.com

1 Faculty of Medicine, Department of Pathology, Autonomous University of Nuevo León, México

2 Department of Pathology, Hospital Universitario La Paz, Faculty of Medicine, Universidad Autonoma de Madrid, Madrid, Spain

3 Sertoli Lab Asociados, Civil Association, Monterrey, Nuevo León, México

References

[1] Mascarenhas MN, Flaxman SR, Boerma T, Vanderpoel S, Stevens GA. National, regional, and global trends in infertility prevalence since 1990: a systematic analysis of 277 health surveys. PLoS Medicine. 2012;**9**:1001356

[2] Viniker DA. Hypothesis on the role of sub-clinical bacteria of the endometrium (bacteria endometrialis) in gynaecological and obstetric enigmas. Human Reproduction Update. 1999;**5**:373-385

[3] Bachir BG, Jarvi K. Infectious, inflammatory, and immunologic conditions resulting in male infertility. Urologic Clinics of North America. 2014;**41**:67-81

[4] Licciardi F, Grifo JA, Rosenwaks Z, Witkin SS. Relation between antibodies to *Chlamydia trachomatis* and spontaneous abortion following in vitro fertilization. Journal of Assisted Reproduction and Genetics. 1992;**9**:207-310

[5] Spandorfer SD, Bongiovanni AM, Fasioulotis S, Rosenwaks Z, Ledger WJ, Witkin SS. Prevalence of cervical human papillomavirus in women undergoing in vitro fertilization and association with outcome. Fertility and Sterility. 2006;**86**:765-767

[6] Van Hamont D, Nissen LH, Siebers AG, Hendriks JC, Melchers WJ, Kremer JA, Massuger LF. Abnormal cervical cytology in women eligible for IVF. Human Reproduction. 2006;**21**:2359-2363

[7] Perino A, Giovannelli L, Schillaci R, Ruvolo G, Fiorentino FP, Alimondi P, Cefalù E, Ammatuna P. Human papillomavirus infection in couples undergoing in vitro fertilization procedures: Impact on reproductive out-comes. Fertility and Sterility. 2011;**95**:1845-1848

[8] Sharara FI, Queenan JT. Elevated serum *Chlamydia trachomatis* IgG antibodies. Association with decreased implantation rates in GIFT. The Journal of Reproductive Medicine. 1999;**44**:581-586

[9] Wang Y, Wang C, Qiao J, Wang L, Liang S. Relationship of cytopathology and cervical infection to outcome of in-vitro fertilization and embryo transfer. International Journal of Gynecology & Obstetrics. 2008;**101**:21-26

[10] Nuñez-Troconis JT. *Mycoplasma hominis* and *Ureaplasma urealyticum* in different gynecologic diseases. Investigación Clínica. 1999;**40**:9-24

[11] Paavonen J, Eggert-Kruse W. *Chlamydia trachomatis*: Impact on human reproduction. Human Reproduction Update. 1999;**5**:433-447

[12] Taylor-Robinson D. T-mycoplasmas and infertiliy. Nature. 1974;**248**:267

[13] Brunham RC, Maclean IW, Binns B, Peeling RW. *Chlamydia trachomatis*: Its role in tubal infertility. The Journal of Infectious Diseases. 1985;**152**:1275-1282

[14] Cohen CR, Manhart LE, Bukusi EA, Astete S, Brunham RC, Holmes KK, et al. Association between *Mycoplasma genitalium* and acute endometritis. Lancet. 2002;**359**:765-766

[15] Anagrius C, Loré B, Jensen JS. *Mycoplasma genitalium*: Prevalence, clinical significance, and transmission. Sexually Transmitted Infections. 2005;**81**:458-462

[16] Ross JD, Jensen JS. *Mycoplasma genitalium* as a sexually transmitted infection: Implications for screening, testing, and treatment. Sexually Transmitted Infections. 2006;**82**:269-271

[17] Baczynska A, Funch P, Fedder J, Knudsen HJ, Birkelund S, Christiansen G. Morphology of human fallopian tubes after infection with *Mycoplasma genitalium* and *Mycoplasma hominis in vitro*—Organ culture study. Human Reproduction. 2007;**22**:968-979

[18] Manhart LE, Holmes KK, Hughes JP, Houston LS, Totten PA. *Mycoplasma genitalium* among young adults in the United States: An emerging sexually transmitted infection. American Journal of Public Health. 2007;**97**:1118-1125

[19] Haedicke J, Iftner T. Human papillomaviruses and cancer. Radiotherapy and Oncology. 2013;**108**:397-402

[20] Ghittoni R, Accardi R, Chiocca S, Tommasino M. Role of human papillomaviruses in carcinogenesis. Ecancer Medical Science. 2015;**9**:526

[21] Forman D, de Martel C, Lacey CJ, Soerjomataram I, Lortet-Tieulent J, Bruni L, et al. Global burden of human papillomavirus and related diseases. Vaccine. 2012;**30** (Suppl 5):F12-F23

[22] Steben M, Duarte-Franco E. Human papillomavirus infection: Epidemiology and pathophysiology. Gynecologic Oncology. 2007;**107** (Suppl 1):S2–S5

[23] Secretaría de Salubridad y Asistencia (SSA-México). CENEVACE. Anuarios de Morbilidad 1984-2010; CONAPO. Proyecciones de población en México 2005-2050

[24] National Institute of Statistic and Geography of Mexico (*Consulte of 2 June, 2015* http://www.inegi.org.mx)

[25] Longworth M, Laimins L. Pathogenesis of human papillomaviruses in differentiating epithelia. Microbiology and Molecular Biology Reviews. 2004;**68**:362-372

[26] Handisurya A, Day PM, Thompson CD, Buck CB, Kwak K, Roden RB, Lowy DR, Schiller JT. Murine skin and vaginal mucosa are similarly susceptible to infection by pseudovirions of different papillomavirus classifications and species. Virology. 2012;**433**:385-394

[27] Dunne EF, Park IU. HPV and HPV-associated diseases. Infectious Disease Clinics of North America. 2013;**27**:765-778

[28] zur-Hausen H. Papillomaviruses and cancer: From basic studies to clinical application. Nature Reviews Cancer. 2002;**2**:342-350

[29] Bhatla N, Puri K, Joseph E, Kriplani A, Iyer VK, Sreenivas V. Association of *Chlamydia trachomatis* infection with Human Papilloma Virus (HPV) and cervical intraepithelial neoplasia—A pilot study. Indian Journal of Medical Research. 2013;**137**:533-539

[30] Serman F. Cáncer cervicouterino: epidemio-logía, historia natural y rol del virus del papiloma humano, perspectivas en prevencion y tratamiento. Rev Chil Obstet Ginecol. 2002;**67**:318-323

[31] Syrjänen K. 2013: Detection of human papillomavirus in lung cancer: Systematic review and meta-analysis. Anticancer Research. 2012;**32**:3235-3250

[32] Badillo-Almaraz I, Zapata-Benavides P, Saavedra-Alonso S, Zamora-Davila D, Rezendez-Pérez D, Tamez-Guerra R, Herrera-Esparza R, Rodríguez-Padila, C. Human Papillomavirus16/18 infections in lung cancer patients in Mexico. Intervirology, DOI: 10.11590003510752013

[33] zurHauasen H : Papillomavirus in the causation of human cancers.Virology.2009;**384**: 260-265

[34] Fei Y, Yang J, Hsieh WC, Wu JY, Wu T, Goan YG, Lee H, Cheng YW.: Different Human papillomavirus 16/18 in Chinese non-small cell lung cancer patients living in Wuhan, China. Japanese Journal of Clinical Oncology. 2006;**36**: 22274-22279

[35] Chatuverdi AK, Engels EA, Pfeiffer RM, Hernandez BY, Xiao W, Kim E, Jiang B, Goodman MT, Sibug-Saber M, Cozen W, et al.: Human Papilloma Virus and rising oropharyngeal cancer incidence in the United States. Journal of Clinical Oncology. 2011;**29**: 4294-4301

[36] Ang KK, Harris J, Wheeler R, Weber R, Rosenthal DI, Nguyen-Tan PF, Westra WH, Chung CH, Jordan RC and LU C. Human Papilloma Virus and survival of patients with oropharyngeal cancer. The New England Journal of Medicine. 2010;**363**: 24-35

[37] Gillison ML, Castellsagué X, Chaturvedi A, Goodman MT, Snijders P, Tommasino M, *Arbyn M, Franceschi S*. Eurogin Roadmap: Comparative epidemiology of HPV infection and associated cancers of the head and neck and cervix. International Journal of Cancer. 2014;**134**: 497-507

[38] Souho T, Benlemlih M, Bennani B.: Human papillomavirus infection and fertility alteration: A systematic review. PLoS One. 2015;10:e0126936

[39] Guizzo S, Ferrari B, Noventa M, Ferrari E, Patrelli TS, Gangemi M, Nardelli GB.: Male and couple fertility impairment due to HPV-DNA sperm infection: Update on molecular mechanism and clinical impact–Systematic review. BioMed Research International. 2014;**230263**: 1-12

[40] Schillaci R, Capra G, Bellavia C, Ruvolo G, Scazzone C, Venezia R, Perino A.: Detection of oncogenic human papillomavirus genotypes on spermatozoa from male partners of in-fertile couples. Fertility and Sterility. 2013;**100**: 1236-1240

[41] Conde-Ferráez L, Chan-May Ade A, Carrillo-Martínez JR, Ayora-Talavera G, González-Losa MR.: Human papillomavirus infection and spontaneous abortion: A case–control study performed in Mexico. European Journal of Obstetrics and Gynecology. 2013;**170**: 468-473

[42] Pérez-Andino J, Buck CB, Ribbeck K.: Adsorption of human papillomavirus 16 to live human sperm. PLoS One. 2009;4: e5847

[43] Foresta C, Garolla A, Zuccarello D, Pizzol D, Moretti A, Barzon L, Palù G.: Human papillomavirus found in sperm head of young adult males affects the progressive motility. Fertility and Sterility. 2010;**93**: 802-806

[44] **Garolla** A, Pizzol D, Bertoldo A, De Toni L, Barzon L, Foresta C.: Association, prevalence, and clearance of human papillomavirus and antisperm antibodies in infected semen samples from infertile patients. Fertility and Sterility. 2013;**99**: 125-131

[45] Yang Y, Jia CW, Ma YM, Zhou LY, Wang SY.: Correlation between HPV sperm infection and male infertility. Asian Journal of Andrology. 2013;**15**: 529-532

[46] Connelly DA, Chan PJ, Patton WC, King A.: Human sperm deoxyribonucleic acid fragmentation by specific types of papilloma-virus. American Journal of Obstetrics & Gynecology. 2001;**184**: 1068-1070

[47] Lee CA, Huang CT, King A, Chan PJ.: Differential effects of human papillomavirus DNA types on p53 tumor-suppressor gene apoptosis in sperm. Gynecologic Oncology. 2002;**85**: 511-516

[48] Gomez LM, Ma Y, Ho C, McGrath CM, Nelson DB, Parry S.: Placental infection with human papillomavirus is associated with spontaneous preterm delivery. Human Reproduction. 2008;**23**: 709-715

[49] Skoczyński M, Gozdzicka-Józefiak A, Kwaśniewska A.: Prevalence of human papillomavirus in spontaneously aborted products of conception. Acta Obstetricia et Gynecologica Scandinavica. 2011;**90**: 1402-1045

[50] Cho G, Min KJ, Hong HR, Kim S, Hong JH, Lee JK, Oh MJ, Kim H.: High-risk human papillomavirus infection is associated with premature rupture of membranes. BMC Pregnancy Childbirth. 2013;**13**: 173

[51] Rintala MA, Grénman SE, Puranen MH, Isolauri E, Ekblad U, Kero PO, Syrjänen SM. Transmission of high-risk human papilloma-virus (HPV) between parents and infant?: A prospective study of HPV in families in Finland. Journal of Clinical Microbiology. 2005;**43**:376-381

[52] Castellsagué X, Drudis T, Cañadas MP, Goncé A, Ros R, Pérez JM, et al. Human Papillomavirus (HPV) infection in pregnant women and mother-to-child transmission of genital HPV genotypes: A prospective study in Spain. BMC Infectious Diseases. 2009;**9**: 74

[53] Freitas A, Mariz F, Silva A, Jesus A. Human papillomavirus vertical transmission: Review of current data. Clinical Infectious Diseases. 2013;**56**:1451-1456

[54] Koskimaa HM, Paaso AE, Welters MJ, Grénman SE, Syrjänen KJ, van der Burg SH, Syrjänen SM. Human papillomavirus 16 E2-, E6- and E7-specific T-cell responses in children and their mothers who developed incident cervical intraepithelial neoplasia during a 14-year follow-up of the Finnish Family HPV cohort. Journal of Translational Medicine. 2014;**12**:44

[55] Murray PR, Rosenthal KS, Pfaller MA. Chlamydia and chlamydophila. Medical Microbiology. 6th ed. Philadelphia, PA: Mosby Elsevier; 2009. p. 441

[56] Al-Younes HM, Brinkmann V, Meyer TF. Interaction of Chlamydia trachomatis serovar L2 with the host autophagic pathway. Infection and Immunity. 2004;**72**:4751-4762

[57] Moulder JW. Interaction of chlamydiae and host cells in vitro. Microbiology Reviews. 1991;**55**:143-190

[58] Taylor-Robinson D, Thomas BJ. The role of *Chlamydia trachomatis* genital tract and associated diseases. Journal of Clinical Pathology. 1980;**33**:205-233

[59] Ness RB, Goodman MT, Shen C, Brunham RC. Serologic evidence of past infection with Chlamydia trachomatis, in relation to ovarian cancer. The Journal of Infectious Disease. 2003;**187**:1147-1152

[60] Gonzales GF, Muñoz G, Sánchez R, Henkel R, Gallegos-Avila G, Díaz-Gutierrez O, Vigil P, Vásquez F, Kortebani G, Mazzolli A, Bustos-Obregón E. Update on the impact of *Chlamydia trachomatis* infection on male fertility. Andrologia. 2004;**36**:1-23

[61] Mazzoli S, Cai T, Addonisio *P, Bechi A, Mondaini* N, Bartoletti R.: Chlamydia trachomatis infection is rel*ated to poor semen q*uality in young prostatitis patients. European Urology. 2009;**57**:708-714

[62] Gdoura R, Kchaou W, Ammar-Keskes L, Chakroun N, Sellemi A, Znazen A, Rebai T, Hammami A. Assessment of Chlamydia trachomatis, **Ure**aplasma urealyticum, Ureaplasma parvum, Mycoplasma hominis, and Mycoplasma genitalium in semen and first void urine specimens of asymptomatic male partners of infertile couples. Journal of Andrology. 2008;**29**:198-206

[63] Stamm WE, Norrby SR. Urinary tract infections: disease panorama and challenges. The Journal of Infectious Diseases. 2001;**183**(Suppl 1):S1–S4

[64] Terán S, Walsh C, Irwin KL. *Chlamydia trachomatis* infection in women: Bad news, good news, and next steps in prevention. Journal of the American Medical Women's Association. 2001;**56**:100-104

[65] Marrazzo J. Syphilis and other sexually transmitted diseases in HIV infection. Topics in HIV Medicine. 2007;**15**(1):11-16

[66] Cunningham KA & Beagley KW. Male genital tract chlamydia infection: Implications for pathology and infertility. Biology of Reproduction. 2008;**79**:180-189

[67] Diquelou JY, Pastorini E, Feneux D, Gicquel JM. The role of *Chlamydia trachomatis* in producing abnormal movements by spermatozoa. Journal de Gynécologie Obstétrique et Biologie de la Reproduction (Paris). 1989;**18**:615-625

[68] Gallegos-Avila G. Infecciones por *Chlamydia trachomatis* y *Mycoplasma sp*. Su relación con la infertilidad masculina. Bol Col Mex Urol. 2003;**18**:106-112

[69] Hosseinzadeh S, Eley A, Pacey AA. Semen quality of men with asymptomatic chlamydial infection. Journal of Andrology. 2004;**25**:104-109

[70] Bezold G, Politch JA, Kiviat NB, Kuypers JM, Wolff H, Anderson DJ. Prevalence of sexually transmissible pathogens in semen from asymptomatic male infertility patients with and without leukocytospermia. Fertility and Sterility. 2007;**87**:1087-1097

[71] De Marzo AM, Platz EA, Sutcliffe S, Xu J, Grönberg H, Drake CG, Nakai Y, Isaacs WB, Nelson WG. Inflammation in prostate carcinogenesis. Nature Reviews Cancer. 2007;7:256-269

[72] Gallegos-Avila G, Sánchez JJ, Chávez-Briones ML, Ramos-González B, Niderhauser-García A, Ancer-Rodríguez J, Ortega-Martínez M, Jaramillo-Rangel G. A role of *Chlamydia trachomatis* in prostate cancer: A prostate biopsies study. In: Berhardt LV, editor. Advances in Medicine and Biology. Vol. 37. NY, USA: Nova Science Publishers, Inc.; 2011. pp. 1-13. ISBN: 978-1-62100-102-7

[73] Razin S. The genus Mycoplasma and related genera (class Mollicutes). In: Dworkin M, Falkow S, Rosenberg E, Schleifer KH, Stackebrandt E, editors. The Prokaryotes. A Handbook on the Biology of Bacteria. Volume 4: Bacteria: Firmicutes, Cyanobacteria. 3rd ed. New York, NY: Springer Science+Business Media, LLC; 2006. p. 836

[74] Baseman JB, Tully JG. Mycoplasmas: Sophisticated, reemerging, and burdened by their notoriety. Emerging Infectious Diseases. 1997;**3**:21-32

[75] Dallo SF, Baseman JB. Intracellular DNA replication and long-term survival of pathogenic mycoplasmas. Microbial Pathogenesis. 2000;**29**:301-309

[76] Uusküla A, Kohl PK. Genital mycoplasmas, including *Mycoplasma genitalium,* as sexually transmitted agents. International Journal of STD & AIDS. 2002;**13**:79-85

[77] Kilic D, Basar MM, Kaygusuz S, Yilmaz E, Basar H, Batislam E. Prevalence and treatment of *Chlamydia trachomatis, Ureaplasma urealyticum,* and *Mycoplasma hominis* in patients with non-gonococcal urethritis. Japanese Journal of Infectious Diseases. 2004;**57**:17-20

[78] Jensen JS. *Mycoplasma genitalium*: The etiological agent of urethritis and other sexually transmitted diseases. Journal of the European Academy of Dermatology and Venereology. 2004;**18**:1-11

[79] Yoon BH, Chang JW, Romero R. Isolation of *Ureaplasma urealyticum* from the amniotic cavity and adverse outcome in preterm labor. Obstetrics & Gynecology. 1998;92:77-82

[80] Denks K, Spaeth EL, Jõers K, Randoja R, Talpsep T, Ustav M, Kurg R. Coinfection of *Chlamydia trachomatis, Ureaplasma urea-lyticum* and human papillomavirus among patients attending STD clinics in Estonia. Scandinavian Journal of Infectious Diseases. 2007;**39**:714-718

[81] Dieterle S. Urogenital infections in reproductive medicine. Andrologia. 2008;**40**:117-119

[82] Zeighami H, Peerayeh SN, Yazdi RS, Sorouri R. Prevalence of *Ureaplasma urealyticum* and *Ureaplasma parvum* in semen of infertile and healthy men. International Journal of STD & AIDS. 2009;**20**:387-390

[83] Volgmann T, Ohlinger R, Panzig B. *Ureaplasma urealyticum*-harmless commensal or underestimated enemy of human reproduction? A review. Archives of Gynecology and Obstetrics. 2005;**273**:133-139

[84] Lukic A, Canzio C, Patella A, Giovagnoli MR, Cipriani P, Frega A, Moscarini M. Determination of cervicovaginal micro-organisms in women with abnormal cervical cytology: The role of *Ureaplasma urealyticum*. Anticancer Research. 2006;**26**:4843-4849

[85] Gnarpe H, Friberg J. T-mycoplasmas as a possible cause for reproductive failure. Nature. 1973;**242**:120-121

[86] Fowlkes DM, Dooher GB, Oleary WM. Evidence by scanning electron microscopy for an association between spermatozoa and T-mycoplasmas in men of infertile marriage. Fertility and Sterility. 1975;**26**:1203-1211

[87] Busolo F, Zanchetta R, Bertolini G.: Mycoplasmic localization patterns on spermatozoa from infertile men. Fertility and Sterility. 1984;**42**: 412-417

[88] Grossgebauer K, Hennig A. Ureaplasma-infected human sperm in infertile men. Archives of Andrology. 1984;**12** Suppl:35-41

[89] Xu C, Sun GF, Zhu YF, Wang YF. The correlation of *Ureaplasma urealyticum* infection with infertility. Andrologia. 1997;**29**:219-226

[90] Núñez-Calonge R, Caballero P, Redondo C, Baquero F, Martinez-Ferrer M, Meseguer MA. *Ureaplasma urealyticum* reduces motility and induces membrane alterations in human spermatozoa. Human Reproduction. 1998;**13**:2756-2761

[91] Blanchard A, Hentchel J, Duffy L, Baldus K. Detection of *Ureaplasma urealyticum* by polymerase chain reaction in the urogenital tract of adults, in amniotic fluid, and in the respiratory tract on newborns. Clinical Infectious Diseases. 1993;**17**(Suppl.1):S148–S153

[92] Teng K, Li M, Yu W, Li H, Shen D, Liu D. Comparison of PCR with culture for detection of *Ureaplasma urealyticum* in clinical samples from patients with urogenital infections. Journal of Clinical Microbiology. 1994;**32**:2232-2234

[93] Tsai S, Wear DJ, Shih JW, Lo SC. Mycoplasmas and oncogenesis: persistent infection and multistage malignant transformation. Proceedings of the National Academy of Sciences of the United States of America. 1995;**92**:10197-101201

[94] Zhang S, Tsai S, Lo SC. Alteration of gene expression profiles during mycoplasma-induced malignant cell transformation. BMC Cancer. 2006;**6**:116

[95] Zhang S, Wear DJ, Lo S. Mycoplasmal infections alter gene expression in cultured human prostatic and cervical epithelial cells. FEMS Immunology and Medical Microbiology. 2000;**27**:43-50

[96] Namiki K, Goodison S, Porvasnik S, Allan RW, Iczkowski KA, Urbanek C, Reyes L, Sakamoto N, Rosser CJ. Persistent exposure to Mycoplasma induces malignant transformation of human prostate cells. PLoS One. 2009;**4**:1-9

[97] Dennis LK, Lynch CF, Turner JC. Epidemiologic association between prostatitis and prostate cancer. Urology. 2002;**60**:315-319

[98] Smith JS, Muñoz N, Herrero R, Eluf-Neto J, Ngelangel C, Franceschi S, et al. Evidence for *Chlamydia trachomatis* as a human papilloma-virus cofactor in the etiology of invasive cervical cancer in Brazil and the Philippines. The Journal of Infectious Diseases. 2002;**185**:324-331

[99] Agrawal T, Vats V, Salhan S, Mittal A. Determination of chlamydial load and immune parameters in asymptomatic, symptomatic and infertile women. FEMS Immunology and Medical Microbiology. 2009:**55**:250-257

[100] de Lucena-Oliveira M, de Amorim MM, de Souza AS, de Albuquerque LC, da Costa AA. Chlamydia infection in patients with and without cervical intraepithelial lesions. Revista Da Associacao Medica Brasileira. 2008;**54**:506-512

[101] Fleming DT, Wasserheit JN. From epidemiological synergy to public health policy and practice: The contribution of other sexually transmitted diseases to sexual transmission of HIV infection. Journal Sexually Transmitted Infections. 1999;**75**:3-17

[102] Luostarinen T, Lehtinen M, Bjørge T, Abeler V, Hakama M, Hallmans G, et al. Joint effects of different human papillomaviruses and *Chlamydia trachomatis* infections on risk of squamous cell carcinoma of the cervix uteri. European Journal of Cancer. 2004;**40**:1058-1065

[103] de Luca G, Marin M, Schelover E, Chamorro E, Vicente L, Albhom M, Alonso JM. Infeccion por Chlamydia trachomatis y Papilomavirus en mujeres con alteraciones citohistologicas de cuello uterino. Medicina (B Aires). 2006;**66**:303-306

[104] European Centre for Disease Prevention and Control. Annual Epidemiological Report on Communicable Diseases in Europe. 2008. http://ecdc.europa.eu/en/publications/Publications/0812_SUR_Annual_Epidemiological_Report_2008.pdf

[105] Samoff E, Koumans EH, Markowitz LE, Sternberg M, Sawyer MK, Swan D, Papp JR, Black CM, Unger ER. Association of *Chlamydia trachomatis* with persistence of high-risk types of human papillomavirus in a cohort of female adolescents. American Journal of Epidemiology. 2005;**162**:668-675

[106] Silins I, Ryd W, Strand A, Wadell G, Törnberg S, Hansson BG, et al. *Chlamydia trachomatis* infection and persistence of human papilloma-virus. International Journal of Cancer. 2005;**116**:110-115

[107] Paba P, Bonifacio D, Di Bonito L, Ombres D, Favalli C, Syrjänen K, Ciotti M. Co-expression of HSV2 and *Chlamydia trachomatis* in HPV-positive cervical cancer and cervical intraepithelial neoplasia lesions is associated with aberrations in key intracellular pathways. Intervirology. 2008;**51**:230-234

[108] Gallegos-Ávila G. Estudio citológico del semen de hombres infértiles con infección genital por Chlamydia y Mycoplasma. Observaciones en cortes semifinos y ultrafinos [thesis]. Universidad Autónoma de Madrid; 2005

[109] Gallegos-Avila G, Ancer-Rodriguez J, Alvarez-Cuevas S, Ramos-González B, Sanchez-Hernández J, Nistal M, Regadera J. Relevancy of semithin section on the analysis of seminal damage, due to infection by Chlamydia and Mycoplasma, in couples with unsuccessful assisted reproduction. In: Ballesca Lagarda JL, Oliva Virgili R, editors. Papers contributed to 9th International Congress of Andrology. MEDIMOND International Proceedings. Barcelona, Spain; 2009, pp. 123-128

[110] Gallegos-Avila G, Ortega-Martínez M, Ramos-González B, Tijerina-Menchaca R, Ancer-Rodríguez J, Jaramillo-Rangel G. Ultrastructural findings in semen samples of infertile men infected with *Chlamydia trachomatis* and mycoplasmas. Fertility and Sterility. 2009;**91**:915-919

[111] Gallegos-Ávila G, Alvarez-Cuevas S, Niderhauser-García A, Ancer-Rodríguez J, Jaramillo-Rangel G, Ortega-Martínez M. Phagocytosis of spermatozoa and leucocytes by epithelial cells of the genital tract in infertile men infected with Chlamydia trachomatis and mycoplasmas. Histopathology. 2009;**55**:232-234

[112] Gallegos-Ávila G, Ancer-Rodríguez J, Ortega-Martínez, Jaramillo-Rangel G. Infection and phagocytosis: Analysis in semen with transmission electron microscopy. In: Méndez-Vilas A, Díaz J, editors. Microscopy: Science, Technology, Applications and Education. No. 4. Vol. 1: Applications in Biology and Medicine Formatex, Microscopy series ed. Badajoz, Spain. 2010. pp. 85-92. ISBN-13: 978-84-614-6191-2

[113] Gallegos-Ávila G, Marcos M, Alvarez-Cuevas S, Niderhauser-García, Ancer-Rodríguez J. Citología seminal en infecciones del aparato genital masculino. In: Regadera J, Noguera R, Hardisson D, editors. Atlas de Histología y del desarrollo del aparato genital masculino. Cap. 29. International Marketing and Communication, Madrid, Spain. 2016. pp. 267-271. ISBN 978-84-7867-490-9

[114] Gallegos G, Ramos B, Santiso R, Goyanes V, Gosalvez J, Fernandez JL. Sperm DNA fragmentation in infertile men with genito-urinary infection by *Chlamydia trachomatis* and *Mycoplasma*. Fertility and Sterility. 2008;**90**:328-334

[115] Gallegos G. Infertility due to C. trachomatis and Mycoplasma is a result of sperm damage fragmentation. Nature Clinical Practice Urology. Research Highlights. 2008;**5**(11):580

[116] Gallegos Ávila MG, Ramos González B, Sánchez Hernández JJ, Niderhauser García A, Ancer Rodríguez J. Aplicación del NBT-Test para evaluar la producción espermática de ROS en la infección seminal por C. trachomatis y su asociación con la fragmentación de la cromatina y el deterioro de la calidad espermática. International Review of Andrology. 2011;**9**:88

[117] Ramos-González B. Fragmentación del ADN espermático en hombres infértiles con infección por Chlamydia trachomatis y Mycoplasma sp. Efecto de la terapia antibiótica y antioxidante [thesis]. Madrid, Spain: Universidad Autónoma de Madrid; 2012

[118] Chávez-Briones ML. Endometritis por Chlamydia trachomatis y Ureaplasma urealyticum en mujeres con infertilidad y aborto [thesis]. Madrid, Spain: Universidad Autónoma de Madrid; 2012

[119] Chávez-Briones ML, Alvarez-Cuevas S, Ramos-González B, Casillas-Vega N, Niderhauser-García A, Ancer-Rodríguez J, Hardisson-Hernáez D, Gallegos-Ávila MG. Endometritis por Chlamydia trachomatis y Ureaplasma urealyticum en mujeres con infertilidad y aborto. Medicina Universitaria. 2013;**5**(Suppl 1):1-124

[120] Gallegos Ávila MG, Ramos González B, Sánchez Hernández JJ, Niderhauser García A, Ancer Rodríguez J. Disminución de la teratozoospermia secundaria a tratamiento antibiótico en pacientes infértiles con infección urogenital ocasionada por *Chlamydia trachomatis* y *Mycoplasma sp.* International Review of Andrology. 2011;**9**:90

[121] Gallegos-Ávila MG, Álvarez-Cuevas S, Sánchez-Hernández JJ, Niderhauser-García A, Casillas-Vega N, Ramos-González B. Resultado del tratamiento del binomio Andro-Ginecológico en la infertilidad conyugal por infección genital interna. Andrology. 2013;**11**:1-14

[122] Alberts CJ, Schim van der Loeff MF, Papenfuss MR, da Silva RJ, Villa LL, et al. Association of Chlamydia trachomatis infection and herpes simplex virus type 2 serostatus with genital human papillomavirus infection in men: the HPV in men study. Sexually Transmitted Diseases. 2013;**40**:508-515

4

Anogenital HPV

Özge Aşkın

Abstract

Human papilloma virus (HPV) is the most common sexually transmitted infection in the world. HPV is associated with various oral, genital and cutaneous conditions, both benign and malignant. HPV infection can be asymptomatic, but it may persist and cause lesions such as warts, dysplasia and cancers depending on low or high risk type of HPV infection. Anogenital warts are the most common clinical presentation of HPV infection. Despite the high incidence of HPV infections, vaccines, precaution methods and treatments are still matters of debate.

Keywords: HPV, anogenital, warts, condyloma acuminata, cancer, vaccines

1. Introduction

Human papilloma virus (HPV) can reside in epithelial basal cells of skin and mucosa. More than 200 genotypes have been identified; nearly 40–50 of these types cause genital infections. HPV 6, HPV 11 and HPV 16 are the most associated with genital warts. The transmission of the virus is by direct contact, but their infectivity is variable due to the number and the type of virus particles and the immune system of the infected human. Trauma, microabrasions and microdefects on the skin and mucosa promote the contagion. Less than 1–2% of infected people have clinically apparent anogenital warts [1, 2].

2. Epidemiology

HPV infection is a common sexually transmitted infection worldwide. HPV may cause several reproductive tract diseases, including genital warts and cervical cancer. The incidence of HPV infections has been steadily increasing especially in the second decade of life. Genital warts affect both males and females, although slightly higher in men according to latest data [3].

The prevalence of HPV infection is estimated currently at 10–15%, with substantial regional variation [4]. The most common benign genital HPV infection is genital warts, caused in about 90% of the cases by nononcogenic HPV types such as 6 and 11. HPV infection is detected for more than 90% of the cases of cervical cancer [3, 4].

3. Etiology and pathogenesis

HPVs are small, circular, double-stranded DNA viruses. The capsid is made up of 72 icosahedral structures. Different types of HPV come from their variable L1 code. L1 encodes primary structural protein in the virus capsid. Genital HPV is associated with a high risk of carcinogenesis, as the viral DNA integrates into the hosts' DNA [5]. All HPVs target epithelia tissues and link their productive life cycles to differentiation of the infected host cell. HPVs are associated with a spectrum of manifestations ranging from unapparent infections to malignant neoplasias. The alpha-papillomaviruses contain viruses that infect mucosal epithelium, some of which are considered high risk (HR) and others low risk (LR) based on their association with cancers. The LR-HPVs can cause benign hyperproliferative lesions such as warts, and the High-risk HPV (HR-HPV) has been linked with progress tohifh-grade neoplasia and invasive malignant cancer [6, 7]. Low-risk HPV types include HPV 6 and 11 that have been associated with benign anogenital warts. At least 12 HR-HPV types, HPV 16, 18, 31, 33, 35, 39, 45, 51, 52, 56, 58 and 59, have been associated with anogenital cancers as well as precursor neoplastic lesions [8]. It is now established that HPV 16 and 18 are the major papillomavirus types responsible for cervical cancer. Two viral proteins, E6 and E7, are essential for the integration into host chromosomes during malignant progression. They interact with p53 protein that regulates DNA damage repair [6, 7]. The high-risk mucosal HPVs, such as HPV 16, 18, 31 and 33, appear to have relation to the function of the E5, E6 and E7 gene products and the regulatory mechanisms that govern their expression. The cellular tumor suppressor gene p16 is an important biomarker for HPV-associated intraepithelial neoplasia. The overexpression of p16 is found in examined LSIL (CIN) lesions, except for those being caused by "low-risk" HPV types. There was no expression in healthy cervical epithelium [7].

Direct genital mucosa contact during sexual intercourse is the classical way of HPV transmission. The risk of male-to-female transmission is lower than that of female-to-male transmission. Five prospective studies have reported a significantly higher female-to-male transmission rate of any type of HPV than that of male-to-female. This may be explained by: (a) more transient infections in men; (b) lower HPV viral load in men; and (c) lower seroconversion rate for HPV infection in men [9]. Concordance of HPV infection between sexual partners is 40–60%. Length of sexual relationship, frequency of intercourse, condom use and number of sexual partners may play a role for the transmission. There is also vertical transmission to newborn from the mother. Contact with vaginal and cervical mucosa, transmission by placental or by amniotic fluid is the way of vertical infection to newborn. The rate of vertical transmission changes between 20 and 30% [10].

HPV enters epidermis through small defects on the skin or mucosa and proceeds to the basal layer of keratinocytes. The infected cells cannot undergo terminal differentiation. After the viral replication, multinucleation, nuclear enlargement, parakeratosis and koilocytes are seen in the upper layer of the epidermis. As the infected cells cornify and are shed, virus particles lead to further infection or transmission [2, 10].

4. Laboratory

A clinical diagnosis can be made in apparent infection. If the lesion is suspicious, biopsy is possible for the differential diagnosis. To detect the HPV in subclinic infections, variable methods are used. HPV testing plays an important role adjunct to the cervical cytology after the Pap-smear categories. Serological tests have been developed for the early diagnosis of cervical cancer and to detect high risk HPV types. HPV-DNA testing includes PCR, southern blot hybridization and fluorescent in situ hybridization (FISH). PCR is highly sensitive in identifying small amounts of viral nucleic acids. The specimen can be taken from cervicovaginal area, vulva, urethra and anal anogenital area for PCR analysis [11]. Cytology and HPV testing are important for detecting cervical dysplasia. Because there is no treatment for asymptomatic HPV in men, routine HPV testing is not recommended in men [10, 11].

5. Clinical presentation

Anogenital warts are the most common clinical presentation of HPV infection. Although warts are benign lesions, they cause a lot of stress and discomfort in patients' social life. Itching, bleeding, discomfort and pain are the rare symptoms, usually they are asymptomatic. Genital warts are highly infectious, and approximately 65% of people whose sexual partner has genital warts will develop warts themselves. The incubation period of HPV infection is estimated 2 weeks to 8 months, with the majority of genital warts appearing 2–3 months after an HPV infection. Approximately 20–30% of genital warts will spontaneously regress within 1 year; however, recurrence of warts is common [12].

5.1. Anogenital warts (condylomata acuminata)

Lesions may be single or multiple, of varying sizes, and are usually asymptomatic. Condylomata acuminata are pale pink papules or nodules with a smooth and velvety surface. The difference from other warts is the lack of hyperkeratosis. They may grow exophytic and cauliflower-like mass. They are highly contagious. HPV 6–11 are the most common types detected in condylomata acuminata. These are low risk types. Many other types have also been described including HPV 2, 30–33, 35, 39, 41–45, 51–56 and 59, many of which are intermediate and high risk types. HPV 16–18 are the most common high risk types and can be found isolated or with HPV 6–11 [1, 13, 14]. The HR-HPV types, most often HPV 16 and 18, are considered to be the primary etiologic agents for cervical cancer and precancerous lesions in women (CIN, VIN, VaIN) [15]. HPV 16 is the main virus type to be associated with the development of VAIN. Also, HPV 16 infection, VIN or condylomata acuminata in the past medical history seemed to be significant factors for early relapse [16]. Multiple studies verified that persistent HPV infection is considered to play a key role in the development of cervical cancer. Cervical intraepithelial neoplasia (CIN) is the prelesion of cervical cancer, and high-grade squamous intraepithelial lesions (HSIL) with HPV infection can develop and progress to cervical cancer over a period of 8–12 years. HPV 16, 58, 52 and 18 are the predominant high risk types correlated with cervical lesion. The distribution of dominant HPV genotypes showed obvious regional differences. HPV 16 is more prevalent in Europe and North America, HPV 31 is more prevalent in South/Central America, HPV 33 and 45 are more prevalent in Africa and HPV 52 and 58 are more prevalent in Asia [17]. In male anogenital area, HPV is responsible for a subset of squamous cell carcinomas and associated precursor lesions (penile intraepithelial neoplasia, Bowenoid papulosis, erythroplasia of Queyrat (EQ)) [15]. The most typical locations in women are the external genitalia, but lesions can also be in the cervix and labia minor. In men, condylomas usually involve the coronal sulcus, glans penis and the penile shaft. Circumcision is reported to reduce HPV prevalence in men; however, the efficacy remains imprecise. Recurrences occur in up to one-third of cases [14, 18]. The warts may coalesce in the rectal and perianal area without practicing anal sex. In this region, cauliflower-like shape is the most typical. Since HPV thrives in the rectum, all patients with anal lesions should undergo anoscopy or proctoscopy [2, 13]. Differential diagnosis should be made with condylomata lata, nevi, acrocordon and pemphigus vegetans [2]. If there are anogenital warts in children, sexual abuse should be considered. It should also be reported to the authorities. However, most of the cases in children warts are caused by nongenital HPV types. The mechanism for perinatal and postnatal transmission includes vertical transmission, autoinoculation, sexual transmission and indirectly through contaminated objects and surfaces. This can be explained by mother with hand warts, or child can transfer warts from his/her hand to his/her own genital or anal area [1, 14].

Histopathological findings in warts are hyperkeratosis with parakeratosis, papillomatosis and marked acanthosis. Keratohyalin granules and koilocytes in the granular layer are characteristic for condylomata acuminata. Rete ridges tend to be elongated and point inward toward the center of the wart, and the dermis will often display an increased vascularization with the presence of thrombosed capillaries [14]. Cytoplasmic vacuolization is specific for condyloma when located within deeper portions of the epidermis such as the stratum spinosum, given that the upper portions of the epithelia of mucosal surfaces normally have some degree of cytoplasmic vacuolization already [15].

5.2. Condylomata plana

Condylomata plana are large flat warts mostly found on the cervix and prepuce. Identification of these warts often was possible only after applying acetic acid or colposcopic procedures. HPV 16–18 are usually responsible, and it is possible to progress in SCC of the genitalia [2].

5.3. Bowenoid papulosis

Bowenoid papulosis is characterized by multiple flat papules, plaques or macules less than 1cm in size in the genital area that may or may not be pigmented. The surfaces of the lesion mostly are flat, dome-shaped, papillomatous and verrucous. The color of the lesions can be shiny flesh-colored, reddish-brown, violaceous or black [19, 20]. It resembles clinically viral wart and histopathologically Bowen's disease. The most common sites affected are the penis and vulva. In females, it is referred to as multifocal vulvar intraepithelial neoplasia [20]. Bowenoid papulosis is associated with HPV 16–18, but in a small number, HPV 31, 33, 35, 39 and 53, or mixed infections, have also been detected. Clinically, it should be differentiated from genital warts, seborrheic keratosis, lichen planus, molluscum contagiosum, Bowen's disease (BD) and melanocytic nevus. Younger age and multiple lesions differentiate it from Bowen's disease, but histologically it can be sometimes impossible to differ. Bowenoid papulosis and Bowen disease are clinical entities with similar histological findings of intraepithelial neoplasia. Bowenoid papulosis shows acrotrichial sparing, less pronounced cellular dysplasia and mitotic figures, which helps its differentiation [13, 20, 21]. The histopathological findings revealed full thickness epidermal atypia, acanthosis, papillomatosis, dyskeratotic cells and clumping cells with mild atypical nuclei [22, 23]. Bowenoid papulosis has a variable course, the lesions can stay for a few weeks or over 10 years, with a median of 8 months, but usually spontaneously resolves. Transformation to invasive carcinoma is rare occurring in <1% of cases, especially in immunocompromised [20, 22]. Women with BP have a risk of cervical dysplasia.

5.4. Buschke-Löwenstein tumor

Buschke-Löwenstein tumor (BLT), also known as giant condyloma acuminatum, was first described by *Buschke* and *Löwenstein* in 1925. It is a slow-growing, locally destructive tumor of the anogenital region, while the characteristic feature of tumor is benign appearance on histopathology [24, 25]. It is a sexually transmitted disease that it is thought to be induced by HPV 6 and 11. The estimated incidence of BLT is about 0.1% in the general population [26]. BLT is clinically seen as expansive, destructive exophytic fungating masses, sometimes with a cauliflower-like morphology. The tumor is located mostly (81–94%) on the penis in men, and the anorectal area is the second common area for BLW and in the urethral lesion is found in 5% of cases in men. In females, vulva is the most affected area (90%) and an anorectal location is less frequent. Suprapubic localization is rarely involved [27]. For the histological diagnosis, large and deeper biopsy should be performed to ensure that no malignant cytological characteristics are missed in superficially biopsied specimens. Microscopic features are thick stratum corneum, marked papillary proliferation, tendency to deep invasion, with displacement of surrounding tissues, negligible cellular atypia and a low mitotic rate [25, 28]. Similar features are also seen in verrucous carcinoma. As distinction between verrucous carcinoma and BLT is difficult, BLT is often regarded as a variant of verrucous carcinoma. Some authors also consider BLT as an intermediate lesion between condyloma acuminatum and VC, referring to it as a condyloma-like precancerous lesion [24, 27]. Although several etiologic factors are implicated in the malignant transformation, the etiology of BLT is not known. HPV type 6 or 11 subtypes that are normally lack of malignant potential have been frequently identified in typical cauliflower-like lesions, suggesting the pathogenic role of the virus in the initiation and progression of the tumor. It remains unknown if viral or host risk factors are the determinant factor. Increased viral gene expression or inability to mount a cytotoxic immune response may change the oncogenic potential of HPV types 6 or 11, causing progression of benign condyloma acuminatum to the invasive giant condyloma phenotype. It is also believed that malignant transformation can be caused by the release of free oxygen radicals by activated inflammatory cells, inducing genetic damage and neoplastic transformation. Regular follow-up is necessary because of the frequent recurrences and possible malignant transformation of BLT [28].

5.5. Bowen's disease

Bowen's disease is an in situ squamous cell carcinoma that rarely progress to invasive carcinoma. The disease is associated with the high-risk HPVP types, mostly HPV 16. Clinically, usually a single, sharply demarcated plaque without spontaneous regression is seen in the genital area. The lesions are generally asymptomatic; however, they may cause pruritus or burning pain. Genital BD usually is found in elderly men, especially on the mucosa of the penis (glans or prepuce). Some authors consider mucosal BD equal to the erythroplasia of Queyrat; however, some of them accept them as different histological patterns [13, 29]. Histological characteristics are atypia and anaplasia of cells from the mucous malpighian body with cellular loss of polarity and presence of some dyskeratotic cells, in both the basal and squamous layers [29].

5.6. Erythroplasia of Queyrat

Erythroplasia of Queyrat is an in situ carcinoma that mainly occurs on the glans penis, the prepuce or the urethral meatus of elderly males. In females, vulva is the common area that is affected. The cause of erythroplasia of Queyrat is largely unknown. But in one study some HPV DNAs are detected; all patients were infected with the carcinogenic EV-associated cutaneous HPV type 8. HPV 16, 39 and 51 are other types that are found [30]. Sharply demarcated, erythematous, velvety and bright reddish plaques are characteristics for EQ. Progression to squamous cell carcinoma is more than 30% and is higher than the BD [13].

5.7. Cervical cancer

Cervical carcinoma, which is caused by malignant transformation of cervical epithelial cells following persistent HPV infection, is one of the most common malignant cancer among women, approximately 10% of all cancers in the female population [31]. The relationship between HPV and cervical cancer is observed in many studies, and the persistent infection of the HPV carcinogenic types is found to be the cause in about 90–100% of the cases. HPV 16 and 18 are the two most common types that are responsible for about 70% of cervical carcinomas and 50% of intraepithelial neoplasia grade 3 [13].

6. Prevention methods

Condoms can be a protective method from HPV infection in a limited way. It can lower the chance of transmitting HPV, but it may not be totally safe because of the infected areas that are not covered by condom. Avoiding sexual intercourse or reducing the number of sex partners can lower the risk for HPV. Abstaining from sexual activity is the most reliable method for preventing genital HPV infection. Pre-exposure vaccination is one of the most effective methods for preventing transmission of HPV. The Cervarix (bivalent) and Gardasil (quadrivalent) vaccines protect against most cases of cervical cancer. These vaccines are safe and effective [32]. Cervical cancer and its precursor lesions can be detected by screening women with screening technologies such as cytology-based screening, application of acetic acid during the inspection and HPV DNA test. By using these methods, cancer or precursor lesion is detected at an early stage, thereby improving the survival. The disease can also be prevented by HPV vaccination against oncogenic HPV types [33].

6.1. Vaccines

HPV infections and associated diseases remain a serious burden worldwide. The incidence of HPV-related carcinomas has been increasing every year. Vaccines have been used for over a decade, but widespread vaccine administration is still problematic for multiple reasons in some countries and areas. Many socioeconomically developed countries have been applying the vaccine programs for females and some of the countries are also starting to include the males between the ages of 9–26 for vaccine programs [34].

In 1991, Zhou et al. were the first to develop an innovative vaccine technology based on noninfective recombinant virus-like particle (VLP) of L1, the so-called major papillomavirus virion protein. The VLPs do not contain the viral DNA, and they are completely noninfectious and nononcogenic. Three HPV vaccines are available on the market: bivalent HPV vaccine, quadrivalent HPV and nine-valent HPV vaccine. In bivalent HPV vaccine, there are the VLP form antigens of oncogenic HPV types 16 and 18. Quadrivalent HPV vaccine contains HPV types 6, 11, 16 and 18 L1 proteins. Antigens of HPV 6, 11, 16, 18, 31, 33, 45, 52 and 58 types are in the nine-valent HPV vaccine [35]. According to the recent 58 studies in nine countries from 2007 to February 2016, it is found that a nearly 90% decrease in HPV infection, anogenital warts and cervical lesions in countries with the highest vaccination rates is seen [36]. Gardasil (quadrivalent) is European Medicines Agency (EMA)-approved for males and females, whereas the EMA-approval for Cervarix (bivalent) is currently limited to females only. Gardasil-9 (ninevalent) is a newly EMA-approved nonavalent vaccine in 2015 [37]. All HPV vaccines are administered as three doses i.m. injections in a 6-month period, with the second and third doses given 2 and 6 months after the first dose. The same vaccine product should be used for the three injections. Vaccine is applied in the age of 11–12 for girls and also can be administered at 9-year-old girls. But if the girls or women aged 13–26 years have not been administered the vaccines, they should receive the vaccine as it is possible. The quadrivalent or 9-valent HPV vaccine is also recommended routinely for boys aged 11–12 years. For the unvaccinated, immunocompromised patients, vaccination is recommended through age 26 years. HPV vaccines cannot be used in pregnant women. Women who have received HPV vaccine should continue cervical cancer screening routinely after 21 years of age [32]. Common adverse effects of HPV vaccines are pain, redness, swelling, syncope, dizziness, nausea, headache, fatigue and fewer. Life-threatening side effects are very low with autoimmune responses [34, 35].

Duration of efficacy is a key question when discussing the HPV vaccines. All three vaccines provide very high immunogenicity with antibody titers that are higher than the natural infections and remain high enough to prevent new infections. Booster doses' necessity is still unknown. Up to now, it has been shown that the duration of vaccines may last 5–9 years. But more studies are needed about these important issues [35, 38]. The development of HPV vaccine is a milestone in the prevention of HPV-related infections and probably in the prevention of cervical cancer. But HPV screening still has a major role in cancer prevention and should be improved in low-income countries. It is clear that early vaccination before exposure provides the best results. The Global Alliance for Vaccination and Immunization (GAVI) has demonstrated that a reasonable price and wide distribution can be achieved. Projects in Rwanda and Bhutan have showed that a well-organized, school-based program can achieve excellent coverage. In countries with screening programs, the prevention of abnormal Papanicolaou tests and treatments for precancerous lesions will lower costs [39].

7. Treatment

Anogenital warts can potentially heal without treatment. Waiting a period of time before starting treatment is an option. However, there is uncertainty around the frequency of spontaneous resolution of lesions, with reports of rates of clearance without treatment ranging between 0 and 50% of people affected. A delay in treatment could result in a worsening of anogenital warts and increase the transmission rates. First-line treatment is not always successful in achieving complete clearance of warts and repeated treatments might be required to eradicate large or persistent lesions. Treatment of the warts does not mean to clear the HPV deoxyribonucleic acid (DNA). Cells that remain infected with HPV DNA can stay dormant (latent) for prolonged periods of time, and there can be a recurrence after months, or even years, after initial infection. Thus, those who do not become HPV DNA negative can also pass on the virus, even after treatment or clearance of lesions. These are the important information that should be given and explained in detail to the patients. A wide range of therapies are presently in use, which are highly variable and can differ dramatically with respect to effectivity, cost, side effects, dosing schedules and duration of treatment [32, 40].

7.1. Topical treatment

7.1.1. Patient-applied treatments

Imiquimod: Imiquimod is a non-nucleoside heterocyclic amine, which acts as an immunomodulator. It increases the cellular levels of interferon alpha (IFN-α), tumor necrosis factor alpha (TNF-α) and interleukin-6 (IL-6) by binding to toll-like receptor 7, which leads to strong antiviral and antitumor effects [41]. It is available as a 5% cream. Its pregnancy category is C. Imiquimod is licensed by the European Medicines Agency (EMA) and the US Food and Drug Administration (FDA) for the topical treatment of external genital and perianal warts (condylomata acuminata) in adults. Patients should apply imiquimod cream a thin layer onto the affected area every other night for three nights weekly. The cream should be left in place for

6–10 hours, and after that the treated area should be washed with soap and water. Application of an excess of cream or prolonged contact with the skin might result in a severe application site reaction. The treatment can be continued until the warts resolve or for up to 16 weeks [42, 43]. Common side effects are itching, erythema, burning, irritation, tenderness, erosion, ulceration and pain. Occasionally, patients may experience systemic side effects such as headaches, muscle aches, fatigue, and general malaise. In the pivotal clinical study, wart clearance was achieved in 56% of patients with imiquimod. More women (77%) than men (40%) cleared their warts, with the male study population comprising predominantly circumsized men. Females had a shorter median time to clearance (8 weeks) compared to males (12 weeks). A low recurrence rate (13%) was found [40].

In 2010, the FDA approved imiquimod 3.75% cream for the treatment of anogenital warts in patients 12 years of age or older. Imiquimod 3.75% should be applied to warts daily for 2-weeks and then with repeat of 2-weeks treatments after a 2-weeks rest period. The cure rates for the 3.75% imiquimod are not as high as the 5% imiquimod; however, the newer product has fewer side effects and is more appropriate for patient compliance [44].

Podofilox: Podofilox is an anti-mitotic drug that causes tissue necrosis. It is purified from podophyllin. This product is available as 0.5% gel or solution. Patients should apply the solution to affected areas twice daily for 3 days, followed by 4 days of no therapy. This weekly cycle can be repeated for up to 4 weeks. Clearance rates (45–77%) are similar to imiquimod, and recurrence rates range from 4 % to 33%. Most common adverse effects are burning, pain, erosion, itching and inflammation. Podofilox is contraindicated in pregnancy [32, 42].

Sinecatechins: Sinecatechins are extracts of green tea leaves from Camellia sinensis that are compounded as a 15% ointment. It contains eight different catechins and other green tea components. The main catechin in sinecatechins ointment is epigallocatechin gallate (EGCG), which has the highest biological activity. Sinecatechins are thought to decrease viral replication. Also they have an anti-oxidant by inhibiting a number of proteins, including enzymes involved in oxidative stress, immunostimulatory activity by blocking the kinases needed in tumor cell signaling and induction of apoptosis. These mechanisms presumably contribute to the therapeutic effect of sinecatechins ointment [45]. Patients should apply a 0.5-cm strand of ointment onto each wart three times daily until the complete clearance of warts. But it should not be used for longer than 16 weeks. Common side effects are: erythema, pruritus, burning, pain, erosion, edema, induration and vesicular eruption. Sinecatechins should not be put on open wounds. Mucosal surfaces should be avoided because of the irritation by sinecatechins. The medication is not recommended for patients with HIV infection, other immunocompromised conditions, or genital herpes because the safety and efficacy of therapy has not been evaluated. The pregnancy category of this product is C [32, 44]. Ten percent of sinecatechins ointment is also effective against genital warts. It is also used three times a day like the 15% form. Efficacy rates from the Phase III trials of sinecatechins 10% ointment are higher than those achieved with podophyllotoxin 0.5% or imiquimod 5% and 3.75%. Sinecatechins 10% ointment has lower recurrence rates relative to other patient-applied therapies; therefore, it presents a botanically based alternative to currently available treatments for external anogenital warts [46].

7.1.2. Clinician-applied treatments

Podophyllin: Podophyllin is available as a 25% solution. The preparation causes wart regression and necrosis by stopping mitosis. The solution is typically applied once weekly until complete clearance up to 3–6 weeks. Because of the corrosive nature and the toxicity of the treatment, when podophyllin is overapplied or occluded, it is recommended to limit the application area to less than 10 cm^2 of warts per treatment, limiting the amount applied to less than 0.5 mL per treatment. Podophyllin should not be used in pregnant women or breastfeeding [42, 43].

Trichloroacetic (TCA): Trichloroacetic acid may be compounded in different concentration, generally 60–90%. It is a caustic that erodes the skin and mucous membranes, but generally is not absorbed systemically.TCA is applied in the office with a cotton tip applicator, with repeated applications up to three times weekly until the warts have resolved. It is more effective in few small, moist lesions. The initial response rate is 70–81%, but recurrence rate is up to 36%. TCA also can be used to treat vaginal and anal lesions. TCA treatment is delivered in a controlled manner to provide limited local destruction. A small amount should be applied only to the warts and allowed to dry until the white frosting develops. It destroys the warts by chemical coagulation of proteins. The application of TCA is accompanied by a burning sensation that lasts for 2–5 min. A neutralizing agent (sodium bicarbonate) should be at reach in case of excess application or spills. Dermal injury or scarring is rare. Common side effects are local and include pain, ulceration and crust formation [47, 48].

7.2. Ablative treatments

Cryotherapy: Cryotherapy is a process in which the abnormal tissue is frozen by using of a cooling agent such as through the use of a nitrous oxide or liquid nitrogen. Freezing causes permanent dermal and vascular damage. This leads to the initiation of an immune repair response which causes necrosis and clearance of the destroyed cells. This treatment is most effective when used for multiple small warts on the penile shaft or vulva. Treatment should be repeated every 1–2 weeks. Clearance rates range from 71 to 79%, with recurrence rates of 38–73% at 6 months. Cryotherapy has been used to treat external genital warts without adverse effects during pregnancy [40, 42]. Application of this treatment is easy, and it has a rapid destructive effect. It also has an advantage in treating bulky lesions, grouped lesions and lesions on hair-bearing areas. It does not have systemic side effects and only affects tissue to which it is directly applied. Common side effects include local tissue destruction, such as painful blistering, ulceration, infection, rarely scarring and loss of pigmentation. Another disadvantage of cryosurgery is that subclinical lesions cannot be treated in the surrounding skin. Multiple outpatient visits are required for the clearance of warts, and the pain associated with its application can limit its repeated use in certain patients and localizations [40, 47].

Electrosurgery: There are two types of electrosurgery: electrocautery and electrical surgery. Local anesthesia is needed to perform electrosurgery. In electrocautery, electricity flows only through the instrument producing heat that is applied to the lesion. In the alternating-current form of electrosurgery, electricity flows from the instrument through the patient to a grounding plate. The alternating current systems produce cutting, coagulation, or a blend of both. Electrotherapy is particularly effective for treating smaller warts located on the shaft of the penis, the rectum or the vulva or for pedunculated lesions, but is not recommended for the larger warts because of the permanent scarring [43, 47]. Clearance rates with electrosurgery range from 90 to 96%, and recurrence rates of 18% have been reported. The smoke resulting from this procedure may contain HPV particles. To prevent the transmission to the oropharynx, use of smoke evacuation equipment and a mask is recommended [42].

Surgical excision: Surgical excision may be the most cost-effective treatment for genital warts. This method is more effective when warts are large, pedunculated or exophytic. The advantage of this method is to preserve intact tissue for histologic examination and offers quick results. Pain, scarring, slow healing and pigment changes are the disadvantages [42]. Especially for treatment of BLT, wide surgical excision by Mohs technique is recommended as the most important therapeutic intervention [25].

Carbon dioxide laser therapy: Carbon dioxide laser therapy relies upon the use of a concentrated beam of infrared light energy, which will heat and cauterize the affected area. The intense light energy has the added benefit of providing immediate cauterization of any ligated vessels, ensuring a virtually bloodless procedure. Side effects are generally mild and limited to the burning of tissue surrounding the lesion. The deep penetrating effect of the laser often allows for a greater and more complete viral attack than seen with other surgical treatment options. This makes the laser treatment a better choice for immunosuppressed individuals, and for pregnant women with extensive lesions which are unresponsive to TCA or cryotherapy. Laser therapy is typically considered to be less effective than other forms of surgical treatment, with clearance rates ranging between 23 and 52%. Recurrence rates are also high as 77%. Laser treatment is also more complex and costly than electrosurgery or cryotherapy. A CO_2 laser requires maintenance and additional training to perform correctly [40, 47].

7.3. Other treatments

Interferons: Interferons are a class of small (15–28 kDa) protein and glycoprotein cytokines (15–28 kDa) produced by T cells, fibroblasts and other cells in response to viral infection and other biologic and synthetic stimuli. Interferon has been used in the treatment of genital warts for its immunomodulatory, antiproliferative and antiviral properties. Interferon could be used either locally or systemically. Local administrations are mainly composed of intralesional injections and topical applications. Interferon tends to be a well-tolerated form of therapy. According to different administration, topical interferon appears to be much more effective than both systemically used interferon and placebo in either improving the complete response rate or reducing the recurrence rate for the treatment of genital warts [41, 49]. Combining interferon with other treatments increases the effectiveness of treatment. In one study, the addition of subcutaneously administered interferon α-2b to laser-treated patients with chronic therapy-resistant genital lesions significantly enhanced the chance of eliminating these warts, and it was fairly well tolerated. It is also suggested that gel form of interferon can help treat intravaginal warts. However, because of its high cost and inconsistent effect, interferon is best considered to the genital warts that are resistant to other treatments [47].

Cidofovir: Cidofovir is a monophosphate nucleotide analogue. Cidofovir is converted to the active cidofovir diphosphate that is a competitive inhibitor and an alternative substrate for viral DNA polymerases. As cidofovir acts directly on viral DNA, it has been found effective on immunocompromised people and thus could potentially afford greater clinical benefit for people with HIV infection than with other treatments available. Cidofovir has been formulated as a 1% gel and is applied topically to lesions overnight, three times a week for up to 16 weeks [43, 50].

5-Fluorouracil: Use of topical 5-FU is indicated for therapy-resistant condylomata. It can be applied to the affected extragenital area once or twice for 10 weeks. It appears to be as effective as continued regimens but better tolerated [51].

Zinc: Zinc is an immunoregulator that stimulates the leucocytes and natural killer cells. Oral and topical form of zinc has been found effective in the treatment of warts. It has been shown that there is a deficiency of zinc in patients with multiple or recurrent warts. Oral zinc sulfate given in a dose of 10 mg/kg/day has been used, with approximately 84–87% patients showing complete resolution of warts in 2 months in two randomized placebo-controlled trials [41]. In a study, the podophyllin-, imiquimod- and cryotherapy-treated patient is combined with 400 mg oral zinc sulfate for 8 weeks. And it is shown that oral zinc sulfate combination therapy appears to reduce the relapse rate of vulvar warts [52]. Topical 5 and 10% zinc solution has been used in cutaneous warts, three times a day for 4 weeks with only 5 and 11% responses [41].

H2 receptor blockers: Cimetidine is a H2 receptor blocker that can be used in the treatment of warts especially in children. It blocks the type 2 histamine receptors on suppressor T cells and augments cell-mediated immunity. It increases mitogen-induced lymphocyte proliferation and the levels of IFNγ and IL-2 and inhibits suppressor T cells. It decreases the levels of IL-18. It has been used in a dose of 20–40 mg/kg/day for 3–4 months with response ranging from 30 to 87% [41]. In a study that included four children with extensive condylomata acuminata of the genital and perigenital areas, high doses of cimetidine have been found effective to eradicate the condyloma and avoid recurrence in two and as primary treatment in two. All patients were treated with 30–40 mg/kg cimetidine daily in three divided doses during a 3-month period. So it is suggested that cimetidine can be considered as first-line therapy and is useful for primary and adjunctive treatment of condyloma in young children [53].

Photodynamic therapy: Photodynamic therapy (PDT) with 5-aminolevulinic acid (ALA) is a new technique based on the interaction of light, photosensitizer and oxygen. ALA is a topical used photosensitizer with few side effects. It is the first compound in the porphyrin synthesis pathway. ALA is selectively absorbed by tumor cells and rapidly proliferating cells and transformed to endogenous protoporphyrin IX (PpIX) after the exogenous application of ALA. The PpIX is then activated by red light, leading to the formation of singlet oxygen, which leads to the killing or destruction of tumor cells and proliferative cells. Cells infected by human papillomavirus are proliferative cells; ALA is selectively absorbed by these cells and can be killed by the radiation of red light. This means ALA-PDT treatment can destroy visible and invisible infected tissues and reduce the number of the viral load and the recurrence rate [54]. The common side effects in patients treated with ALA-PDT mainly include mild burning and/or stinging restricted to the applied area [41].

7.4. Treatments in pregnancy

Patients who have condyloma acuminata during pregnancy are a risky group. During pregnancy, vaginal secretions contacting the skin and mucous membranes are more abundant, meaning that the vulva will remain in a moist and immersed state. In pregnancy, hormones and reduced immunoresponsiveness can promote the growth of HPV-induced lesions. The warts are characterized by fast-growing and a reduced tolerance and poor compliance to treatment. Only a few treatments have been tested and recommended in pregnancy [55]. Podofilox (podophyllotoxin), podophyllin and sinecatechins should not be used during pregnancy. Trichloroacetic acid, cryotherapy, electrocautery and surgical excision, including laser treatment, are recommended treatments. But the resolution might be incomplete or poor until pregnancy is complete. Significant side effects have been observed for some of these methods, including local ulceration and scar formation, which may reduce a patient's compliance with treatment requirements. Medicine could potentially cause fetal malformation, and laser treatment and surgical excision may cause uterine contraction, or even abortion [32, 55]. The safety of imiquimod has not been established, but a small number of patients worldwide have been treated with imiquimod and found to be effective and promising. No adverse fetal outcomes or fetal and neonatal abnormalities were observed. No complications were observed in the postpartum and follow-up period [56]. Photodynamic therapy with topical ALA seems to be safe and effective in the treatment of condyloma acuminata in pregnancy. In case reports, it demonstrated high clearance rate of warts, was well-tolerated by patients and showed no adverse effects on mothers or fetuses [57]. Cryotherapy appears to be the best choice. During the cryotherapy procedure, liquid nitrogen freezes the tissue and thereby causes necrosis; the treatment also stimulates specific immune responses, such as an immunomodulatory action of T lymphocytes against the remaining viable wart tissue. It is also a simple and inexpensive procedure, rarely causes scarring or depigmentation, and is safe for use in pregnancy. The transmission (transplacental, perinatal or postnatal) of virus to the baby is not completely understood. So the necessity of cesarean section in the presence of genital warts is also unclear. Cesarean delivery is indicated for women with anogenital warts if the pelvic outlet is obstructed or if vaginal delivery would result in excessive bleeding [32]. Prophylactic cesarean delivery is not recommended to prevent the respiratory papillomatosis in infants and children, because it is reported that only 7 infants of 1000 in mothers with external genital warts developed respiratory papillomatosis, and cesarean delivery did not reduce this risk [42].

7.5. Treatment in immunosuppressive patients

Patients with significant immunosuppression (patients with HIV infection, immunosuppressive therapy to suppress transplant rejection, or other concomitant disease) might have larger or more numerous lesions, might not respond to therapies and might have more frequent recurrences after treatment. They are also at increased risk of squamous cell carcinoma, which may be clinically similar to genital warts. Lesions that ulcerate, grow rapidly, or are atypical should be biopsied to rule out squamous cell carcinoma [32, 42]. Cryotherapy, electrosurgery, excision and laser therapy can be applied to these patients.

8. Conclusion

Genital warts, also known as condylomata acuminata, are one of the most common forms of sexually transmitted diseases affecting the general population. Most infections do not result in the manifestation of genital warts. Genital warts are not themselves cancerous, but warts caused by high risk types of HPV are predisposed to oncogenic transformation. Because of the contagiousness and the progression to precancerous lesions, HPV infections should be underestimated. Selection of a treatment modality may depend on the patient, all the propriate choices should be explained to patients, and they should be informed what risks can be seen. Given the strikingly high prevalence of genital warts among the population, and the lack of adequate therapies, HPV vaccines may play a significant role in reducing the burden of disease by preventing viral infection and transmission.

Author details

Özge Aşkın

Address all correspondence to: ozgee_karakus@hotmail.com

Department of Dermatology, Memorial Atasehir Hospital, Istanbul, Turkey

References

[1] Habif TP. Clinical Dermatology. 5th ed. Hanover: Mosby Elsevier; 2010. p. 419

[2] Burgdorf WHC, Plewig G, Wolff HH, Landthaler M, editors. Braun-Falco's Dermatology. 3rd ed. Heidelberg: Springer; 2009. p. 84

[3] Suligoi B, Vittori G, Salfa MC, Timelli L, Corsini D, et al. Prevalence and incidence of external genital warts in a sample of Italian general female population. BMC Infectious Diseases. 2017;**17**(1):126. DOİ: 10.1186/s12879-017-2202-6

[4] Colpani V, Bidinotto AB, Falavigna M, Giozza SP, Benzaken AS, et al. Prevalence of papillomavirus in Brazil: A systematic review protocol. BMJ Open. 2016;**6**(11):e011884. DOI: 10.1136/bmjopen-2016-011884

[5] Araldi RP, Assaf SM, Carvalho RF, Carvalho MA, Souza JM, et al. Papillomaviruses: A systematic review. Genetics and Molecular Biology. 2017; 40(1):1-21. DOI: 10.1590/1678-4685-GMB-2016-0128

[6] Galloway DA, Laimins LA. Human papillomaviruses: Shared and distinct pathways for pathogenesis. Current Opinion in Virology. 2015;**14**:87-92. DOİ: 10.1016/j.coviro.2015.09.001

[7] Egawa N, Egawa K, Griffin H, Doorbar J. Human papillomaviruses; epithelial tropisms, and the development of neoplasia. Viruses. 2015;**7**(7):3863-3890. DOI: 10.3390/v7072802

[8] Alhamlan FS, Al-Qahtani AA, Al-Ahdal MN. Current studies on human papillomavirus in Saudi Arabia. The Journal of Infection in Developing Countries. 2015;**9**(6):571-576. DOI: 10.3855/jidc.6538

[9] Liu M, He Z, Zhang C, Liu F, Liu Y, et al. Transmission of genital human papillomavirus infection in couples: A population-based cohort study in rural China. Scientific Reports. 2015;**5**:10986. DOI: 10.1038/srep10986

[10] Erickson BK, Alvarez RD, Huh WK. Human papillomavirus: What every provider should know. The American Journal of Obstetrics and Gynecology. 2013;**208**(3):169-175. DOI: 10.1016/j.ajog.2012.09.007

[11] Modibbo F, Iregbu KC, Okuma J, Leeman A, Kasius A, et al. Randomized trial evaluating self-sampling for HPV DNA based tests for cervical cancer screening in Nigeria. Infectious Agents and Cancer. DOI: 10.1186/s13027-017-0123-z

[12] Anic GM, Giuliano AR. Genital HPV infection and related lesions in men. Preventive Medicine. 2011;**53**(Suppl 1):S36-S41. DOI: 10.1016/j.ypmed.2011.08.002

[13] Leto Md, Santos Junior GF, Porro AM, Tomimori J. Human papillomavirus infection: Etiopathogenesis, molecular biology and clinical manifestations. Anais Brasileiros de Dermatologia. 2011;**86**(2):306-317

[14] Cardoso JC, Calonje E. Cutaneous manifestations of human papillomaviruses: A review. Acta Dermatovenerologica Alpina, Pannonica et Adriatic. 2011;**20**(3):145-154.

[15] Vyas NS, Pierce Campbell CM, Mathew R, Abrahamsen M, Van der Kooi K, et al. Role of histological findings and pathologic diagnosis for detection of human papillomavirus infection in men. Journal of Medical Virology. 2015;**87**(10):1777-1787. DOI: 10.1002/jmv.24238

[16] Lamos C, Mihaljevic C, Aulmann S, Bruckner T, Domschke C, et al. Detection of human papillomavirus infection in patients with vaginal intraepithelial neoplasia. PLoS One. 2016;**11**(12):e0167386. DOI: 10.1371/journal.pone.0167386

[17] Zhao J, Guo Z, Wang Q, Si T, Pei S, et al. Human papillomavirus genotypes associated with cervical precancerous lesions and cancer in the highest area of cervical cancer mortality, Longnan, China. Infectious Agents and Cancer. 2017;**12**:8. DOI: 10.1186/s13027-017-0116-y

[18] Zhu YP, Jia ZW, Dai B, Ye DW, Kong YY, et al. Relationship between circumcision and human papillomavirus infection: A systematic review and meta-analysis. Asian Journal of Andrology. 2017;**19**(1):125-131. DOI: 10.4103/1008-682X.175092

[19] Tschandl P, Rosendahl C, Kittler H. Cutaneous human papillomavirus infection: Manifestations and diagnosis. Current Problems in Dermatology. 2014;**45**:92-97. DOI: 10.1159/000355966

[20] Peng WS, Tan C. Bowenoid papulosis in a linear distribution. Postepy Dermatol Alergol. 2016;**33**(2):146-148. DOI: 10.5114/ada.2016.59161

[21] Shastry V, Betkerur J, Kushalappa. Bowenoid papulosis of the genitalia successfully treated with topical tazarotene: A report of two cases. The Indian Journal of Dermatology. 2009;**54**(3):283-286. DOI: 10.4103/0019-5154.55643

[22] Nayak SU, Shenoi SD, Bhat ST, Shivamurthy A. Bowenoid papulosis. The Indian Journal of Sexually Transmitted Diseases. 2015;**36**(2):223-225. DOI: 10.4103/0253-7184.167196

[23] Shimizu A, Kato M, Ishikawa O. Bowenoid papulosis successfully treated with imiquimod 5% cream. The Journal of Dermatology. 2014;**41**(6):545-546. DOI: 10.1111/1346-8138.12510

[24] Pinto AR, Guedes-Martins L, Marques C, Cabral JM. Buschke-Lowenstein tumor. Acta Médica Portuguesa. 2012;**25**(5):345-347

[25] Sandhu R, Min Z, Bhanot N. A gigantic anogenital lesion: Buschke-Lowenstein tumor. Case Reports in Dermatological Medicine. 2014;**2014**:650714. DOI: 10.1155/2014/650714

[26] Patel R, Kaloucava S. A case of penile Buschke-Lowenstein tumor in a developing country. Clinical Case Reports. 2017;**5**(3):257-259. DOI: 10.1002/ccr3.805

[27] Ahsaini M, Tahiri Y, Tazi MF, Elammari J, Mellas S, et al. Verrucous carcinoma arising in an extended giant condyloma acuminatum (Buschke-Löwenstein tumor): A case report and review of the literature. Journal of Medical Case Reports. 2013;7:273. DOI: 10.1186/1752-1947-7-273

[28] Martin JM, Molina I, Monteagudo C, Marti N, Lopez V, Jorda E. Buschke-Lowenstein tumor. Journal of Dermatological Case Reports. 2008;**2**(4):60-62. DOI: 10.3315/jdcr.2008.1019

[29] Ishioka P, Yamada S, Michalany NS, Hirata SH. Dermoscopy of Bowen's disease: Pigmented variant on the penis. Anais Brasileiros de Dermatologia. 2012;**87**(3):482-484.

[30] Wieland U, Jurk S, Weissenborn S, Krieg T, Pfister H, Ritzkowsky A. Erythroplasia of queyrat. Coinfection with cutaneous carcinogenic human papillomavirus type 8 and genital papillomaviruses in a carcinoma in situ. Journal of Investigative Dermatology. 2000;**115**(3):396-401

[31] Mehta AM, Mooij M, Brankovic I, Ouburg S, Morre SA, Jordanova ES. Cervical carcinogenesis and immune response gene polymorphisms: A review. Journal of Immunology Research. 2017;**2017**:8913860. DOI: 10.1155/2017/8913860

[32] Workowski KA, Bolan GA, Centers for Disease Control and Prevention. Sexually transmitted diseases treatment guidelines, 2015. The MMWR Recommendations and Reports. 2015;**64**(RR-03):1-137

[33] Ekwunife OI, O'Mahony JF, Gerber Grote A, Mosch C, Paeck T, Lhachimi SK. Challenges in cost-effectiveness analysis modelling of HPV vaccines in low- and middle-income countries: A systematic review and practice recommendations. Pharmacoeconomics. 2017;**35**(1):65-82. DOI: 10.1007/s40273-016-0451-7

[34] White MD. Pros, cons, and ethics of HPV vaccine in teens—Why such controversy? The Translational Andrology and Urology. 2014;**3**(4):429-434. DOI: 10.3978/j.issn.2223-4683.2014.11.02

[35] Angioli R, Lopez S, Aloisi A, Terranova C, De Cicco C, et al. Ten years of HPV vaccines: State of art and controversies. Critical Reviews in Oncology/Hematology. 2016;**102**:65-72. DOI: 10.1016/j.critrevonc.2016.03.020

[36] Wathion N. HPV vaccines are safety to use. Tidsskr Nor Laegeforen. 2017;**137**(1):13-14. DOI: 10.4045/tidsskr.16.1095

[37] Kolben TM, Dannecker C, Baltateanu K, Goess C, Starrach T, et al. HPV vaccination: Attitude and knowledge among German gynecologists. Geburtshilfe Frauenheilkd. 2016;**76**(10):1074-1080

[38] Nicol AF, Andrade CV, Russomano FB, Rodrigues LL, Oliveira NS, Provance DW Jr. HPV vaccines: A controversial issue? Brazilian Journal of Medical and Biological Research. 2016;**49**(5):e5060. DOI: 10.1590/1414-431X20155060

[39] Pils S, Joura EA. From the monovalent to the nine-valent HPV vaccine. Clinical Microbiology and Infection. 2015;**21**(9):827-33. DOI: 10.1016/j.cmi.2015.05.001

[40] Yanofsky VR, Patel RV, Goldenberg G. Genital warts: A comprehensive review. Journal of Clinical and Aesthetic Dermatology. 2012;**5**(6):25-36

[41] Thappa DM, Chiramel MJ. Evolving role of immunotherapy in the treatment of refractory warts. Indian Dermatology Online Journal. 2016;**7**(5):364-370

[42] Karnes JB, Usatine RP. Management of external genital warts. American Family Physician. 2014;**90**(5):312-318

[43] Thurgar E, Barton S, Karner C, Edwards SJ. Clinical effectiveness and cost-effectiveness of interventions for the treatment of anogenital warts: Systematic review and economic evaluation. Health Technology Assessment. 2016;**20**(24):v-vi, 1-486. DOI: 10.3310/hta20240

[44] Scheinfeld N. Update on the treatment of genital warts. Dermatology Online Journal. 2013;**19**(6):18559

[45] Balaji G. Sinecatechins: A better prospect for treating anogenital warts. The Indian Journal of Sexually Transmitted Diseases. 2014;**35**(1):75-76. DOI: 10.4103/0253-7184.132415

[46] Gupta AK, Daigle D. Sinecatechins 10% ointment: A green tea extract for the treatment of external genital warts. Skin Therapy Letter. 2015;**20**(1):6-8

[47] Scheinfeld N, Lehman DS. An evidence-based review of medical and surgical treatments of genital warts. Dermatology Online Journal. 2006;**12**(3):5

[48] von Krogh G, Lacey CJ, Gross G, Barrasso R, Schneider A. European course on HPV associated pathology: Guidelines for primary care physicians for the diagnosis and management of anogenital warts. Sexually Transmitted Infections. 2000;**76**(3):162-168

[49] Yang J, Pu YG, Zeng ZM, Yu ZJ, Huang N, Deng QW. Interferon for the treatment of genital warts: A systematic review. BMC Infectious Diseases. 2009;**9**:156. DOI: 10.1186/1471-2334-9-156

[50] Hengge UR, Tietze G. Successful treatment of recalcitrant condyloma with topical cidofovir. Sexually Transmitted Infections. 2000;**76**(2):143

[51] Krebs HB. Treatment of genital condylomata with topical 5-fluorouracil. Dermatologic Clinics. 1991;**9**(2):333-341

[52] Akhavan S, Mohammadi SR, Modarres Gillani M, Mousavi AS, Shirazi M. Efficacy of combination therapy of oral zinc sulfate with imiquimod, podophyllin or cryotherapy in the treatment of vulvar warts. The Journal of Obstetrics and Gynaecology Research. 2014;**40**(10):2110-2113. DOI:10.1111/jog.12457

[53] Franco I. Oral cimetidine for the management of genital and perigenital warts in children. The Journal of Urology. 2000;**164**(3 Pt 2):1074-1075

[54] Zhang Z, Lu XN, Liang J, Tang H, Yang YS, et al. Evaluation of photodynamic therapy using topical aminolevulinic acid hydrochloride in the treatment of condylomata acuminate. International Journal of Clinical and Experimental Medicine. 2015;**8**(4):6517-6521

[55] Yang LJ, Zhu DN, Dang YL, Zhao X. Treatment of condyloma acuminata in pregnant women with cryotherapy combined with proanthocyanidins: Outcome and safety. Experimental and Therapeutic Medicine. 2016;**11**(6):2391-2394

[56] Ciavattini A, Tsiroglou D, Vichi M, Di Giuseppe J, Cecchi S, Tranquilli AL. Topical Imiquimod 5% cream therapy for external anogenital warts in pregnant women: Report of four cases and review of the literature. The Journal of Maternal-Fetal and Neonatal Medicine. 2012;**25**(7):873-876. DOI: 10.3109/14767058.2011.600795

[57] Yang YG, Zou XB, Zhao H, Zhang YJ, Li HJ. Photodynamic therapy of condyloma acuminata in pregnant women. Chinese Medical Journal (English Edition). 2012;**125**(16): 2925-2928

5

Microbicides for the Prevention of HPV, HIV-1, and HSV-2: Sexually Transmitted Viral Infections

Naveed Shahzad, Roman Farooq, Bilal Aslam and Muhammad Umer

Abstract

Sexually transmitted diseases (STDs) can be transmitted through genital-genital, oro-genital, or anogenital contacts and remain to be a public health concern worldwide. Approximately one million people around the world are believed to be newly infected with sexually transmitted infections (STIs) each day. Numerous causative agents including bacteria, viruses, protozoa, yeast, and fungi are responsible for STIs; however, viruses exhibit more serious risks, probabilities and outcomes of STDs than other organisms. The most lethal viral STIs are human immunodeficiency virus-1 (HIV), herpes simplex viruses 1 and 2 (HSV-1 and HSV-2), and human papillomavirus (HPV), which are responsible for major sexually transmitted viral infections including AIDS, herpes simplex, and genital warts, respectively. Despite the fact that several prevention strategies such as vaccination, abstinence from sex, limiting sex partners, the use of condoms and a range of therapeutic drugs have drastically reduced the risk of contracting STIs, these three infections continue to spread at an alarming rate. The high incidence and lack of effective vaccine, instigated scientists to look for alternate, cheap, and efficient strategies for controlling these deadly viruses. Microbicide are relatively new approach that may be helpful in preventing STIs transmission when applied inside the genitals before inter course. Like other interventions, microbicides are used as prophylactic measures against STIs. Therefore, an excellent safety and efficacy profile analysis is mandatory before their approval for human use. Although no safe and efficacious microbicide is yet available, many candidates including nonoxynol-9, Savvy, cellulose sulfate, Carraguard, VivaGel, tenofovir gel, and PRO 2000 have shown promising in vitro activity and many more are under development. However, very few of them have moved to large-scale phase III trials. This chapter aims to provide a brief overview of various microbicides along with their mechanism of actions and recent updates on safety and effectiveness trials.

Keywords: HPV, HIV-1, HSV-2, sexually transmitted infections (STIs), microbicides, prevention of STIs

1. Introduction

Sexually transmitted diseases (STDs) or venereal diseases (VDs) being responsible for millions of deaths worldwide have proven to be a major burden on human health [1]. Approximately 19 million new cases of STDs are reported in the United States every year [2]. More strikingly, according to Centers for Disease Control and Prevention (CDC) recent press release, the largest increase in STD cases was observed from 2014 to 2015. STDs are caused by more than 30 different pathogens including bacteria, viruses, parasites, yeast, and fungus commonly known as sexually transmitted infections (STIs) (**Figure 1**). Among all known STIs, viruses exhibit more serious risks, probabilities, and outcomes of sexually transmitted diseases. Viral STIs include human immunodeficiency virus-1 (HIV), herpes simplex viruses 1 and 2 (HSV-1 and HSV-2), human papillomavirus (HPV), hepatitis B virus (HBV), and molluscum contagiosum virus (MCV) causing acquired immunodeficiency syndrome (AIDS), herpes simplex, genital warts, viral hepatitis, and molluscum contagiosum, respectively. However, HPV, HIV-1, and HSV-2 targeting the mucosa of the penis, vulva, rectum, and urinary tract account for major sexually transmitted viral infections. In order to understand the wreckage caused by these infections, it is imperative to understand the biology and pathogenesis of the abovementioned sexually transmitted viruses.

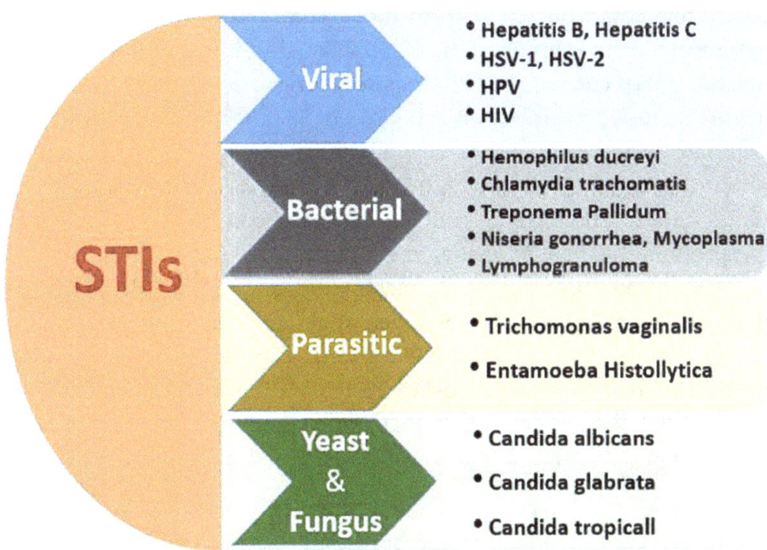

Figure 1. Sexually transmitted infections (STIs).

1.1. Biology of human papillomavirus

Human papillomaviruses (HPVs) named for warts (papillomas) are the most common sexually transmitted infectious agents both in men and women across the globe, particularly in undeveloped countries. It is believed that nearly all men and women acquire HPV infection at least once at some stage of their lives [2]. However, sexual transmission being the major route of HPV infection, the probability of getting HPV infection in adulthood is high due to increased sexual activity. The HPV prevalence falls with the increasing age probably as a consequence of decreased sexual activity and establishment of immune response against the virus [3].

HPV is a small, nonenveloped, and double-stranded DNA virus having genome size of 8 kbp. The circular genome of HPV encodes six early and two late overlapping open reading frames (ORFs) and a noncoding long control region (LCR) [4]. Upon infection, the virus first transcribes six early proteins (E1, E2, E4, E5, E6, and E7), which are mainly involved in viral DNA replication and HPV-mediated pathogenesis. Late structural proteins L1 and L2, which make up the viral capsid, are transcribed during later phases of virus replication [5]. The early genes are expressed within the basal surface of the epithelium while late genes in supra-basal layer of the epithelium. The LCR located upstream of early and late genes contains various promoter and transcriptional regulatory sequences which act as binding sites for several viral and host transcription factors [6].

Based on L1 gene nucleotide sequence, the HPVs are classified into genera, species, and types. To date, almost 151 types of HPV have been identified and divided into five genera known as *alpha, beta, gamma, mu,* and *nu* [7]. HPV types are further categorized into cutaneous and mucosal types. While cutaneous HPV types target keratinocytes in the hand and feet skin, mucosal types infect the inner lining of the respiratory, digestive (mouth, throat, esophagus), and anogenital tracts. The cutaneous HPVs mostly belong to beta and gamma genera, whereas mucosal types are included in alpha genus [8]. About 30 HPV types have been reported to be transmitted through sexual contact, thereby infecting mucosa of the genitalia [9]. The genital HPV types are further categorized into high risk (HR) and low risk (LR) based on the severity of clinical manifestation. The LR-HPVs such as subtypes 6, 11, 42, 44, 51, 53, and 83 induce warts or hyperproliferative benign lesion on genital. On the other hand, HR-HPV subtypes including 16, 18, 31, 33, 35, 39, 45, 51, 52, 56, 58, 59, 68,73, and 82 are linked with premalignant and malignant cervical, penile, vulvar, vaginal, anal, and head and neck carcinomas [10]. Notably, majority of the LR-HPV infections are caused by HPV 6 and 11 subtypes, while subtypes 16 and 18 are responsible for most of the HR-HPV infections [11, 12]. In fact, HPV 16 and 18 are the most lethal subtypes, which together account for 70% cases of cervical cancer, the fifth most commonly diagnosed type of cancer and leading cause of cancer deaths [13].

The HPV lesions are believed to commence from the basal keratinocytes, which are exposed to HPV infection as a consequence of microabrasions or trauma during sexual intercourse [9, 14]. The virus then binds to specific cell surface receptors and is subsequently internalized in to the cells where it establishes episomal or integrated persistent infection, a pivotal step in cervical cancer causation. Various viral proteins are expressed during the replication cycle of HPV that control the transcription as well as replication of virus and induce cell proliferation. The E5, E6, and E7 are the essential proteins which help the virus during initiation and progression of cervical cancer [15]. These oncoproteins interfere with cell cycle and other regulatory pathways and induce genome instability mainly by inhibiting key tumor suppressor proteins such as p53 and pRB [16]. The p53 being the guardian of genome is targeted by HPV E6 protein for proteasomal degradation, while E7 competes with pRB protein releasing the E2F transcription factor, which helps the transcription of genes that drive cell cycle further on. Likewise, HPV oncoproteins maneuver host cell in such a way to keep them in a condition favorable for virus replication. For example, overexpression of E1 and E2 proteins has been evidenced to push the cell in S and G2 phases that stably maintain viral episomes [17]. HPV has also been described to alter numerous cell regulatory pathways; for instance, E6 and E7 are believed to be involved in beta-catenin nuclear accumulation leading to activation of Wnt signaling pathway that is one of the major deregulated signal transduction pathways in cancer [18]. Another salient example elaborating the role of HPV proteins in carcinogenesis was described by Accardi et al. who proved that HPV16 E6 and E7 proteins jointly dissociate Na^+/H^+ exchange regulatory factor-1 (NHERF-1), which is involved in the regulation of various cellular processes including signaling and transformation. The degradation of NHERF-1 leads to activation of the PI3K/AKT signaling pathway, which is known to be a major player involved in carcinogenesis [19].

1.2. Biology of herpes simplex virus

Herpes, from the ancient Greek meaning to creep or crawl, is the name ascribed to the infections caused by a large family of DNA viruses called *Herpesviridae*. The members of this virus family are known to equally infect human and animals. Among the described human herpes viruses, closely related herpes simplex virus-1 (HSV-1) and herpes simplex virus-2 (HSV-2) that show 70% genomic homology are considered to be most contagious human herpes viruses and are transmitted via sexual contact [20]. HSV-1 may be transmitted by oral to oral or oral to genital contact, thereby causing oral or genital herpes, while HSV-2 is exclusively transmitted by sexual contact and is responsible for genital infections only [21]. Mostly oral and genital herpes are symptomless; however, complications can cause painful blisters or ulcers at the site of infection. Both of these viruses are widespread in human population. In 2012, it was estimated that 67% human population under the age of 50 were living with HSV 1 infection while 11% with HSV-2 [22].

The HSV virion is structurally divided into four parts: an electron dense core containing the viral genome, an icosapentahedral capsid, a tegument comprising a protein cluster, and a glycoprotein-based envelope [23]. The genome of HSV-1 and HSV-2 is a complex large double-stranded DNA molecule which is divided into two unique regions: the long unique (U_L) and the short unique regions (U_S). The U_L transcribes 56 viral genes whereas U_S merely 12 [24]. The translated proteins from these genes are involved in making virus components, controlling virus replication and infectivity. The virus gets entry into the nerve cells in the lower layer of the skin as a consequence of interaction between numerous viral glycoproteins and host cell receptors mainly heparan sulfate [25]. Upon internalization, the virion is dismantled, and capsid is routed to the nuclear pore ejecting its DNA into the nucleus where transcription of viral genes takes place with the help of RNA polymerase II [26]. The HSV replication involves sequential production of different viral proteins. At first, immediate early proteins are synthesized that regulate viral gene expression during replication. The enzymes carrying out viral replication are also products of early gene transcription. The late transcribed genes predominantly encode proteins required for capsid and envelop formation [24].

The primary HSV infection occurs in the epithelial cells from where virus ascends to the sensory nerve terminal at peripheral site. Then by retrograde axonal transport virus enters the trigeminal nerve ganglion and establishes latency resulting in long-time persistence [27]. During the latency phase, virus expresses latency-associated transcript (LAT) which regulates the host cell genome in order to maintain the virus reservoir in the host without any clinical manifestation [28]. Furthermore, HSV evades host immune response either by mimicking the human interleukin 10 (HIL-10) or by downregulation of the major histocompatibility complexes I and II (MHC I and II) in the contaminated cell, thus ensuring virus survival in latency [29]. The HSV encodes a HIL-10 homologous protein that blocks the production of pro-inflammatory cytokines such as IFN-γ, IL-1α, GM-CSF, IL-6, and TNF-α, thereby reducing the natural killer cells and cell-mediated response against virus [30]. Likewise, for the downregulation of MHCI-II, HSV encodes ICP47 protein that blocks the presentation of MHC-class-1 proteins on the cell surface by retaining the newly synthesized MHC molecules in the endoplasmic reticulum [31]. The lack of MHC expression on the surface of infected cells results in the absence of T-cell activation ultimately helping virus to hide from the immune system. In some infected persons, viral reactivation occurs sporadically due to some triggering factors such as physical or emotional stress, fever, ultraviolet light, tissue damage, and other immune-compromising events [32]. Upon activation, virus travels from the dorsal root ganglion in conjunction with sensory nerve cells to the epidermal-dermal junction. During virus activation phase, a transition in the gene expression takes place, and virus expresses multiple lytic genes which direct the elevated viral replication and host cell death on the other hand [28]. The active virus is ultimately transported to the skin again where virus sheds and initiates new cutaneous or mucosal sores.

1.3. Biology of human immunodeficiency virus

Human immunodeficiency viruses (HIV) are members of *Retroviridae* family, which cause disease in both genders of almost all ages. Though two closely related HIV types (HIV-1 and HIV-2) have been described, however, HIV-1 is more virulent and is responsible for majority of HIV-related infections [33]. This virus is known to infect cells of the immune system including macrophages and dendritic and CD4$^+$T cells, thereby destroying them and impairing host immune function [34]. If left untreated, HIV infection may lead to a devastating disease called acquired immunodeficiency syndrome (AIDS). It is estimated that during 2015 alone, 36.7 million people got infected with HIV, while 1.1 million died of HIV-related causes worldwide.

The HIV is a tiny enveloped virus consisting of two copies of positive sense RNA molecules, which are accompanied by several nucleocapsid proteins and enzymes, for instance, proteases and integrases [35]. The genome of HIV is complex and for the most part marked as 5'LTR-gag-pol-env-LTR'3 [36]. However, six other genes—*tat, rev, nef, vif, vpr,* and *vpu* are also encoded by virus genome. The *gag* (group antigens) and *env* genes encode major nucleocapsid and structural proteins, while pol transcribes enzymes such as reverse transcriptase required for virus replication [35]. In fact, the *gag, pol,* and *env* proteins act as precursor and cleaved by proteases to give rise several other proteins. The remaining six genes are considered as accessory genes which are required for efficient virus replication and for regulation of viral gene expression [37]. Among these six accessory proteins, *nef* and *vif* are of extreme importance as they help virus in immune evasion and deal with antiviral activity of host APOBEC3G protein. The *nef* reduced the antigen presentation on the HIV-infected cells, thereby hiding from the immune system, while *vif* neutralized the infectivity of APOBEC3G protein, which degrades the viral RNA in the infected cell [38].

The HIV targets CD4+ T cells, macrophages, and dendritic and microglial cells for its multiplication. The life cycle of the virus begins with the virus attachment to CCR5 and CXCR4 receptors through its trimeric glycoprotein complex made up of gp120, gp160, and gp41. The surface proteins of HIV fuse with host cell membrane releasing viral genome inside the cells. The virus ssRNA is converted into complementary DNA (cDNA) by utilizing virus enzymes that are the part of mature HIV virion. The complementary part of the cDNA is synthesized and then transported to the nucleus where it integrates into host genome as provirus again with the help of virus-encoded integrase enzyme [39]. The integrated genome is transcribed into mRNA which is utilized simultaneously to produce viral proteins as well as the viral genome. The viral-encoded proteins tet and rev regulate the expression of HIV genes. For the synthesis of HIV virion, structural protein gp 160 is transported to the cell membrane where all virus components are assembled and finally bud off from the cell [40].

The destruction of CD4+ T cell is the mainstay mechanism of HIV-mediated pathogenesis. The HIV reduces the number of CD4+ T cells by several mechanisms. Programmed cell death or apoptosis is among the most prominent mechanisms underlying HIV-mediated destruction of CD4+ T cells [41]. The increased apoptosis of CD4+ T cells in HIV infection could be due to direct viral cytotoxicity or due to signaling events triggered by viral proteins. The apoptosis in HIV-infected patients is not limited to infected T cells only, but uninfected cells are also destroyed by the so-called bystander mechanism. While several viral proteins are believed to play a role in apoptosis of bystander CD4+ T cells, interactions between viral Env glycoprotein expressed on surface of infected T cells and specific receptors and coreceptors on the surface of neighboring uninfected T cells have been proposed as the major mechanism responsible [42]. The bystander apoptosis reduces the number of T cells to an alarming level making the person more likely to get other opportunistic infections including viruses and bacteria that put the life in serious danger [43].

2. Conventional methods for the prevention of STIs

Ever since their discovery, successful prevention and treatment of STIs, including HIV-1, HSV-2, and HPV, have been a high-priority research area. To date, several recommendations with varying effectiveness have been put forward by researchers and healthcare providers in order to limit STIs. The focal point of these described strategies is the prevention, i.e., blocking the acquisition of STIs. The STI prevention approaches are mainly based on reducing the risk factors, deployment of physical barriers, prophylactic immunization against sexually transmitted agents, efficient and timely diagnosis of STIs, and treatment of active infection [44, 45]. There has been remarkable progress in the diagnosis and treatment of STIs; however, the discussion on them would be beyond the scope of this chapter. Nevertheless, other preventive measures against STIs particularly HIV-1, HSV-2, and HPV will be discussed thoroughly in the coming sections of this chapter.

2.1. Curtailing risk factors for STIs

The act of sexual intercourse in humans is known to create small unnoticeable microabrasions which in turn pave the way for entry of numerous STIs. The epidemiological synergy has also hinted that the presence of some STIs favors the acquisition of other STIs. For instance, the existence of chlamydia, herpes, gonorrhea, and syphilis in an infected person makes him/her more likely to acquire HIV infection [46]. It is also worth mentioning that multiple STI coinfections prove to be more harmful than the single STI [47]. Therefore, the paramount approach in treating STDs would be to combat the transmission of STIs altogether. This could only be achieved by reducing risk factors, such as unprotected sex, early age sex, and multiple sex partners that increase the chances of catching various STIs [48].

The most reliable way of controlling STDs is the complete abstinence from any type of sex particularly during teen ages and comprehensive sex education [49]. Nevertheless, this does not seem to be a practical approach. However, limited number of sex partners and long-term sexual relationship with a single uninfected individual are believed to be most pragmatic ways in this regard [50]. Talking with partners about sexual health prior to sexual activities also mitigate the risk of getting STIs. Some important considerations before, during, or after sexual intercourse such as washing ahead of performing sex, avoiding sex when drunk, and circumvent unharmful sex positions have significantly reduced the STI burden [51]. Recently, male circumcision has been reported as a vital mean of reducing STI risk. Three separate clinical trials have demonstrated that circumcision can reduce the HIV acquisition by 60% [52, 53]. Moreover, male circumcision was also found to be effective against other STIs including HPV and HSV-2 [54].

2.2. Putting the physical barriers to STIs

The use of physical barriers, including male and female condoms, is not only among the most commonly used birth control methods but also serves to curtail the spread of STIs effectively. Male condoms are classified into natural or synthetic categories based on the material they are made of. Natural membrane condoms usually derived from lamb cecum are primarily meant for pregnancy prevention rather stopping STIs. In fact, the pores in the natural condoms are large enough to let the passage of small STI-causing organisms, particularly viruses [55]. On the other hand, the efficacy of synthetic condoms in the prevention of STIs has been proved by various epidemiological and laboratory studies [55]. Synthetic condoms are either made of latex or other nonlatex material such as polyurethane or polyisoprene. Latex condoms are flexible, broadly available, and least expensive among all types of condoms. They are exceedingly effective in preventing the sexual transmission of plethora of STIs, including HPV, HIV-1, and HSV-2 [56–58]. The failure of latex condoms to safeguard STIs or unintended pregnancy is usually due to inconsistent or incorrect use [59]. The nonlatex condoms are particularly suitable for those allergic to latex. Polyurethane condoms are relatively thin and odorless. They provide comparable protection as of latex condoms against various STIs [60]. However, polyurethane condoms are at higher risk of breakage during intercourse. Both latex and nonlatex condoms' efficiency of protecting STIs can be enhanced by using some germicidal spray on them [61].

Female condoms are usually made up of thin plastic polyurethane material and have rings on the both ends. The ring inside the vagina covers up the cervix with a plastic sheet while outer ring is open and resides outside the vagina covering the vulva. Like male condoms, these are designed to avoid pregnancy as well as to prevent the infection spread during sexual process [62]. Female condoms are usually recommended to sex partner when male condoms cannot be used appropriately. Contradictory reports have been presented regarding efficiency of female condoms. One systemic review based on different randomized control trials revealed that female condoms are good in avoiding pregnancy but not in protection from STIs [63]. On the contrary, another randomized control trial concluded that female condoms' efficacy is comparable with male condom [64]. As a matter of fact, the female condom efficiency like male condom varies according to their use. In the nutshell, it has been estimated that female condoms are more efficient if used consistently with accuracy [65].

Another way of protecting pregnancy and STD in females is the use of cervical diaphragms. Diaphragm is a dome-shaped bowl made of thin and flexible rubber that sits over the cervix. In order to use it as a contraceptive, spermicide is placed into the bowl and edges of the diaphragm before inserting into the vagina [66]. After sex, the diaphragms are left inside the vagina at least for 6–24 h. There is ample epidemiological and biological data suggesting that diaphragm use can reduce the risk of acquiring some of the STDs including gonorrhea, chlamydia, and trichomoniasis [57]. However, diaphragm has been proved to be ineffective in reducing the risk of acquiring HIV infection. Moreover, spermicide use along with diaphragm increases the risk of bacterial urinary tract infections [67]. It is therefore recommended that targeted clinical trials must be conducted before approval of diaphragms as a method for STI prevention.

2.3. Immunization against HPV, HIV-1, and HSV-2

Vaccines prime individuals' immune response to build up adaptive immunity, thereby protecting them from subsequent infection. Preexposure vaccination probably is the most effective means of preventing transmissible infection including STIs [51]. Unfortunately, except for HPV, no vaccine is approved for other sexually transmitted viral infection. However, vaccines against HIV-1 and HSV-2 are under developmental phase. **Table 1** enlists and describes characteristics of all proposed vaccines for HPV, HIV-1, and HSV-2.

HPV vaccine being a major public health breakthrough is administered in both males and females before reaching the age where HPV risk is maximum. Up till now, three HPV vaccines under the trade name of Cervarix, Gardasil, and Gardasil 9 have been approved by FDA [68]. The Cervarix is bivalent vaccine designed against HPV types 16 and 18 that are responsible for 70% cervical cancer. In addition to HPV 16 and 18, Gardasil provides protection against HPV 6 and 11, which cause 90% of genital warts [69]. The Gardasil got approved from FDA in 2006 while Cervarix in 2009. Recently in 2014, another vaccine Gardasil 9 was approved and is meant to protect against 9 HPV types: 6, 11, 16, 18, 31, 33, 45, 52, and 58 (FDA press release). All these vaccines are administered in a series of three doses at the ages of 16–26. However, they can be administered up to the age of 45. The effectiveness of all these vaccines has been assessed clinically in many randomized controlled trials, and all these trials

Virus	Vaccine name/ pharmaceutical company	Vaccine type	For which type	Clinical status
HPV	Gardasil/Merck & Co.	Recombinant	HPV 16, 18, 6, and 11	FDA approved (2006)
	Cervarix/ GlaxoSmithKline	Recombinant	HPV 16, 18	FDA approved (2009)
	Gardasil 9/Merck & Co.	Recombinant	HPV 6, 11, 16, 18, 31, 33,45, 52, and 58	FDA approved (2014)
	GEN-003/Genocea	HSV subunit vaccine	HSV-1 and HSV-2	Phase II
	HerpV/Agenus	Peptide vaccine	HSV-1 and HSV-2	Phase II completed
HSV	Vical HSV-2 (therapeutic vaccine)/ Vical	DNA vaccine	HSV-2	Phase II
	Shingrix/ GlaxoSmithKline	Subunit vaccine	HSV-2	Phase III
	HSV-529/Sanofi	Live attenuated vaccine	HSV-2	Phase I
	gD2t/ GlaxoSmithKline	Synthetic vaccine	HSV-2	Phase II completed
	AGS-004/Argos	Therapeutic vaccine	HIV-1	Phase IIb
HIV	GTU multi-HIV+ Lipo5	DNA+ lipopeptide vaccine	HIV-1	Phase II
	VAC-3S InnaVirVax	Peptide based	HIV-1	Phase II

Table 1. The list and characteristics of all available/proposed vaccines against HPV, HIV-1, and HSV-2.

endorsed the safety of these vaccines [70, 71]. Likewise, HPV vaccine is safe and is associated with no or mild side effects such as fever, nausea, and headache. The available HPV vaccines have noticeably reduced the incidence of genital warts, cervical intraepithelial neoplasia, as well as cervical cancer worldwide [72].

Several preventive and therapeutic antiherpes vaccines are under different developmental stages, but no vaccine has been approved so far. Most of these vaccines target HSV-2 rather than HSV-1. Nonetheless HSV-2 vaccine would also be effective against HSV-1 because of homology between two viruses. Nowadays, several approaches have been used by academic institutes, government agencies, and pharmaceutical companies who are engaged in developing and testing HSV vaccines. Most of the endeavors are based on the concept of using virus glycoproteins to design subunit vaccine. The largest clinical trials were conducted on "Herpevac" vaccine which employs virus glycoprotein D-2 (gD2) as immunogen. These trials showed that vaccine provided significant protection against HSV-1 but not HSV-2 [73]. A replication-defective HSV-2 vaccine (HSV529) has also entered phase I trials [74]. One live attenuated vaccine has produced marvelous results in the mouse model. However serious concerns have been noticed regarding the safety of this vaccine. One of the important points for the failure of HSV-2 vaccine is the nonavailability of suitable animal model for HSV. Due to spontaneous reactivation in the genital tract, guinea pigs are considered a better model than mice [75]. For the last decade, almost three anti HSV-2 vaccines, namely, GEN-003, HerpV, and gD/UL46, have entered phase I/phase II clinical trials. These vaccines were designed to stimulate T-cell immunity.

It has now been more than a quarter century that researchers are engaged in finding an effective measure that can provide a significant degree of protection against HIV infection. Some promising advances regarding HIV vaccine development have been witnessed during last two decades, but an effective and safe HIV vaccine is still needed. In fact, HIV being an RNA virus exhibit high mutation rate and hence increased genetic variability. This particular aspect of HIV biology is the main reason hindering HIV vaccine development efforts [76]. A range of approaches are being tested for developing an effective HIV vaccine such as protein subunit vaccines, viral vectors encoding for HIV proteins, DNA vaccines, as well as prime-boost strategy that uses a canarypox viral vector encoding HIV Env, Gag, and Pol proteins to prime the immune system followed by a mixture of same protein subunits as booster dose [77]. All these approaches employed one of the three scientific concepts that include induction of neutralizing antibodies, cell-mediated immunity, and exploration of combination approaches [76]. The vaccines being developed for HIV prevention have been subjected to clinical trials for safety and efficacy analysis. The VAX003 and VAX004 were the first efficacy trials of bivalent HIV vaccine, conducted by in men who have sex with men (MSM) and injection drug users [78]. These phase III trials show that vaccine was not effective in preventing HIV disease progression [79]. Similarly, two trials—HVTN 502 and HVTN 503 also called "Step Study" of *Adenovirus* vector-based HIV vaccine—failed to prove the efficacy of vaccine. HVTN 505 vaccination trials were also stopped in 2013 because initial results revealed that the vaccine was ineffective in preventing HIV infections [80]. However, the encouraging results were obtained in RV144 trials of HIV vaccine where it has noticed that vaccine reduced the infection in 31% cases [81]. This was the only trial that showed somewhat positive results.

3. Microbicides for the prevention of STIs

As mentioned in preceding discussion, a range of preventive strategies with varying degrees of efficacy and efficiency have been employed to curtail the transmission of HPV, HIV-1, and HSV-2 infections. However, these three deadly viruses continue to spread at alarming rates. Increasing incidence and failure in the development of effective HIV-1 and HSV-2 vaccines have instigated scientists to explore alternate research avenues. As STI spread is directly correlated with socioeconomic status of subjects, economically disadvantaged population being at high risk, there is also a dire need for cheaper options.

Microbicides are antimicrobial compounds claimed to be helpful in controlling the transmission of STIs upon self-administration inside the vagina and rectum. Some of the microbicides have been witnessed to provide considerable protection against STIs including HIV-1, HPV, and HSV-2 [82]. However, it is not clear whether microbicides render anticontraceptive effect too. Ideal microbicides are colorless, odorless, and tasteless compounds available in different biological formulations such as gels, creams, rings, suppositories, pessaries, films, and invisible condoms. Other criteria for microbicides to be ideal are safety and effectiveness in preventing broad range of STIs. Moreover, its repeated use should cause minimal or no symptoms in the vagina or rectum. The microbicides as STI-controlling measure are advantageous in many ways. In comparison to other interventions, microbicides are cheap, offered over the counter, and available in many formulations [83]. They can be easily applied by women themselves and do not create a physical barrier to intimate contact. Similarly sex worker can apply them without prior information to their clients. Moreover they are safe and nonirritating.

Currently, more than 50 potential microbicide agents have been identified. However, very few of them proved to be effective and have gone under advance phase III clinical trials [84]. The coming section of this chapter will provide a comprehensive review of various microbicides, along with their mechanism of action and current status of clinical trials, in order to highlight their strengths and shortcomings.

3.1. Stages in microbicide development

Drug development is a long-term work, which can even be of a decade or more sometimes. The microbicide development would have to follow the same protocols of drug development as any other drugs do [85]. The development of drug starts with the insight of the researchers to a new potential compound or chemical that can hinder or stop the cascade of destruction by the infection or to eliminate the pathogen as well. So once the potential candidate from many compounds is isolated for research and development of drug, then every aspect of it is practically assessed like its absorbance, distribution, destabilization, mechanism of action, dosage and side effects, etc. Then comes the preclinical testing of the drug, which can be in vitro or in vivo. Once the pre-clinical testing is complete, the clinical trials of the drug will show how it works in the real system. There are four phases of the clinical trials from 1 to 4 depending upon the no. of volunteers assigned to it, the duration of the phase, and the purpose of testing. Phase I of clinical trials is to assess safety and dosage, and almost 70% of the drugs pass this phase. Phase II clinical trial is to judge efficacy and side effects of the drug and could take up to 2 years, and 33% of the drugs pass it. In phase III, efficacy and adverse reactions are monitored, and about 25–30% move to the next level [86]. In phase IV, several thousands of volunteers are involved, and safety and efficacy of the drug are observed. If the drug shows the satisfactory results in all phases of trials, then it got reviewed by the drug regulatory authority that then monitors the marketing and follows active surveillance. The developmental phases of microbicides are summarized in **Figure 2**.

3.2. Microbicide mechanism of STI prevention

Microbicides exert their antimicrobial function by a range of mechanisms which can be divided broadly into four categories: vaginal defense enhancers, inactivation of virus in the vagina, virus attachment and fusion inhibiters, and virus replication inhibitors. **Figure 3** enlists some categories of microbicides and their mechanism of action altogether.

	Description	Time Line	No. of Volunteers
Ideas	Hypothesis	-	-
Pre- clinical testing	Lab and Animals	2-6 Years	-
Phase 1	Multiple Studies (Early Safety)	2 – 12 Weeks	25-200
Phase 2	Expanded Safety	6- 12 Months	200-800
Phase 2b	Safety and Effectiveness	Up to 3 Years	1500-3000
Phase 3	Effectiveness	1- 4 Years	3,000-10,000
Regulatory approval	Regulatory Approval	1-2 Years	-
Introduction (Phase 4)	Post Marketing Studies	-	-

Microbicide development phases

Figure 2. Phases of microbicide development.

3.2.1. Vaginal defense enhancers

Naturally, the acidic pH of the vagina provides an established defense against invading infections. Some organisms such as lactobacilli being natural inhabitant of the vagina play a pivotal role in maintaining thc low vaginal pH [87]. This organism also releases some antimicrobial compounds, for instance, lactic acid, hydrogen peroxide, bacteriocins, and biosurfactants, which keep the vagina protected from pathogens. However, semen and some bacterial

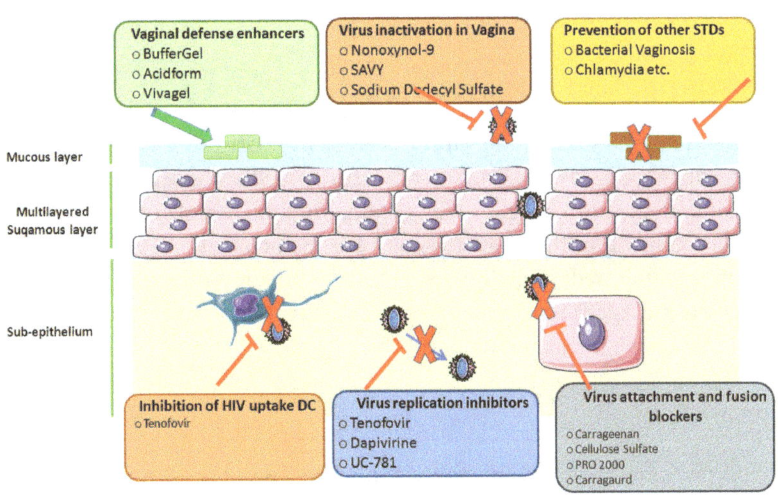

Figure 3. Categories of microbicides along with their mechanism of action.

infections increase the pH, thereby making the vagina more likely to catch infections including STIs [88]. Some acid-buffering microbicides can reduce the pH of the vagina to make it protected again from STIs. The pH-reducing microbicides include AcidForm and BufferGel. The microorganism such as *Lactobacillus crispatus* replacing missing *Lactobacillus* could also be important in enhancing vaginal defense [89].

3.2.1.1. BufferGel

BufferGel is a polymer of buffering Carbopol which is osmotically balanced with some physiological salts. They are not irritating for the genital surfaces and therefore can be used along with condoms or diaphragms. It helps to maintain the acidic pH of the vagina even in the presence of semen, thereby reducing the germ flow inside the female genital tract. The BufferGel has been reported to reduce the bacterial population in the vagina other than *Lactobacillus,* thus maintaining the natural milieu of the vagina [90]. The phase I clinical trials for BufferGel showed satisfactory results, and the agent was tolerated well by subjects [91, 92]. These trials also endorsed the potential of BufferGel to avoid pregnancy and to check the transmission of HIV-1, HPV, HSV-2, and chlamydia infections. However, phase III trial results failed to exhibit required performance level; therefore further production of BufferGel was abandoned [93].

3.2.1.2. AcidForm

AcidForm is another buffering gel used as spermicidal and microbicide. The mode of action of this gel is to maintain the vaginal acidity for a long period of time, hence protecting the vaginal and cervical epithelium from pathogens. This buffering gel is reported to be effective against HSV, chlamydia, gonorrhea, HPV, and HIV-infected leukocytes. Besides the protection from STIs, it can also act as contraceptive [94]. AcidForm trials for assessment of safety and bactericidal activity showed that it may augment mucosal defense. However, AcidForm was associated with more irritation than placebo and lower levels of antimicrobial (lactoferrin) and anti-inflammatory (IL-1ra) [95]. Currently, AcidForm has cleared phase I safety trials, while phase III trials are in progress for this buffering microbicide [96, 97].

3.2.2. Inactivation of virus in the vagina

First-generation detergents and surfactants, for example, Nonoxynol-9, sodium dodecyl sulfate (SDS), and Savvy (1% C31G), kill viral infection by disrupting their outmost coverings, i.e., envelope or capsid, thereby causing their destruction [98]. These types of microbicides are equally dangerous for the normal cells of the genital mucosa. Initial clinical trials showed their ineffectiveness in controlling the transmission of STIs including HIV-1. On these grounds, further trials were abandoned. Nonetheless, broad-spectrum viral inactivating topical microbicides are a promising agent for fight against STIs; therefore, efforts to develop novel drugs as well as combination regimes are ongoing.

3.2.2.1. Nonoxynol-9

Nonoxynol-9 (Nonylphenoxypolyethoxyethanol or N-9) was one of the earliest known spermicidal compounds that have been clinically evaluated as topical microbicides against HIV transmission [99]. Nonoxynol-9 is the active ingredient in most of the spermicidal and is available over the counter in the form of creams, jellies, foams, gel, film, and suppositories. In various clinical trials, Nonoxynol-9 was proved to be a good spermicidal but not effective against STIs. Two phase III clinical trials in Africa demonstrated that Nonoxynol-9 does confer any protection against HIV in comparison to the placebo. In addition, its use increases the risk of genital diseases and even contracting HIV [100]. It was lately revealed that N-9 induces superficial de-epithelialization and high rate of petechial hemorrhages, thereby making the genital mucosa prone to other infections [101]. On these grounds, the World Health Organization (WHO) recently asked to include the sentence "this product does not block STIs" in the labeling of that compound [84].

3.2.2.2. *Savvy (1% C31G)*

Savvy or C31G (Cellegy Pharmaceuticals, Quakertown, PA, USA) is another spermicidal and antimicrobial surfactant containing acetyl betaine and myristamine oxide. The mode of action of Savvy is not much different from the N-9 but with less side effects. Moreover it has the ability to be quickly dissolved and spread on the genital mucosa [90]. At very low concentration like 0.001%, it has shown very minimum toxicity in preclinical trials and even no toxicity at 0.003% to mammalian cells as measured by MTT assay [99]. Several in vitro studies have suggested that C31G (Savvy) has the ability to disrupt the outer membrane of HIV [104]. Although, in phase I trials, Savvy proved to be safe in use, its production was stopped several years ago due to ineffective results in phase III clinical trials in Ghana and Nigeria [84].

3.2.2.3. *Sodium lauryl sulfate*

Because of the limitations of N-9, efforts have been directed toward the development of second-generation microbicidal agents with broader activity and lower toxicity. Sodium lauryl sulfate (SLS) is an anionic surfactant and has recently been tested as novel microbicidal agent that demonstrated significant lethal activity against a broad spectrum of STD pathogens, including HIV-1 [102]. This agent behaves as a liquid at room temperature and converts into gel form at body temperature to protect the STI transmission [103, 104]. Therefore it can be used as invisible condoms. Two phase II trials in Cameron revealed that SLS is safe to use intravaginally for long period of time and can be moved on to phase III trials [105].

3.2.3. *Virus attachment and fusion-blocking microbicides*

Second-generation microbicides are designed to block the entry of STI-causing pathogens into the susceptible host cells. These agents usually interfere with viral entry process by altering or blocking cellular receptors that are the first attachment sites for the pathogens. Receptor-blocking microbicides act both by nonspecific and specific mechanisms. The former mechanism blocks the attachment of multiple organisms, while latter mechanism hinders the entry of specific organism, for example, targeting CD4 receptors for the blockage of HIV entry [106].

3.2.3.1. *Carrageenan*

The carrageenan is an unbranched sulfated polysaccharide belonging to polyanoin class and extracted from red algae. It is chemically similar to heparan sulfate, which is used as receptor by many pathogens to initiate the entry. These entry inhibitors work through electrostatic interaction with the viral surface proteins. The negatively charged polyanoin molecules may neutralize the positively charged surface of virus, for instance, HIV, thereby blocking attachment and entry into the healthy target cells [107].

It is in rife commercial use as a thickener in a number of products including cosmetics, food products, sexual lubricants, and infant feeding formulas. It has also been reported as an extremely potent inhibitor for a broad range of sexually transmitted infections [84]. This tropical microbicide has been proven to block HPV infectivity in vitro, even when diluted a million-fold. Carrageenan prevents the binding of HPV virions to the host cells and is observed to be more potent than heparin, a form of cell-free heparan sulfate that has been regarded as a highly effective HPV inhibitor. Carrageenan can also block HPV infection through a second, post-attachment heparan sulfate-independent effect. Besides HPVs carrageenan can inhibit HSV-2 and some strains of HIV-1 in vitro [108].

Two preparations of carrageenan, polynaphthalene sulfonate (PRO 2000) and Carraguard, have been introduced. Both the products strongly bind to STI pathogens including HIV-1, HPV, and HSV-2. Both of the carrageenan preparations have been proven to be safe in phase I clinical trials albeit in low doses. However, in phase III trials, these products proved to be ineffective; therefore, further trials were abandoned [109].

3.2.3.2. Cellulose sulfate

Polyanion cellulose sulfate is another long-chain sulfated polysaccharide that is being developed as a contraceptive and microbicidal agent. It has manifested in vitro activity against a broad spectrum of sexually transmitted pathogens. Moreover, inhibitory effect was marked up to 8 h after initiation of infection [84]. Cellulose sulfate has antimicrobial activity in vitro against various sexually transmitted pathogens including *Neisseria gonorrhoeae, Chlamydia trachomatis,* and HIV-1. It has been shown to bind with HIV-1 gp120 and block its interaction with D4+ receptors [110]. Phase I safety studies revealed that cellulose sulfate is safe and well tolerated [111]. However, in phase III trials, it failed to protect against HIV and tends to increase the risk of infection [111].

3.2.3.3. VivaGel

VivaGel belongs to dendrimers that are new members of polyanoin family and are highly branched nanoscale macromolecules having various surface features. These macromolecules have recently been described as microbicides with considerable safety and effectiveness [112]. Dendrimers utilize polyvalent interactions for binding and initiating biologic activity. VivaGel™ (SPL7013) is a commercial polyanion dendrimer developed by Starpharma (Melbourne, Australia). It is a water-based vaginal product in the form of mucoadhesive gel containing 3% w/w active ingredient and is administered in the vagina alone or mixed in Carbopol buffered gel that is used to maintain the physiological pH of the vagina [113]. It was developed for specific binding to surface proteins of virus, thereby blocking their attachment with the receptors of host cells. For instance, in the case of HIV, it binds with gp120 protein which virus use to attach CD4+ T cells. Several trials have been conducted to evaluate the safety and efficacy of this product. These studies unanimously describe that SPL7013 is non-toxic and safe to use even at very high concentrations of (1000 μg/ml) [112, 114]. Likewise, in vitro trials showed effectiveness in inhibition of HIV-1 and HSV-2 infections in human cell lines as well as macaque PBMCs. Recognizing its potential, the FDA included VivaGel™ in Fast Track status since January 2006 for the prevention of HIV indication. Recently in 2016, Starpharma announced the completion of enrollment for phase III trial of VivaGel effectiveness in preventing the bacterial vaginosis and several STIs including HIV and HSV-2. Trial results are now expected in the first quarter of 2017.

3.2.4. *Virus replication inhibitors*

Unlike previously described microbicides, third-generation microbicides work by interfering with a specific step of virus replication cycle when administered locally on the mucosa. The most widely studied examples of virus replication blocker are antiretroviral (ARV) microbicides, which can be divided into nucleoside reverse transcriptase inhibitors (NRTI) and non-nucleoside reverse transcriptase inhibitors (NNRTI). Both of these ARV microbicides block the activity of HIV reverse transcriptase enzyme that is required for the conversion of RNA into DNA, an essential step required for integration of HIV into the host genome [115]. This blockage ultimately reduces the number of HIV virions in the infected cell. These next-generation microbicides are formulated in the form of long-acting vaginal ring, film, or gels. In addition to other benefits, the reverse transcriptase inhibitor class of microbicides is also cost-effective. Some of the ARV examples being tested include tenofovir, dapivirine, and UC-781.

3.2.4.1. *Tenofovir*

Tenofovir is a highly acclaimed antiretroviral drug which obstructs the virus growth inside the host cells. It is usually taken in the form of pills, and it has become a necessary component of the three-drug cocktail for antiretroviral therapy approved by the FDA [116]. However, it has also been prepared in the form of gels to be used as topical microbicides. The gel preparation of tenofovir is currently under assessment as a tropical microbicide for the prevention of HIV infection in high-risk populations, and several safeties and efficacy-related trials are underway.

A study known as "CAPRISA 004" completed by scientists at the Centre for the AIDS Programme of Research in South Africa (CAPRISA) in 2010 revealed that 1% tenofovir gel application before and after sex was 39% efficient in reducing a woman's risk of getting infected with HIV and 51% effective in preventing genital herpes infections [117]. Moreover in this study, the protective effect against HIV increased with gel adhesiveness and increased use of tenofovir. For example, 54% reduction in HIV infections was observed in women who used gel in more than 80% of their sex acts, whereas those who used the gel in less than half of their sex acts had a 28% reduction in HIV infections. The efficacy of tenofovir gel for the prevention of HIV was also evaluated in another study known as VOICE. Unlike CAPRISA, this study reported that tenofovir preparation does stop the transmission of HIV-1 [118]. However, poor adherence was employed by the participants of this trial.

Another trial on tenofovir gel known as "The FACTS 001" was conducted to evaluate the reproducibility of the CAPRISA 004 trial results. The results of this trial were announced on February 24, 2015. Disappointingly, the study did not confirm the pericoital tenofovir gel effectiveness. In this trial, the gel only showed a protective effect when used consistently and covered most of the sex acts, but most women in this trial were unable to use it in this manner. However, the gel appeared to be acceptable and easy to apply for most of the women [119]. Very recently, the use of tenofovir on the genital mucosa has been linked with some toxic effects such as suppression of anti-inflammatory mediators, increased T-lymphocyte infiltration of the mucosa, and induced mitochondrial dysfunction, which were noticed [105]. These unexpected results led to tenofovir gels being dropped from a large ongoing clinical trial.

3.2.4.2. UC-781

UC-781 is a hydrophobic thiocarboxanilide nonnucleoside reverse transcriptase inhibitor (NNRTI) developed as antiretroviral drug having high affinity for HIV reverse transcriptase. This agent eagerly crosses membrane barriers and inactivates reverse transcriptase even before entry into the cell, thereby acting as potent antiretroviral agent. However the production of it as antiretroviral drug was abandoned due to poor bioavailability. Later on, this agent was developed in the form of tropical formulation. Phase I safety trials confirmed its safety for vaginal application at lower concentrations [120]. Recently UC-781 in the form of vaginal ring has been reported to provide strong protection against HIV transmission. Moreover no toxicity was observed in this study [121]. Further large-scale clinical trials are required before the UC-781 microbicide gel formulation reported to be successful in the prevention of HIV-1 sexual transmission.

3.2.4.3. Dapivirine

Dapivirine being nonnucleoside reverse transcriptase inhibitor has been reported to act as microbicide against various STIs, particularly HIV-1. It is reported to have dual mode of action against HIV-1; it inhibits both viral entry and reverse transcription stopping the conversion of viral RNA to proviral DNA. Because of dapivirine's tight binding and lipophilic characteristics, it may be active against both cell-free and cell-associated HIV [122]. Dapivirine is the only microbicide used in human in the form of vaginal rings and believed to be nontoxic [123]. The phase III clinical trials (the ASPIRE study) showed a 27% reduction in HIV-1 acquisition upon using dapivirine vaginal rings [124]. The protection effect was more pronounced in the women aged 21 or more; however, no significant protection was observed for women under age 21 [10]. Another phase III trial for efficacy evaluation of dapivirine is in progress.

4. Conclusion and future prospects

Microbicides offer an accessible, easy-to-use, and low-cost option for the control of sexually transmitted infections and hence have been an area of high interest for scientists and researchers around the world. However, progress in this area has been dismal, and very few microbicide drugs have so far been able to enter the market. With ever-growing epidemic of STIs, particularly in less developed areas of the world, there is an immediate need to gear up concerted efforts for the development and discovery of novel microbicide compounds. Moreover, it is imperative that efforts should be made to develop novel delivery methods to improve the efficacy of existing microbicides. Results from recent trials can guide for more development of more rationally, accurately, behaviorally, and socially accepted and single solution maximum potential STIs.

Author details

Naveed Shahzad[1]*, Roman Farooq[2], Bilal Aslam[2] and Muhammad Umer[3]

*Address all correspondence to: hnaveed.shahzad@gmail.com

1 School of Biological Sciences, University of the Punjab, Lahore, Pakistan

2 Department of Microbiology, Government College University Faisalabad, Pakistan

3 National Institute for Biotechnology and Genetic Engineering, Faisalabad, Pakistan

References

[1] Newman L, Rowley J, Vander Hoorn S, Wijesooriya NS, Unemo M, and Low N. Global estimates of the prevalence and incidence of four curable sexually transmitted infections in 2012 based on systematic review and global reporting. PLoS One. 2015;**10**(12):e0143304

[2] Satterwhite CL, Torrone E and Meites E. Sexually transmitted infections among US women and men: Prevalence and incidence estimates. Sexually Transmitted Diseases. 2013;**40**:187-193

[3] Chan PK, Chang AR, Yu MY, Li WH, Chan MY, Yeung AC, Cheung TH, Yau TN, Wong SM, Yau CW and Ng HK. Age distribution of human papillomavirus infection and cervical neoplasia reflects caveats of cervical screening policies. International Journal of Cancer. 2010;**126**(1):297-301

[4] Zhi-Ming Z, Carl CB. Papillomavirus genome structure, expression, and post-transcriptional regulation. Frontiers in Biosciences. 2006;**1**(11):2286-2302

[5] Graham SV. Human papillomavirus: Gene expression, regulation and prospects for novel diagnostic methods and antiviral therapies. Future Microbiology. 2010;**5**(10):1493-1506

[6] Woolridge T, Laimins LA. Regulation of human papillomavirus type 31 gene expression during the differentiation-dependent life cycle through histone modifications and transcription factor binding. Virology. 2008;**374**(2):371-380

[7] Hanse UB, Robert DB, Zigui C, Koenraad VD, Harald ZH, Ethel-Michele DV. Classification of papillomaviruses (PVs) based on 189 PV types and proposal of taxonomic amendments. Virology. 2010;**401**(1):70-79

[8] Zur-Hausen H. Papillomaviruses in human cancers. Proceeding of the Association of American Physicians. 1999;**111**:581-587

[9] Harro CD, Pang YS, Roden RBS, Hildesheim A, Wang Z, Reynolds MJ, Mast TC, Robinson R, Murphy BR, Karron RA, Dillner J, Schiller JT, Lowy DR. Safety and immunogenicity trial in adult volunteers of a human papillomavirus 16 L1 virus-like particle vaccine. Journal of the National Cancer Institute. 2001;**93**:284-292

[10] Stanley M. Pathology and epidemiology of HPV infection in females. Gynecology and Oncology. 2010;**117**:5-10

[11] Allen M, Kalantari M, Ylitalo N, Pettersson B, Hagmar B, Scheibenplug L, Johansson B, Petterson U, Gyllensten U. HLA DQ-DR haplotype and susceptibility to cervical carcinoma: Indications of increased risk for development of cervical carcinoma in individuals infected with HPV 18. Tissue Antigens. 1996;**48**:32-37

[12] Bontkes HJ, Van MD, DeGruijl TD, Duggan-Keen MF, Walboomers JM, Stukart MJ, Vereheijen RH, Helmerhorst TJ, Meijer CJ, Scheper RJ, Stevens FR, Dyer PA, Sinnott P, Stern PL. HPV 16 infection and progression of cervical intraepithelial neoplasia: Analysis of HLA polymorphism and HPV 16 E6 sequences variants. International Journal of Cancer. 1998;**78**:166-171

[13] Winer RL, Hughes JP, Feng Q, O'Reilly S, Kiviat NB, Holmes KK, Koutsky LA. Condom use and the risk of genital human papillomavirus infection in young women. New England Journal of Medicine. 2006;**354**(25):2645-2654

[14] Giroglu T, Florin L, Schäfer F, Streek RE, Sapp M. Human papillomavirus infection requires cell surface heparan sulfate. Journal of Virology. 2001;**75**:1565-1570

[15] Torrisi, A, Del M, Onnis GL, Merlin F, Bertorelle R, Minucci D. Colposcopy, cytology and HPV testing in HIV-positive and HIV-negative women. European Journal of Gynecology and Oncology. 2000;**21**:168-172

[16] Ashrafi GH, Haghshenans M, Marchetti B, Campo MS. E5 protein of human papilloma virus 16 down regulates HLA Class I and interacts with heavy chain via its first hydrophobic domain. International Journal of Cancer. 2006;**119**(9):2105-2112

[17] Reinson T, Henno L, Toots M, Ustav M Jr, Ustav M. The cell cycle timing of human papillomavirus DNA replication. PLoS One. 2015;**10**(7):e0131675

[18] Rampias T, Boutati E, Pectasides E, Sasaki C, Kountourakis P, Weinberger P, Psyrri A. Activation of Wnt signaling pathway by human papillomavirus E6 and E7 oncogenes in HPV16-positive oropharyngeal squamous carcinoma cells. Molecular Cancer Research. 2010;**8**:433-443

[19] Accardi R, Rosa R, Mariafrancesca S, Tarik G, Shahzad N, Miranda T, Lawrence B, Cesare I, Bakary SS, Rosa AC, Stephan JR, Massimo T. E6 and E7 from human papillomavirus type 16 cooperate to target the PDZ protein Na/H exchange regulatory factor 1. Journal of Virology. 2011;**85**:8208-8216

[20] Susanna LL, Ruchi MN, Oliver L, Aaron AR, Robert CC, Stuart CR, David MK, Jeffrey C, David MK, Thomas CQ. Global diversity within and between human herpes virus 1 and 2 glycoproteins. Journal of Virology. 2015;**89**(16):8206-8218

[21] Schillinger JA, Xu F, Sternberg MR, et al. National seroprevalence and trends in herpes simplex virus type 1 in the United States, 1976-1994. Sexually Transmitted Diseases. 2004;**3**:1753-1760

[22] Looker KJ, Magaret AS, May MT, Turner KME, Vickeman P, Gottlieb SL. Correction: Global estimates of prevalent and incident herpes simplex virus type 2 infections in 2012. PLoS One. 2015;**10**(5):e0128615

[23] Geoffrey AC, Anindya D, Duncan WW. Herpes simplex virus DNA packaging without measurable DNA synthesis. Journal of Virology. 1998;**72**(4):2745-2751

[24] Thomas C. Mettenleiter herpesvirus assembly and egress. Journal of Virology. 2002; **76**(4):1537-1547

[25] Patricia GS, Richard L. Herpesvirus entry: An update. Journal of Virology. 2003;**77**(19): 10179-10185

[26] Knipe DM. The role of viral and cellular nuclear proteins in herpes simplex virus replication. Advances in Virus Research. 1989;**37**:85-103

[27] Antinone SE, Smith GA. Retrograde axon transport of herpes simplex virus and pseudorabies virus: A live-cell comparative analysis. Journal of Virology. 2010;**84**(3):1504-1512

[28] Michael P, Nicoll, Hann W, Shivkumar M, Harman LER, Coleman HM, Proenca JT, Efstathiou S. The HSV-1 latency-associated transcript functions to repress latent phase lytic gene expression and suppress virus reactivation from latently infected neurons. Public Library of Science Pathogens. 2016;**12**(4): e1005539

[29] Powrie F, Menon S, Cofman RL. Interleukin-4 and interleukin-10 synergize to inhibit cell-mediated immunity in vivo. Europian Journal of Immunology. 1993;**23**:2223

[30] Moore KW, Waal MR, Coffman RL, O'Garra A. Interleukin-10 and the interleukin-10 receptor. Annual Review of Immunology. 2001;**19**:683-765

[31] Oosten LE, Koppers-Lalic D, Blokland E, Mulder A, Ressing ME, Mutis T, van Halteren AG, Wiertz EJ, Goulmy E. TAP-inhibiting proteins US6, ICP47 and UL49.5 differentially affect minor and major histocompatibility antigen-specific recognition by cytotoxic T lymphocytes. International Immunology. 2007;**19**:1115-1122

[32] Fishman JA. Overview: Cytomegalovirus and the herpes viruses in transplantation. American Journal of Transplantation. 2013;13(3):1-8

[33] Osmanov S, Pattou C, Walker N, Schwardländer B, Esparza J, WHO-UNAIDS Network for HIV Isolation and characterization. Estimated global distribution and regional spread of HIV-1 genetic subtypes in the year. Journal of Acquired Immune Deficiency Syndrome. 2000;**29**:184-190

[34] Koppensteiner H, Werner RB, Schindler M. Macrophages and their relevance in human immunodeficiency virus type I infection. Retrovirology. 2012;**9**:82

[35] Antoinette C, Kuyl VD. HIV infection and HERV expression: A review. Retrovirology. 2012;**9**(6):4690-4696

[36] Nasioulas, G, Paraskevis D, Magiorkinis E, Theodoridou M, Hatzakis A. Molecular analysis of the full-length genome of the HIV-1 subtype I: Evidence of A/G/I recombination. AIDS Research and Human Retroviruses. 1999;**15**:745-758

[37] Kleinman CL, Doria M, Orecchini E, Giuliani E, Galardi S, Jay ND, Michienzi A. HIV-1 infection causes a down-regulation of genes involved in ribosome biogenesis. PLoS One. 2014;**9**(12):e113908

[38] Bogerd HP, Doehle BP, Wiegand HL, Cullen BR. A single amino acid difference in the host APOBEC3G protein controls the primate species specificity of HIV type 1 virion infectivity factor. Proceedings of the National Academy of Sciences USA. 2004;101:3770-3774

[39] Zheng YH, Lovsin N, Peterlin BM. Newly identified host factors modulate HIV replication. Immunology Letters. 2005;**97**(2):225-234

[40] Checkley MA, Luttge BG, Freed EO. HIV-1 Envelope Glycoprotein Biosynthesis, Trafficking, and Incorporation. Journal of Microbiology. 2011;**410**(4):582-608

[41] Tateyama M, Oyaizu N, McCloskey TW, Than S, Pahwa S. CD4 T lymphocytes are primed to express Fas ligand by CD4 cross-linking and to contribute to CD8 T-cell apoptosis via Fas/FasL death signaling pathway. Blood. 2000;**96**:195-202

[42] Himanshu G, Jonathon M, Anjali J. HIV-1 induced bystander apoptosis. Viruses. 2012;**4**(11):3020-3043

[43] Finkel TH, Tudor-Williams G, Banda NK, Cotton MF, Curiel T, Monks C. Apoptosis occurs predominantly in bystander cells and not in productively infected cells of HIV- and SIV-infected lymph nodes. Nature Medicine. 1995;**1**(2):129-134

[44] Fenton KA, Korovessis C, Johnson AM, McCadden A, McManus S, Wellings K. Sexual behaviour in Britain: Reported sexually transmitted infections and prevalent genital chlamydia trachomatis infection. The Lancet. 2001;**358**(9296):1851-1854

[45] Garnett GP, Rottingen JA. Measuring the Risk of HIV Transmission. AIDS. 2001;**15**(5): 641-643

[46] Freeman EE, Weiss HA, Glynn JR, Cross PL, Whitworth JA, Hayes RJ. Herpes simplex virus 2 infection, increases HIV acquisition in men and women: Systematic review and meta-analysis of longitudinal studies. AIDS. 2006;**20**(1):73-83

[47] Lingappa JR, Baeten JM, Wald A, Hughes JP, Thomas KK, Mujugira A, Partners in Prevention HSV/HIV Transmission Study Team. Daily acyclovir for HIV-1 disease progression in people dually infected with HIV-1 and herpes simplex virus type2: A randomised placebo-controlled trial. The Lancet. 2010;**375**(9717):824-833

[48] Kelly JA, Lawrence JS, Hood HVand Brasfield TL. Behavioral intervention to reduce AIDS risk activities. Journal of Consulting and Clinical Psychology. 1989;**57**:60-67

[49] Stanger-Hall KF, Hall DW. Abstinence-only education and teen pregnancy rates: Why we need comprehensive sex education in the U.S. Public Library of Science One. 2011; **6**(10): e24658

[50] Lucia FO, Susie H, Abigail H, Curtis D. Multiple sexual partners, and young adults' sexual relationships: Understanding the role of gender in the study of risk. The Journal of Urban Health. 2006;**83**(4):695-708

[51] Marrazzo JM, Cates W. Interventions to prevent sexually transmitted infections, including HIV Infection. Clinical Infectious Diseases. 2011;**53**(3):S64-S78

[52] Gray RH, Kigozi G, Makumbi F, Watya S, Nalugoda F, Kiwanuka N, Moulton LH, Chaudhry MA, Chen MZ, Sewankambo NK, Mangen FW, Bacon MC, Williams CFM, Opendi P, Reynolds SJ, Laeyendecker O, Quinn TC, Wawer M. Male circumcision for HIV prevention in men in Rakai, Uganda: A randomised trial. The Lancet. 2007;**369**(9562): 657-66

[53] Bailey RC, Moses S, Parkeretal CB. Male circumcision for HIV prevention in young men in Kisumu, Kenya: A randomised controlled trial. The Lancet. 2007;**369**(9562):643-656.

[54] Tobian AA, Serwadda D, Quinn TC. Male circumcision for the prevention of HSV-2 and HPV infections and syphilis. New England Journal of Medicine. 2009;**360**:1298-1309

[55] Carey RF, Lytle CD, Cyr WH. Implications of laboratory tests of condom integrity. Sexually Transmitted Diseases. 1999;**26**(4):216-220

[56] Wald A, Langenberg AG, Link K, Izu AE, Ashley R, Warren T, Tyring S, Douglas JM Jr, Corey L. Effect of condoms on reducing the transmission of herpes simplex virus type 2 from men to women. JAMA. 2001;**285**(24):3100-3106

[57] Weller SC, Davis BK. Condom effectiveness in reducing heterosexual HIV transmission. Cochrane Database of Systematic Reviews. 2001;(3). Art. No.: CD003255. DOI: 10.1002/14651858.CD003255

[58] Smith DK, Herbst JH, Zhang X, Rose CE. Condom effectiveness for HIV prevention by consistency of use among men who have sex with men in the United States. Journal of Acquired Immune Deficiency Syndrome. 2015;68(3):337-344

[59] Steiner MJ, Cates WJ, Warner L. The real problem with male condoms is nonuse. Sexually Transmitted Diseases. 1999;**26**:459-462

[60] Warner L, Stone KM, Macaluso M, Buehler JW, Austin HD. Condom use and risk of gonorrhea and Chlamydia: A systematic review of design and measurement factors assessed in epidemiologic studies. Sexually Transmitted Diseases. 2006;**33**:36-51

[61] CDC. Male Latex Condoms and Sexually Transmitted Diseases. Atlanta, GA: CDC; 2002

[62] Green Y. CDC promotes the female condom for HIV/STD prevention. American Journal of Public Health. 2001;**91**(11):1732

[63] Vijayakumar G, Mabude Z, Smit J, Beksinska M, Lurie M. A review of female-condom effectiveness: Patterns of use and impact on protected sex acts and STI incidence. International Journal of STD & AIDS. 2006;**17**:652-659

[64] Minnis AM, Padian NS. Effectiveness of female controlled barrier methods in preventing sexually transmitted infections and HIV: Current evidence and future research directions. Sexually Transmitted Infections. 2005;**81**:193-200

[65] Hoffman S,Exner TM, Leu CS,Ehrhardt AA, Stein Z. Female-condom use in a gender-specific family planning clinic trial. American Journal for Public Health. 2003;**93**(11):1897-1903

[66] Gallo MF, Macaluso M, Warner L, Fleenor ME, Hook EW, Brill I, Weaver MA. Bacterial vaginosis, gonorrhea, and chlamydial infection among women attending a sexually transmitted disease clinic: A longitudinal analysis of possible causal links. Annals of Epidemiology. 2012;**22**:213-220

[67] Litza JA, Brill JR. Urinary tract infections. Primary Care. 2010;**37**(3):491-507

[68] Shahzad N, Muhammad U, Memoona R, Bilal A. Preventive strategies against human papillomaviruses, human papillomavirus. Research in a Global Perspective; 2016. InTech, DOI: 10.5772/62831

[69] Koutsky LA, Ault KA, Wheeler CM. A controlled trial of a human papillomavirus type 16 vaccine. New England Journal of Medicine. 2002;**347**(21):1645-1651

[70] Munoz N, Manalastas R, Pitisuttihum P, Tresukosol D, Monsonego J, Ault K, Clavel C, Luna J, Myers E, Hood S, Bautista O, Bryan J, Taddeo F, Esser M, Vuocolo S, Haupt R, Barr E, Saah A. Safety, immunogenicity, and efficacy of quadrivalent HPV (types 6, 11, 16, 18) recombinant vaccine in adult women between 24 and 45 years of age: A randomized, double-blind trial. The Lancet. 2009;**373**:1921-1922

[71] Petaja T, Keranen H, Karppa T, Kawa A, Lantela S, Siitari-Mattila M. Immunogenicity and safety of human papillomavirus (HPV)-16/18 AS04-adjuvanted vaccine in healthy boys aged 10-18 years. Journal of Adolescent Health. 2009;**44**(1):33-40

[72] Cutts FT, Franceschi S, Goldie S, et al. Human papillomavirus and HPV vaccines: A review. Bull World Health Organ. 2007;**85**:719-726

[73] Belshe RB, Heineman TC, Bernstein DI, Abbie RB, Marian E, Robbert M, Carolyn DD, Deal. Correlate of immune protection against HSV-1 genital disease in vaccinated women. The Journal of Infectious Diseases. 2014;**209**(6):828-836

[74] Petro C, González PA, Cheshenko N, Jandl T, Khajoueinejad N, Bénard A. Herpes simplex type 2 virus deleted in glycoprotein D protects against vaginal, skin and neural disease. eLife. 2015;**4**:06054

[75] Amandeep G, Michael R, Steven RB. Bacterial toxin modulation of the eukaryotic cell cycle: Are all cytolethal distending toxins created equally? Frontier in Cellular and Infectious Microbiology. 2012;**2**:124

[76] Benmira S, Bhattacharya V, Schmid ML. An effective HIV vaccine: A combination of humoral and cellular immunity? Current HIV Research. 2010;**8**(6):441-449

[77] Cohen YZ, Dolin R. Novel HIV vaccine strategies: Overview and perspective. Therapeutic Advances in Vaccines. 2013;**1**(3):99-112

[78] Flynn NM, Forthal DN, Harro CD, Judson FN, Mayer KH, Para MF. Placebo-controlled phase 3 trial of a recombinant glycoprotein 120 vaccine to prevent HIV-1 infection. Journal of Infectious Diseases. 2005;**191**(5):654-665

[79] Pitisuttithum P, Gilbert P, Gurwith M, Heyward W, Martin M, van Griensven F, Hu D, Tappero JW, Choopanya K, Bangkok M, Vaccine Evaluation Group. Randomized, double-blind, placebo-controlled efficacy trial of a bivalent recombinant glycoprotein 120 HIV-1 vaccine among injection drug users in Bangkok, Thailand. The Journal of Infectious disease. 2006;**194**(12):1661-1671

[80] Day TA, Kublin JG. Lessons learned from HIV vaccine clinical efficacy trials. Current HIV Research. 2013;**11**(6):441-449

[81] Rolland M, Gilbert P. Evaluating immune correlates in HIV type 1 vaccine efficacy trials: What RV144 may provide. AIDS Research and Human Retroviruses. 2012;**28**(4):400-404

[82] Lederman MM, Offord RR, Hartley O. Microbicides and other topical strategies to prevent vaginal transmission of HIV. Nature Reviews Immunology. 2006;**6**:371-382

[83] Bonaventura CTM. New biomedical technologies and strategies for prevention of HIV and other sexually transmitted infections. Journal of Sexually Transmitted Diseases. 2016; Article ID 7684768, 10 pages

[84] Onkar S, Tarun G, Goutam R, Amit KG, Microbicides for the treatment of sexually transmitted HIV infections. Journal of Pharmaceutics. 2014;**2014**:18, Article ID 352425. DOI: 10.1155/2014/352425

[85] Stone A. Regulatory Issues in Microbicide Development. WHO; 2009

[86] Nunn AA, McCormack S, Crook AM, Pool R, Rutterford C, Hayes R. Microbicides development programme: Design of a phase III trial to measure the efficacy of the vaginal microbicide PRO 2000/5 for HIV prevention. Trials. 2009;**10**:99

[87] O'Hanlon DE, Moench TR, Cone RA. Vaginal pH and microbicidal lactic acid when lactobacilli dominate the microbiota. PLoS One. 2013;**8**(11):e80074

[88] Patricia SF, Sarah JH, Adrienne RB, Gustavo FD, Robin JS. Preclinical evaluation of lime juice as a topical microbicide candidate. Retrovirology. 2008;**5**:3. DOI: 10.1186/1742-4690-5-3

[89] Fichorova RN, Tucker LD, Anderson DJ. The molecular basis of nonoxynol-9-induced vaginal inflammation and its possible relevance to human immunodeficiency virus type 1 transmission. The Journal of Infectious Diseases. 2001;**184**(4):418-428

[90] Turpin JA. Considerations and development of topical microbicides to inhibit the sexual transmission of HIV. Expert Opinion on Investigational Drugs. 2002;**11**:1077-1097

[91] Janneke VW, Andrew F, Clifton K, Sanjay M, Sungwal R, Newton K, Zvavahera C, Smita J, Taha T, Nancy P, Robert B, Kenrad N. Phase 1 trial of the topical microbicide buffer-Gel: Safety results from four international sites. Journal of Acquired Immune Deficiency Syndromes. 2001;**26**(1):21-27

[92] Mayer KH, Peipert J, Fleming T, Fullem A, Moench T, Cu-Uvin S, Bentley M, Chesney M, Rosenberg Z. Safety and tolerability of buffergel, a novel vaginal microbicide, in Women in the United States. Clinical Infectious Diseases. 2001;**32**(3):476-482

[93] Roberts L, Liebenberg L, Barnabas S, Passmore JA. Vaginal microbicides to prevent human immunodeficiency virus infection in women: Perspectives on the female genital tract, sexual maturity and mucosal inflammation. Best Practice & Research in Clinical Obstetrics & Gynaecology. 2012;**26**(4):441-449

[94] Milani M, Barcellona E, Agnello A. Efficacy of the combination of 2 g oral tinidazole and acidic buffering vaginal gel in comparison with vaginal clindamycin alone in bacterial vaginosis: A randomized, investigator-blinded, controlled trial. European Journal of Obstetrics Gynecology & Reproductive Biology. 2003;**109**(1):67-71

[95] Marla JK, Colleen AC, Yungtai L, Mark HE, Congzhou L, David NF, Betsy CH. Phase I randomized safety study of twice daily dosing of acidform vaginal gel: Candidate antimicrobial contraceptive. PLoS One. 2012;**7**(10):e46901

[96] Amaral E, Perdigao A, Souza MH, Mauck C, Waller D, Zaneveld L, Faundes A. Vaginal safety after use of a bioadhesive, acid-buffering, microbicidal contraceptive gel (ACIDFORM) and a 2% nonoxynol-9 product. Contraception. 2006;**73**:542-547

[97] Bayer LL, Jensen JT. ACIDFORM: A review of the evidence. Contraception. 2014;**90**:11-18

[98] Klebanoff SJ, Kazazi F. Inactivation of human immunodeficiency virus type1 by theamineoxidase-peroxidase system. Journal of Clinical Microbiology. 1995;**33**(8):2057

[99] Stafford MK, Ward H, Flanagan A, Rosenstein IJ, Taylor-Robinson D, Smith JR. Safety study of nonoxynol-9 as a vaginal microbicide: Evidence of adverse effects. Journal of Acquired Immune Deficiency Syndrome and Human Retrovirology. 1998;**17**:327-331

[100] Roddy RR, Zekeng L, Ryan KA, Tamoufe U, Weir SS, Wong EL. A controlled trial of nonoxynol 9 film to reduce male-to-female transmission of sexually transmitted diseases. New England Journal of Medicine. 1998;**339**:504-510

[101] Damme LV, Ramjee G, Alary M, Vuylsteke B, Chandeying V, Rees H, Sirivongrangson P, Mukenge-Tshibaka L, Ettiegne-Traore V, Uaheowitchai C, Karim SS, Masse B, Perriens J, Laga M. Group effectiveness of COL-1492, a nonoxynol-9 vaginal gel, on HIV-1 transmission in female sex workers: A randomised controlled trial. The Lancet. 2002;**360**:971-977

[102] Ajayi BO, Otajevwo FD. Extrachromosomal DNA length and antibiograms of Staphylococcus aureus and Pseudomonas aeruginosa isolated from tears of HIV/AIDS patients after curing with sodium dodecyl sulphate. Global Journal of Health Science. 2012;**4**(1):229-236

[103] Cutler B, Justman J. Vaginal microbicides and the prevention of HIV transmission. Lancet Infectious Diseases. 2008;**8**:685-697

[104] Lakshmi YS, Kumar P, Kishore G, Bhaskar C, Kondapi AK. Triple combination MPT vaginal microbicide using curcumin and efavirenz loaded lacto-ferrin nanoparticles. Sciences. 2016;**6**:25479

[105] Kabamba BA, Hazel TM, Grace ML, Chakauya Cand Khati M. Progress and perspectives on HIV-1 microbicide development. Virology. 2016;**497**:69-80

[106] Johnson LK, McNeil S. Megatietal.,"Non-propagating, recombinant vesicular stomatitis virus vectors encoding respiratory syncytial virus proteins generate potent humoral and cellular immunity against RSV and are protective in mice,". Immunology Letters. 2013;**150**(2):134-144

[107] Marais D, Gawarecki D, Allan B, et al. The effectiveness of Carraguard, a vaginal microbicide, in protecting women against high-risk human papillomavirus infection. Antiviral Therapy. 2011;**16**(8):1219-1226

[108] Skoler-Karpoff S, Ramjee G, Ahmed K, Altini L, Plagianos MG, Friedland B, Govender S, De Kock A, Cassim N, Palanee T, Dozier G, Maguire R, Lahteenmaki P. Efficacy of Carraguard for prevention of HIV infection in women in South Africa: A randomised, double-blind, placebo-controlled trial. The Lancet. 2008;**6**(372):1977-1987

[109] Chirenje ZM, Masse BR, Maslankowski LA. Utility of colposcopy in a phase 2 portion of a microbicide clinical trial of BufferGel and 0.5% PRO 2000 gel. Journal of the International AIDS Society. 2012;**15**(2):17376

[110] Neurath AR, Strick N, Jiang S, Li YY, Debnath AK. Anti-HIV-1 activity of cellulose acetate phthalate: Synergy with soluble CD4 and induction of "dead-end" gp41 six-helix bundles. BMC Infectious Diseases. 2002;**2**:6

[111] Agarwal HK, Kumar A, Doncel GF, Parang K. Synthesis, antiviral and contraceptive activities of nucleoside-sodium cellulose sulfate acetate and succinate conjugates. Bioorganic & Medicinal Chemistry Letters. 2010;**20**(23):6993-6997

[112] McCarthy TD, Karellas P, Henderson SA, Giannis M, O'Keefe DF, Heery G, Paull JR, Matthews BR, Holan G. Dendrimers as drugs: Discovery and preclinical and clinical development of dendrimer-based microbicides for HIV and STI prevention. Molecular Pharmacology. 2005;**2**:312-318

[113] Richard R, Susan LR, Lawrence RS. VivaGel™ (SPL7013 Gel): A candidate dendrimer -microbicide for the prevention of HIV and HSV infection. International Journal of Nanomedicine. 2007;**2**(4):561-566

[114] Patton DL, Sweeney YT, McCarthy TD. Preclinical safety and efficacy assessments of dendrimer-based (SPL7013) microbicide gel formulations in a nonhuman primate model. Antimicrobial Agents and Chemotherapy. 2006;**50**:1696-1700

[115] Wei SH, Stephen HH. HIV-1 reverse transcription. Cold Spring Harbor Perspectives in Medicine. 2012;**2**(10):a006882

[116] Mira D, Geetha L, Dikshit RK. Antiretroviral drugs: Critical issues and recent advances. Indian Journal of Pharmacology. 2012;**44**(3):288-298

[117] Karim AQ, Karim SS, Frohlich JA. Effectiveness and safety of tenofovir gel, an anti-retroviral microbicide, for the prevention of HIV infection in women. Science. 2010;**329**(5996):1168-1174

[118] Sokal DC, Karim AQ, Sibeko. Safety of tenofovir gel, a vaginal microbicide, in South African women: Results of the CAPRISA 004 Trial. Antiviral Therapy. 2013;**18**(3):301-310

[119] Salim SA, Quarraisha AK, Cheryl B. Antibodies for HIV Prevention in young women. Current opinion in HIV and AIDS. 2015;**10**(3):183-189

[120] Schwartz JL, Kovalevsky G, Lai JJ, Ballagh SA, McCormick T, Douville K, Mauck CK, Callahan MM. A randomized six-day safety study of an antiretroviral microbicide candidate UC781, a non-nucleoside reverse transcriptase inhibitor. Sexually Transmitted Diseases. 2008;**35**(4):414-419

[121] McConville C, Smith JM, McCoy CF, Srinivasan P, Mitchell J, Holder A, Otten RA, Butera S, Doncel GF, Friend DR, Malcolm RK. Lack of in vitro-in vivo correlation for a UC781-releasing vaginal ring in macaques. Drug Delivery and Translational Research. 2015;**5**:27-37

[122] Garg AB, Nuttall J, Romano J. The future of HIV microbicides: Challenges and opportunities. Antiviral Chemistry and Chemotherapy. 2009;**19**(4):143-150

[123] Nel A, Bekker LG, Bukusi E, Hellstrm E, Kotze P, Louw C, Martinson F, Masenga G, Montgomery E, Ndaba N, Straten A, Niekerk N, Woodsong C. Safety, acceptability and adherence of dapivirine vaginal ring in a microbicide clinical trial conducted in multiple countries in Sub-Saharan Africa. PLoS One. 2016;**11**:e0147743

[124] Baeten JM, Palanee-Phillips T, Brown E, Schwartz K, Soto-Torres LE, Govender V, Mgodi FNM et al. Use of a vaginal ring containing dapivirine for HIV-1 prevention in women. New England Journal of Medicine. 2016;**375**(22): 2121-2132

6

HIV Infection and Infertility

Thana Khawcharoenporn and Beverly E. Sha

Abstract

Human immunodeficiency virus (HIV) infection has become a chronic and manageable disease since the availability of combination antiretroviral therapy (cART). Persons living with HIV are living longer with better quality of life. Given that worldwide many HIV-infected individuals are in the reproductive age, fertility and reproductive desire have emerged as clinically important issues among this population. Biological changes caused by HIV, including systemic illnesses, stress, and weight loss, may affect the function of reproductive organs and result in infertility. Newly diagnosed HIV infection may cause psychological trauma and decrease in sexual drive and sexual activity. Several HIV/acquired immune deficiency syndrome (AIDS)-related comorbidities have been reported to be associated with infertility. These include orchitis, acute epididymitis, and pelvic inflammatory disease caused by opportunistic pathogens and coinfections with sexually transmitted infections (STIs) acquired through a similar route of transmission as HIV. The common STIs caused by *Neisseria gonorrhoeae, Chlamydia trachomatis, Ureaplasma urealyticum, Treponema pallidum*, herpes simplex virus-2, and *Trichomonas vaginalis* can damage the reproductive system and cause infertility. Hypogonadism especially in men with AIDS is one of the important endocrine disorders that causes infertility. Although cART provides significant benefits in reducing morbidity and mortality among HIV-infected persons, some antiretroviral drugs, including nucleoside reverse transcriptase inhibitors, are toxic to cellular mitochondria and may affect the mitochondrial biogenesis of sperm and oocytes. HIV-infected individuals may have limited access to reproductive care given the severity of their disease, cost of care, stigmatization, and lack of specific HIV infection/infertility knowledge among their providers.

In the post–cART era, reproductive care has become an important issue to be co-managed with HIV care. Reproductive care includes not only comprehensively managing HIV infection but also minimizing the risk of horizontal HIV transmission in serodiscordant couples, providing suitable options for unprotected timed intercourse, intrauterine insemination with partner or donor sperm, in vitro fertilization with intracytoplasmic sperm injection (IVF/ICSI), embryo donation, and adoption. This chapter reviews potential effects of HIV infection, related opportunistic infections, and physical and psychological comorbidities on fertility; the impact of cART on fertility; and the management of reproductive issues among HIV-infected individuals.

Keywords: HIV, AIDS, Infection, Infertility

1. Introduction

There were approximately 37 million people living with human immunodeficiency virus (PLWHIV) globally at the end of 2014.[1] The course of HIV infection has changed from a deadly disease to a chronic and manageable disease since the introduction of combination antiretroviral therapy (cART) in the 1990s. The estimated life expectancy of a 20-year-old PLWHIV has increased from 30 years during 1996–1999 to 46 years during 2006–2008 according to the UK Collaborative HIV Cohort Study.[2] The increased life expectancy along with improved quality of life has led to increase in reproductive desire among this population.[3] Fertility of PLWHIV can be affected by HIV infection and associated infections. Infections can physically impact the anatomical structure and biological function of the reproductive system, whereas stress and psychiatric disorders related to HIV infection may lessen sexual drive and frequency of sexual intercourse. In addition, socioeconomic factors including limited financial means, difficulty accessing HIV care, and stigmatization can contribute to social withdrawal and reduced reproductive potential among PLWHIV. Management of reproductive health along with cART has become a necessary component of comprehensive HIV care in the post–cART era. The etiologies and epidemiology of HIV-related infertility, factors that may impact fertility, and management options and considerations for infertility among HIV-infected individuals are reviewed in this chapter.

2. Epidemiology of HIV-related infertility

The data on the magnitude and burden of HIV-related infertility derive mostly from studies conducted among HIV-infected women. A previous study using data from case–control studies and theoretical predictions from a model of the proximate determinants of fertility and HIV incidence in African countries demonstrated the 25–40% lower rate of fertility among HIV-infected women compared to HIV-negative women.[4] In a prospective cohort study from the United States during 1994–2002, women with HIV were less likely to conceive than uninfected women (pregnancy rates 7.4 vs.15.2 per 100 person-years, respectively).[5] Using demographic and health surveys between 2003 and 2007, the Joint United Nations Program on HIV/AIDS (UNAIDS) estimated that the global age-specific fertility ratio for HIV-infected women in the reproductive age group of 20–44 years is 0.53 to 0.76 compared to that of women without HIV.[6] A survey study conducted at HIV fertility clinics in the United Kingdom demonstrated a 40% prevalence of tubal factor infertility among HIV-infected women.[7] Despite the infertility in women living with HIV, pregnancy rates among this population have increased steadily over the past 10 years to between 4 and 6 pregnancies per 100 person-years, varying by region due to the advances in HIV treatment and mother-to-child transmission prevention.[8] This may reflect an increase in reproductive desire and/or unexpected pregnancies and indicate the need for reproductive health care, fertility management, and family planning along with HIV comprehensive care among PLWHIV.

3. HIV effects on fertility

There are several factors associated with HIV infection that can potentially affect fertility in PLWHIV. These factors can be categorized into biological factors, psychological factors, and social factors (Figure 1).

Factors associated with infertility

Biological factors

- Advanced age
- Degree of immunosuppression
- Poor adherence to cART
- Systemic illnesses
- Stress
- Weight loss
- Protracted anovulation and amenorrhea (women)
- Impairment of sperm parameters (men)
- Loss of germ cells within testes (men)
- Primary and secondary hypogonadism
- Sexually-transmitted infections
- Opportunistic infections
- Other genital tract infections
- NRTIs toxicity

Psychological factors

- Feeling of guilt and shame
- Being afraid of HIV transmission
- Awareness of challenges in pregnancy, birth and parenting in the context of HIV infection
- Concerns about personal health and cART efficacy

Social factors

- Financial problems
- Limited reproductive care access
- Social norms and values of reproductive care and HIV/AIDS
- HIV stigmatization
- Lack of knowledge among caring physicians
- Limited availability of assisted reproductive therapy

Note: AIDS, acquired immune deficiency syndrome; cART, combination antiretroviral therapy; HIV, human immunodeficiency virus; NRTIs, nucleoside reverse transcriptase inhibitors.

Figure 1. Factors associated with infertility among people living with human immunodeficiency virus

3.1. Biological factors

Demographic characteristics that have been reported to be associated with low rates of pregnancy among HIV-infected women include advanced age, white ethnicity (compared to black ethnicity), having CD4 cell count of less than 100 cells/mm^3, and poor adherence to cART.[8-10] Systemic illnesses from HIV and its related comorbidities, stress, and weight loss generally impact the reproductive potential of both sexes.[3] HIV-infected women are more likely than non-HIV-infected women to have protracted anovulation and amenorrhea.[11-14] The number of ovulatory cycles was found to correlate with the severity of immunosuppression and having an AIDS diagnosis. Although there have been no reports of ovarian aging or failure,[15] HIV-infected women may have reduced ovarian reserve.[16] In HIV-infected men, impairment of sperm parameters affecting fertility has been described. The impairment includes lower ejaculation volume, sperm count, and progressive motility (defined as the percent of sperm with forward motility) despite normal morphology compared to non-HIV-infected men.[17-19] Sperm concentration levels, total count, and motility were found to positively correlate with the height of the CD4 cell count, indicating the adverse effect of worsening immunodeficiency on these sperm parameters.[19] Other studies demonstrated that the semen of HIV-infected men was more viscous and contained fewer motile sperm but more round cells.[20] In addition, a study of testicular specimens from autopsy samples (1981–1998) revealed progressive loss of germ cells within the testes with prolonged survival with AIDS.[21] Although recent data indicate that cART significantly decreased total sperm count and progressive motility and increased the proportion of abnormal sperm forms,[22] these adverse effects are balanced by the overwhelming benefits of cART for immune reconstitution, morbidity and mortality reduction, and overall improvement of sperm characteristics associated with higher CD4 cell counts.

3.1.1. Hypogonadism and HIV/AIDS

Hypogonadism was recognized as a relatively common condition early in the HIV epidemic and characterized by a low level of testosterone among HIV-infected men. Hypogonadism can be categorized into primary hypogonadism, which is a disorder of the testes, and secondary hypogonadism, which is a disorder of the pituitary or hypothalamus. Hypogonadism can be associated with various signs and symptoms, including muscle wasting, weight loss, low bone mineral density, and decreased libido.[23] During the early course of HIV disease, men tend to have normal serum testosterone levels. As the disease progresses to AIDS, low serum testosterone levels become more frequent, particularly in those with more advanced immunosuppression (e.g., CD4 cell count less than 100 cells/mm^3). Early in the HIV epidemic, 30–50% of symptomatic HIV-infected men had low total serum testosterone levels, which significantly correlated with weight loss and CD4 cell depletion.[24-26] The prevalence of hypogonadism in HIV-infected men has decreased with cART initiation occurring at earlier stages of HIV infection. Effective HIV therapy can normalize testosterone levels over time.[27] Most cases of decreased testosterone levels in HIV-infected men are related to secondary hypogonadism.[24, 28] Other characteristics that have been reported to be associated with low testosterone levels include older age, a detectable HIV RNA level of greater than 10,000 copies/

mL, injection drug use, hepatitis C coinfection, high body mass index, and insulin resistance.[28-31] In addition, several medications commonly used among HIV-infected individuals can affect testosterone levels through varied mechanisms. Systemic glucocorticoids and megestrol acetate can cause hypogonadism by suppressing the hypothalamic–pituitary–gonadal axis, whereas a high dose of ketoconazole (at least 400 mg per day) directly inhibits steroidogenesis. Psychotropic medications can cause hyperprolactinemia and testosterone deficiency, whereas chronic use of alcohol, opiates, and marijuana can impair testosterone production.[32, 33]

Primary hypogonadism	Secondary hypogonadism
Congenital abnormalities	**Congenital abnormalities**
· Klinefelter's syndrome	· Congenital GnRH deficiency
· Other chromosomal abnormalities (e.g., 46, XY/XO; 47, XYY)	· Leptin or leptin receptor mutation
· Mutation in the FSH and LH receptor genes	· Gonadotropin subunit mutations
· Cryptorchidism	
· Disorders of androgen biosynthesis	
· Myotonic dystrophy	
· Congenital anorchia	
· Varicocele	
Acquired diseases	**Acquired diseases**
· Infectious orchitis	· Hyperprolactinemia
· Radiation	· Gonadal steroids
· Alkylating and antineoplastic agents	· Glucocorticoids
· Ketoconazole	· Continuous opiate administration
· Glucocorticoids	· Critical illness
· Dibromochloropropane	· Chronic systemic illness
· Trauma	· Anorexia nervosa
· Testicular torsion	· Diabetes mellitus
· Bilateral orchiectomy	· Obesity
· Autoimmune damage	· Pituitary adenoma
· Chronic systemic diseases	· Metastatic tumor damaging pituitary gland
· Cirrhosis	· Sarcoidosis
· Chronic kidney disease	· Hemochromatosis
· Idiopathic	· Tuberculous meningitis
	· Pituitary apoplexy
	· Trauma
	· Idiopathic

Note: FSH, follicle-stimulating hormone; GnRH, gonadotropin-releasing hormone; LH, luteinizing hormone.

Table 1. Causes of hypogonadism in males

HIV-infected men with symptomatic hypogonadism may present with loss of facial and body hair, decreased muscle mass and strength, diminished libido, impotence, testicular atrophy, gynecomastia, depression, low energy, and poor concentration.[34] Diagnosis of hypogonadism is made based on a clinical suspicion and low serum testosterone levels (generally less than 300 ng/dL). The screening test of choice is the serum total testosterone concentration (free plus protein-bound fractions). However, in some cases, the total testosterone levels may be normal, whereas the free levels may be low because of the higher sex hormone-binding globulin levels among HIV-infected persons. Thus, in a patient with suspected testosterone deficiency and serum total testosterone concentration in the lower half of the normal range (less than 500 ng/dL), the free testosterone levels should be assessed.[34] Testosterone levels should not be evaluated during an acute illness because of the transient decline of androgen levels related to the acute event. To distinguish between primary and secondary hypogonadism, follicle-stimulating hormone (FSH) and luteinizing hormone (LH) levels need to be measured. The elevated FSH and LH levels suggest primary hypogonadism, whereas normal or low levels of FSH and LH are consistent with secondary hypogonadism. Further evaluation should be geared toward diagnosing the possible causes of primary and secondary hypogonadism in HIV-infected men as detailed in Table 1.

3.1.2. Comorbid diseases and HIV/AIDS

3.1.2.1. Sexually Transmitted Infections (STIs)

The impact of STIs on fertility among PLWHIV depends on the local prevalence of the STIs. Given the common route of transmission of causative agents and immunosuppressive status caused by HIV, STIs tend to be more prevalent, to be more severe, to take longer to resolve, and to be more prone to treatment failure in HIV-infected persons compared to the general population. Common causative pathogens for STIs among PLWHIV include bacteria, such as *Neisseria gonorrhoeae, Chlamydia trachomatis, Ureaplasma urealyticum, Mycoplasma hominis, Mycoplasma genitalium, Treponema pallidum, Haemophilus ducreyi,* and *Klebsiella granulomatis;* viruses, such as hepatitis B and C viruses, herpes simplex virus (HSV), and human papillomavirus (HPV); and protozoa, such as *Trichomonas vaginalis*. The underlying pathogenesis for STI-related infertility is direct damage and subsequent anatomical and functional abnormalities of the genital organs, including the testes and epididymis in men and cervix, uterus, fallopian tubes, and ovaries in women. A previous study demonstrated that the DNA of STI pathogens was detected in semen of 45 of 241 asymptomatic men seeking an infertility investigation (19%) and was associated with a decrease in sperm concentration, motile sperm concentration, total sperm count, and neutral alpha-glucosidase concentration.[35]

Gonorrhea is a STI caused by *N. gonorrhea* and commonly manifests as urethritis in both sexes and pelvic inflammatory disease in women. The reported complications related to fertility of gonorrhea include urethral strictures and subsequent impairment of testicular functions in men.[36] Similarly, *C. trachomatis* can cause urethritis in both sexes and pelvic inflammatory disease in females. Epidemiologic data suggest that *C. trachomatis* may be associated with tubal obstruction and subsequent infertility in women.[37] The impact of Mycoplasma, that is, *U.*

urealyticum, M. hominis, and *M. genitalium,* on fertility is uncertain. *U. urealyticum* may cause infertility through its effects on sperm chromatin and DNA, whereas *M. genitalium* can attach to spermatozoa and can be transported to the female genital tract.[38, 39] Syphilis is caused by *T. pallidum* and is more prevalent among PLWHIV. Orchitis, epididymitis, and testicular mass have been reported as manifestations of syphilis in HIV-infected men.[40, 41] Although *H. ducreyi* and *K. granulomatis* do not directly affect the reproductive tract, they both cause ulcers and lymphadenopathy around the genital area, which may affect reproductive potential.

Chronic viral hepatitis B and C can cause impairment in sperm concentration, motility, morphology, and viability, whereas HPV primarily affects sperm motility.[42] The presence of HSV DNA in semen has been associated with decreased sperm concentration and reduced motility.[43] In HIV-infected women, chronic HPV infection increases the risk of cervical cancer development and possibly leads to infertility. An important protozoan *T. vaginalis* is the cause of vaginitis, endometritis, adnexitis, and pyosalpinx in women, which can lead to infertility and preterm birth and low birth weight of the newborn.[44] In men, it is associated with complications including urethritis, prostatitis, epididymitis, and infertility through inflammatory damage or interference with sperm function.[44]

3.1.2.2. Opportunistic Infections (OIs)

HIV-infected persons are at increased risk for opportunistic infections (OIs) depending on their degree of immunosuppression. Tuberculosis is a common OI in HIV-tuberculosis endemic locales and its prevalence is higher among PLWHIV compared to non-HIV-infected persons, regardless of the CD4 cell count. Genital tract infection caused by *Mycobacterium tuberculosis* contributes to infertility and poorer reproductive health outcomes in both sexes.[3] Salmonellosis, toxoplasmosis, and cryptococcosis can manifest as disseminated infections involving the genital organs. Although cytomegalovirus (CMV) can cause orchitis and epididymitis in HIV-infected men, there are no data on its effect on sperm characteristics.[42] Candidiasis is frequently reported among HIV-infected persons with CD4 cell counts less than 200 cells/mm^3. It is the cause of balanitis in men and vaginitis and cervicitis in women, which may affect fertility.

3.1.2.3. Other infections

Other infectious causes of orchitis in both HIV-infected and non-HIV-infected men include bacteria, such as *Escherichia coli, Klebsiella pneumoniae, Pseudomonas aeruginosa, Staphylococcus* spp., and *Streptococcus* spp., and viruses, such as mumps, varicella, coxsackievirus, and echovirus.[45] These infections may also contribute to infertility.

3.1.3. Antiretroviral agents

Nucleoside reverse transcriptase inhibitors (NRTIs) remain key components of recommended cART regimens. They inhibit HIV-1 reverse transcriptase, which reduces viral replication and improves disease control. However, these medications also inhibit mitochondrial DNA (mtDNA) synthesis and cause a decrease in polypeptides involved in electron transport, which can result in cell injury.[46] The degree of mitochondrial toxicity is specific to each NRTI. Theoretically, an HIV-infected person's fertility may be affected by NRTI use via the damage to mitochondrial biogenesis of gametes.[3] This is supported by the mtDNA depletion observed in sperm and oocytes of HIV-infected patients taking NRTIs and in low oocyte mtDNA in patients with ovarian insufficiency.[47-49] Data from epidemiologic studies are conflicting regarding the impact of cART on fertility. A prospective cohort from the United States reported the lower likelihood of conception associated with antiretroviral therapy among HIV-infected women,[5] whereas a more recent study from Africa demonstrated significantly higher pregnancy rates among HIV-infected women on cART compared to those not on cART.[50] However, these two studies were conducted in different settings and time, and specific behavioral and biological mechanisms were not explored. Zidovudine (azidothymidine, AZT) is the NRTI drug that has been studied the most. In animal studies, AZT has been shown to suppress cell division in the preimplantation mouse embryo, causing reduction in inner cell mass proliferation, greater number of resorptions, and fewer fetuses.[51, 52] A previous study demonstrated that exposure to NRTI transplacentally caused significant fetal mitochondrial damage in experimental monkeys.[53] Unfortunately, there have been no studies examining fertility effect of NRTIs in humans.

3.2. Psychological factors

Decrease in sexual activity after a new diagnosis of HIV infection is usually observed and may be accompanied by the feeling of guilt and shame and aggravated by the stigma related to HIV infection.[54] Individuals recently diagnosed with HIV infection reported to have decreased desire for or interest in sex relations. They also reported to use condom more consistently during sexual intercourse to avoid transmission of HIV to their partners.[55] Previous studies indicated that HIV-infected women often chose to avoid pregnancy.[56, 57] However, another study revealed that high-risk behaviors, unplanned pregnancies, and pregnancy termination remain prevalent among this population.[58] In the pre–cART era, there was a significant increase in the pregnancy termination rate from 3.5 to 6.3 per 100 women-years following a new HIV diagnosis in the United Kingdom and Ireland[56] and 47% of pregnancies were voluntarily terminated following a new HIV diagnosis in an Australian study.[57] The reasons for pregnancy termination may include challenges of pregnancy, birth and parenting in the context of HIV infection, concerns about increased risks of complications related to pregnancy and delivery, and risk of HIV transmission to the newborn. A previous study reported that unplanned pregnancy, lower CD4 cell count, and having an HIV-infected current partner were factors associated with the decision to terminate a pregnancy.[59] Following the introduction of cART with overall improvement in health and immune status of HIV-infected women, the rates of elective pregnancy termination after a HIV diagnosis were 22%-26% decreased from the pre–cART period.[60, 61] With the success of cART in preventing mother-to-child HIV transmission, HIV infection was reported to have no effect on desire for pregnancy among young urban African Americans aged 15–24 years.[62] Reproductive desire among PLWHIV may now be associated with personal health, cART, concern about HIV transmission, and social factors. Some HIV-infected persons have an increased desire for children as a way of concealing their HIV-infected status and improving their feelings of self-worth. Others stated that their HIV diagnosis increased their desire for children at an earlier age and some chose to have children following advances in HIV care.[63-65]

3.3. Social factors

The HIV/AIDS epidemic has a significant impact on the economic and political stability of a nation. Awareness of HIV/AIDS at the population level may affect the age of sexual debut, frequency of sexual intercourse, safer sex and contraceptive practices, perceived value of marriage, social norms, and fertility intentions and choices of PLWHIV.[3] The dramatic improvement in the life expectancy of PLWHIV and reduction in HIV transmission rates following treatment of the infected partner have changed ethical considerations regarding childbearing in HIV-infected individuals. Early in the HIV/AIDS epidemic, pregnancy in HIV-infected women was considered morally problematic, whereas recently, the Ethics Committee of the American Society for Reproductive Medicine stated that it is ethical for health care providers to assist PLWHIV who seek pregnancy when optimal precautions to prevent HIV transmission are utilized.[66] Despite more opportunities for access to reproductive care, PLWHIV still face multiple obstacles. First, the severity of their disease, level of immunosuppression, presence of OIs, and other comorbid diseases may impair their fertility. Second, their HIV provider may have limited knowledge to counsel them on reproductive health issues, and infertility specialists may have limited expertise in providing care for HIV-infected persons. Third, HIV stigmatization could potentially preclude them from establishing reproductive care. Finally, assisted fertility therapy (AFT) is technically complicated in regard to HIV transmission prevention and costliness and may not be available in all settings.[3]

4. Fertility management

Fertility management for PLWHIV should be comprehensive and involve cART, specific management for factors associated with infertility, and AFT while minimizing the risk of horizontal and vertical transmission of HIV.

4.1. Combination antiretroviral therapy

With advances in the development of antiretroviral agents, cART has become more potent and effective, more tolerable and convenient to administer, and less toxic. Current guidelines recommend that PLWHIV should receive cART when they are willing and able to commit to treatment and understand the benefits and risks of therapy and the importance of adherence, regardless of the CD4 cell count level.[67] The benefits of early cART among persons with a CD4 cell count above 500 cells/mm^3 were demonstrated in a recent large-scale randomized trial that showed a reduction in mortality, AIDS-related events, and non–AIDS-related events in those started on cART immediately versus waiting until the CD4 cell count fell below 350 cells/mm^3.[68] The currently recommended initial cART regimens consist of a backbone of two NRTIs and any one drug from the following drug classes: non-NRTI, protease inhibitor with a booster, or integrase inhibitor with or without a booster.[67, 69, 70] The initial cART regimens recommended by different consensus guidelines are shown in Table 2. A patient-specific regimen from these lists will be chosen based on convenience of administration, adverse reactions, local availability, cost, and health plan coverage. The goals of cART are immunologic response, defined as an increase in CD4 cell count, and virologic response, defined as HIV RNA suppression below the lower limit of detection. By extending life expectancy and improving overall health, immunity, and quality of life from cART, cART is expected to improve fertility outcomes. Achieving a sustained virologic response is particularly important to reduce the risk of HIV horizontal and vertical transmission during conception attempts, pregnancy, and delivery.

DHHS 2015	**EACS 2015**	**WHO 2013**
ABC + 3TC + DTG	ABC + 3TC + DTG	TDF + FTC/3TC + EFV
TDF + FTC + DTG	TDF + FTC + DTG	
TDF + FTC + EVG/c or TAF + FTC + EVG/c	TDF + FTC + EVG/c	
TDF + FTC + RAL	TDF + FTC + RAL	
TDF + FTC + DRV/r	TDF + FTC + DRV/r	
	TDF + FTC + RPV	

Note: 3TC, lamivudine; ABC, abacavir; DHHS, the U.S. Department of Health and Human Services; DRV/r, ritonavir-boosted darunavir; DTG, dolutegravir; EACS, European AIDS Clinical Society; EFV, efavirenz; EVG/c, cobicistat-boosted elvitegravir; FTC, emtricitabine; RAL, raltegravir; RPV, rilpivirine; TAF, tenofovir alafenamide; TDF, tenofovir disoproxil fumarate; WHO, World Health Organization.

Table 2. Recommended first-line combination antiretroviral therapy regimens based on consensus guidelines

4.2. Specific management for factors associated with infertility

4.2.1. Management of biological factors

Immunosuppression and wasting syndrome can be improved by cART. In addition, PLWHIV who are taking cART with sustained immunologic and virologic responses will have reduced incidences of OIs, such as tuberculosis, salmonellosis, toxoplasmosis, cryptococcosis, CMV infection, and candidiasis. NRTIs selected for the backbone of a cART regimen should have the least toxicity on mitochondria to minimize the impact on oocytes and sperm. These "safer" NRTIs include tenofovir, abacavir, lamivudine, and emtricitabine.[67, 69, 70] Good general health and less physical stress are associated with normal ovulation and menstrual cycles in HIV-infected women, whereas cART improves overall sperm parameters among HIV-infected men. STIs, OIs, and other infections should be promptly diagnosed and treated to prevent damage to the genital organs. It is important that sex partners of patients with STIs should be counseled, tested, and treated accordingly.

Hypogonadism should be recognized early, correctly diagnosed, and treated in HIV-infected men. Testosterone treatment is indicated in men with low serum concentrations of testosterone and any of the following signs or symptoms including low libido and/or hypogonadal symptoms, low bone mineral density, low body mass, or weight loss despite virologic response to cART. Prior to initiation of testosterone replacement therapy, patients should be evaluated for coexisting depression and psychosocial stressors along with baseline laboratory studies including complete blood count, a metabolic panel, lipid panel, and a prostate-specific antigen (PSA). Long-term effects of suppression of the hypothalamic–pituitary–gonadal axis, promoting malignancy of the prostate gland and cardiovascular diseases, in those older than 60 years should be carefully monitored. Patients with a history of prostate cancer, a palpable prostate nodule, or an elevated PSA should not be prescribed testosterone replacement therapy.[34, 71] The routes of testosterone administration should be based on the patient's preference and include transdermal patch, gel, and intramuscular injection. For injections, the initial dose is 200 mg every 2 weeks or 100 mg every week. The dose can be titrated based on testosterone levels measured midway between injections aiming for the mid-normal reference range. Testosterone replacement therapy should continue as long as there are symptomatic benefits and no adverse effects.

4.2.2. Management of psychological and social factors

Knowledge about HIV and its epidemiology, routes of transmission, clinical course, long-term prognosis, and benefit of cART is critical to PLWHIV in reducing HIV transmission to their sexual partners and improvinge their adherence and outcomes. A previous study demonstrated that increased reproductive intention was associated with patient optimism regarding cART efficacy.[72] To overcome the challenges in pregnancy, birth, and parenting, PLWHIV should be informed about the recent advances in antenatal, perinatal, and postnatal care to prevent HIV transmission to their newborns. Family planning counseling should be provided to prepare them for child rearing and to cope with any problems they may face. Issues on reproductive care access for PLWHIV are very new for many developing countries, because the main goals for HIV care in these countries are currently improving access to HIV testing and treatment. Financial burdens, medical coverage, and availability of centers that can provide AFT need to be considered when developing and implementing local, regional, and national policies or guidelines for the reproductive care of PLWHIV. In the meantime, physicians who care for PLWHIV should update their knowledge to optimally assess and manage fertility issues among persons with HIV infection. HIV stigmatization may be reduced by campaigns and specific interventions that are appropriate and feasible for each locale.

4.3. Assisted fertility therapy

Relevant issues to be considered regarding fertility treatment in PLWHIV include risk of HIV horizontal transmission in serodiscordant heterosexual couples and methods to reduce HIV transmission. Generally, the rate of HIV heterosexual transmission is approximately 1 per

500 to 1 per 1,000 episodes of unprotected sexual intercourse.[3] However, the risk of transmission can increase significantly if there are genital tract infections from STIs or OIs, trauma with sex, lack of male circumcision, and high plasma HIV RNA levels in seropositive persons.[73, 74] Thus, a thorough evaluation is needed before AFT. History including a detailed history of their HIV infection and any associated complications, recent CD4 cell counts and HIV RNA levels, past and current cART regimens, history of antiretroviral drug resistance, ongoing HIV risk behaviors, and fertility problems should be obtained. Physical examination should focus on signs relevant to causes of infertility, genital organs, and Pap smear in women. An HIV-infected partner should be treated with cART until HIV RNA suppression has been achieved prior to AFT. Partners who have STIs need to be treated to reduce transmission risks of HIV and STI-associated pathogens. Trauma during sexual intercourse should be avoided or minimized, and safer sex practices should be encouraged outside the conception attempts. Proposed algorithm for fertility management among HIV-infected couples is shown in Figure 2.

Post-exposure prophylaxis (PEP) with cART in uninfected partners may be used after the unprotected sexual intercourse (conception attempt). Although there have not been well-designed studies in human that assess the efficacy of this intervention, the benefits of HIV transmission reduction have been shown in an animal study and a retrospective study of health care workers exposing to body fluids of HIV-infected persons.[75, 76] The recommended PEP regimens that are also safe if the pregnancy does occur are combined tenofovir, emtricitabine, and ritonavir-boosted atazanavir, ritonavir-boosted darunavir, or raltegravir.[77] PEP should be initiated as soon as possible after HIV exposure but within 48 hours and should be continued for 28 days. Because of its demonstrated efficacy, tenofovir–emtricitabine (TDF/FTC) once daily for pre-exposure prophylaxis (PrEP) administered to the seronegative partner is now the preferred approach to reduce the risk of HIV transmission among serodiscordant couples. Among heterosexual couples, pericoital tenofovir vaginal gel was the first PrEP intervention that showed a 39% efficacy at reducing HIV acquisition among high-risk South African women.[78] Several other randomized controlled trials have demonstrated the benefit of PrEP at reducing HIV acquisition among HIV-negative at-risk individuals including 1) the iPrEx study that demonstrated 44% reduction in the incidence of HIV among men who have sex with men taking daily oral TDF/FTC,[79] 2) the Partners-PrEP study that demonstrated 75% and 67% reduction in the incidence of HIV among serodiscordant couples taking daily oral TDF or TDF/FTC, respectively, in Africa,[80] and 3) the TDF2 study that demonstrated 62% reduction in the incidence of HIV among heterosexual men and women taking daily oral TDF/FTC in Botswana.[81] Pharmacokinetic data suggest that PrEP should begin at least 1 week before unprotected sex for optimal benefit. The uninfected partners who choose to take PEP and/or PrEP need to be regularly screened and monitored for HIV infection and adverse effects of the drugs in PEP and/or PrEP regimens.[67, 77]

In regards to limiting risk of HIV vertical transmission, cART given to HIV-infected women antenatally and avoiding breastfeeding can reduce the rate of transmission from 25–40% to less than 1%.[67] Invasive procedures, such as amniocentesis, chorionic villus sampling, and use of fetal scalp electrodes, should be avoided in HIV-infected women because these can

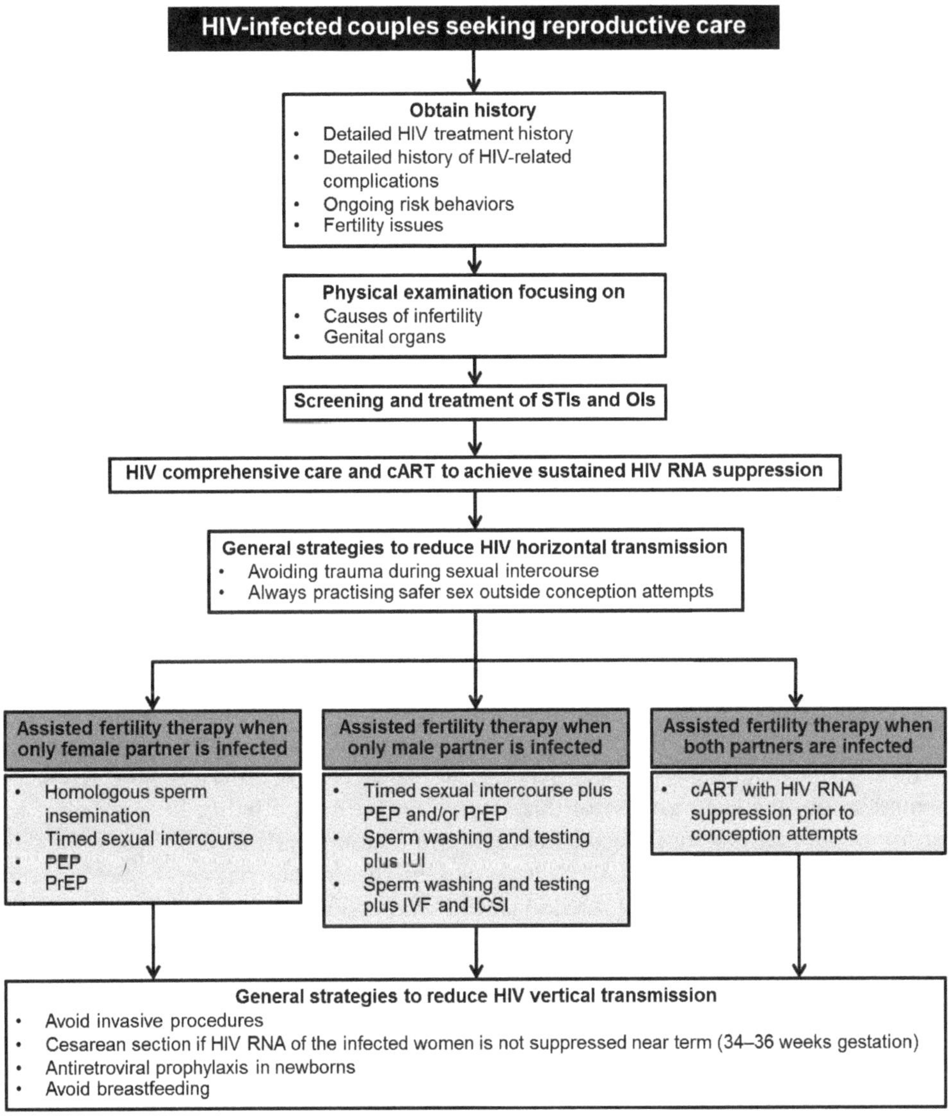

Note: cART, combination antiretroviral therapy; HIV, human immunodeficiency virus; ICSI, intracytoplasmic sperm injection; IUI, intrauterine insemination; IVF, in vitro fertilization; OIs, opportunistic infections; PEP, post-exposure prophylaxis; PrEP, pre-exposure prophylaxis; RNA, ribonucleic acid; STIs, sexually transmitted infections.

Figure 2. Proposed algorithm of fertility management in HIV-infected couples

increase the risk of fetal/infant exposure to maternal body fluids. Cesarean section instead of normal vaginal delivery can further reduce the risk of maternal-infant transmission in HIV-infected pregnant women whose HIV RNA has not been suppressed following cART. United States guidelines use a HIV RNA level of >1,000 copies/mL at 34–36 weeks gestation as a threshold for recommending Cesarean section, whereas European guidelines recommend a threshold of >50 copies/mL.[67, 69] Women who achieve virologic suppression near term can proceed with vaginal delivery without increased transmission risk. Antiretroviral prophylactic regimens for newborns of HIV-infected mothers should be prescribed based on the risk of transmission. In general, AZT is recommended for the first 4–6 weeks of life with additional medications added if the mother did not achieve viral suppression. HIV-infected mothers should not breastfeed their babies due to the risk of transmission via breast milk.

4.3.1. *AFT when only the female partner is infected*

If a woman is HIV infected and her male partner is uninfected, HIV transmission can be avoided by using homologous insemination with the male partner's sperm. However, if this option is not feasible, such as the desire to become pregnant naturally, couples should limit unprotected sexual intercourse to the time of ovulation (timed intercourse) using ovulation kits or basal body temperature monitoring to predict ovulation. These measures allow couples to limit the number of unprotected sexual encounters. In addition, the HIV-infected women should be on cART with a suppressed viral load. The male partner may choose to take PEP and/or PrEP to reduce the risk of HIV transmission; however, these options are not as safe as homologous insemination.[82]

4.3.2. *AFT when only the male partner is infected*

Conception between an HIV-infected man and his HIV-uninfected female partner is more complicated. The risk of HIV transmission can be reduced by using timed intercourse when the HIV-infected man's plasma HIV RNA is undetectable on cART. However, the HIV transmission of timed intercourse in this setting has been reported to be associated with inconsistent condom use outside the conception attempt.[83] Thus, the practice of timed intercourse alone to prevent HIV transmission to the female partner is not generally recommended in this setting.[82] Additional PEP and/or PrEP may be used to reduce HIV transmission. A study of serodiscordant couples, in which the woman was treated with oral tenofovir taken shortly before and after each unprotected sexual encounter, showed that none of the women became infected with HIV and pregnancy rates reached 75% after 12 attempts.[84] Based on available data, once-daily TDF/FTC for the women would generally be recommended throughout the conception period in countries where resources are available for PrEP.

Sperm preparation and testing prior to intrauterine insemination (IUI) have been described as methods to reduce the chance of HIV transmission to the uninfected female partner. The sperm preparation involves a three-step process.[3, 82] First, the liquefied semen is filtered through a Percoll gradient. Next, the isolated spermatozoa are washed to eliminate seminal plasma and hyperosmotic gradient media. Finally, a modified swim-up method recovers highly motile spermatozoa from leukocytes. After this process, the final sperm specimen is tested by polymerase chain reaction assays for the presence of HIV. If this final specimen tests negative, it is used for insemination. In men with severe dyspermia, the final swim-up step that removes infected leukocytes cannot be performed and thus the semen should be tested for HIV DNA. Utilizing this process, 1,600 inseminations were performed in 513 HIV-uninfected women and resulted in 228 pregnancies. At 1-year follow-up, none of the children older than 3 months of age and none of the mothers became HIV infected.[85] In addition, studies reviewing worldwide data in 2004 and data from several centers demonstrated no HIV transmission to the uninfected female partners who were inseminated using sperm washing and IUI.[86, 87]

There have been recent data supporting the use of IVF/ICSI to reduce HIV transmission to uninfected women. A 10-year retrospective study of 181 serodiscordant couples undergoing IVF/ICSI, in which sperm was prepared using a modified density-gradient centrifugation and the swim-up method, revealed no HIV infection among the uninfected women and their 170 children.[88] Another study from the Center for Reproductive Assisted Techniques for HIV in Europe reported no evidence of seroconversion in any uninfected partners or children on follow-up.[86] Unfortunately, these techniques are generally prohibitively expensive. Although the data on efficacy and safety of the AFT techniques are encouraging, the potential risk of HIV transmission is not completely eliminated and more studies are required. Until then, serodiscordant couples should also be counseled about other safer options, including using donor sperm, donor embryo, adoption, or not having children.[82] If couples want to have their own biological children, they should be informed about available risk reduction techniques and the availability of centers that can provide effective methods of sperm preparation and testing. Fertility centers should use approved study protocols with informed consent and provide appropriate follow-up of sexual partners and their children.

4.3.3. AFT when both partners are infected

While HIV seroconcordant couples do not have the same concerns about HIV transmission as do HIV serodiscordant couples, the risk of transmission of different strains of HIV between each other or superinfection exists. HIV superinfection in seroconcordant couples has been reported to increase the risk of HIV RNA rebound and decrease in CD4 cell count following immune reactivation.[89] The best way to minimize the risk of superinfection and optimize reproductive outcomes for couples and their offspring is to use cART to achieve HIV RNA suppression in both partners prior to conception attempts.

4.4. Healthcare workers and cross-contamination risks

Healthcare workers are at risk of exposure to blood-borne pathogens, including HIV through patient care. However, if standard universal precautions to prevent the transmission of infectious diseases are followed, the risk of acquiring these pathogens is very small and is not sufficient to deny reproductive services to PLWHIV. To date, there have been no reports of occupational HIV transmission to health care workers performing AFT, suggesting that the risk of transmission is extremely low. Theoretical concerns about contaminating other gametes and embryos stored in the same laboratory from cross-contamination have been raised. To date, no such event has been reported. To avoid this risk, it is recommended that samples from HIV-infected persons be processed in a separate laboratory or designated space within the main laboratory and to use a dedicated storage tank.[82]

5. Conclusions

Reproductive issues have become more relevant among PLWHIV who are living longer and are staying healthier on cART. Fertility outcomes of PLWHIV have been improving for the past decade, although they remain inferior to those of the general population. HIV can impact fertility in many ways that involve biological, psychological, and social factors. Assessing and managing fertility issues in HIV-infected individuals and couples involve the use of cART, diagnosing and correcting causes of infertility, and AFT, which has become more effective and safer. Further studies are needed to address the efficacy and safety of AFT techniques as well as the complex social and ethical challenges of fertility issues of HIV-infected persons. Healthcare workers caring for PLWHIV should be knowledgeable in both HIV infection and reproductive health because they may now be legally and ethically obligated to provide reproductive care and assistance to this population.

Author details

Thana Khawcharoenporn[1*] and Beverly E. Sha[2]

*Address all correspondence to: thanak30@yahoo.com

1 Division of Infectious Diseases, Faculty of Medicine, Thammasat University, Pathumthani, Thailand

2 Division of Infectious Diseases, Rush University Medical Center, Chicago, IL, USA

References

[1] UNAIDS. Fact Sheet 2015. Available at: www.unaids.org/en/resources/campaigns/HowAIDSchangedeverything/factsheet. Accessed 16 December 2015.

[2] May M, Gompels M, Delpech V, Porter K, Post F, Johnson M, et al. Impact of late diagnosis and treatment on life expectancy in people with HIV-1: UK Collaborative HIV Cohort (UK CHIC) Study. BMJ 2011; 343: d6016. doi: 10.1136/bmj.d6016.

[3] Kushnir VA, Lewis W. Human immunodeficiency virus/acquired immunodeficiency syndrome and infertility: emerging problems in the era of highly active antiretrovirals. Fertil Steril 2011; 96: 546–553.

[4] Zaba B, Gregson S. Measuring the impact of HIV on fertility in Africa. AIDS 1998; 12 Suppl 1: S41–S50.

[5] Massad LS, Springer G, Jacobson L, Watts H, Anastos K, Korn A, et al. Pregnancy rates and predictors of conception, miscarriage and abortion in US women with HIV. AIDS 2004; 18: 281–286.

[6] Chen WJ, Walker N. Fertility of HIV-infected women: insights from demographic and health surveys. Sex Transm Infect 2010; 86: ii22–ii27.

[7] Frodsham LC, Boag F, Barton S, Gilling-Smith C. Human immunodeficiency virus infection and fertility care in the United Kingdom: demand and supply. Fertil Steril 2006; 85: 285–289.

[8] Westreich D, Maskew M, Rubel D, MacDonald P, Jaffray I, Majuba P. Incidence of pregnancy after initiation of antiretroviral therapy in South Africa: a retrospective clinical cohort analysis. Infect Dis Obstet Gynecol 2012; 2012: 917059.

[9] Huntington SE, Thorne C, Bansi LK, Anderson J, Newell ML, Taylor GP, et al. Predictors of pregnancy and changes in pregnancy incidence among HIV-positive women accessing HIV clinical care. AIDS 2013; 27: 95–103.

[10] Lancaster KE, Kwok C, Rinaldi A, Byamugisha J, Magwali T, Nyamapfeni P, et al. Incident pregnancy and pregnancy outcomes among HIV-infected women in Uganda and Zimbabwe. Int J Gynaecol Obstet 2015; 131: 255–259.

[11] Chirgwin KD, Feldman J, Muneyyirci-Delale O, Landesman S, Minkoff H. Menstrual function in human immunodeficiency virus-infected women without acquired immunodeficiency syndrome. J Acquir Immune Defic Syndr Hum Retrovirol 1996; 12: 489–94.

[12] Cejtin HE, Kalinowski A, Bacchetti P, Taylor RN, Watts DH, Kim S, et al. Effects of human immunodeficiency virus on protracted amenorrhea and ovarian dysfunction. Obstet Gynecol 2006; 108: 1423–1431.

[13] Ellerbrock TV, Wright TC, Bush TJ, Dole P, Brudney K, Chiasson M. Characteristics of menstruation in women infected with HIV. Obstet Gynecol 1996; 87: 1030–1034.

[14] Harlow SC, Schuman P, Cohen M, Ohmit SE, Cu-Uvin S, Lin X, et al. Effect of HIV infection on menstrual cycle length. J Acquir Immune Defic Syndr 2000; 24: 68–75.

[15] Seifer DB, Golub ET, Lambert-Messerlian G, Springer G, Holman S, Moxley M, et al. Biologic markers of ovarian reserve and reproductive aging: application in a cohort study of HIV infection in women. Fertil Steril 2007; 88: 1645–1652.

[16] Coll O, Fiore S, Floridia M, Giaquinto C, Grosch-Wörner I, Guiliano M, et al. Pregnancy and HIV infection: a European consensus on management. AIDS 2002; 16 Suppl 2: S1–S18.

[17] White DJ, Mital D, Taylor S, St John JC. Sperm mitochondrial DNA deletions as a consequence of long term highly active antiretroviral therapy. AIDS 2001; 15: 1061–1062.

[18] Bujan L, Sergerie M, Moinard N, Martinet S, Porte L, Massip P, et al. Decreased semen volume and spermatozoa motility in HIV-1-infected patients under antiretroviral treatment. J Androl 2007; 28: 444–452.

[19] Nicopoullos JD, Almeida PA, Ramsay JW, Gilling-Smith C. The effect of human immunodeficiency virus on sperm parameters and the outcome of intrauterine insemination following sperm washing. Hum Reprod 2004; 19: 2289–2297.

[20] Crittenden JA, Handelsman DJ, Stewart GJ. Semen analysis in human immunodeficiency virus infection. Fertil Steril 1992; 57: 1294–1299.

[21] Shevchuk MM, Pigato JB, Khalife G, Armenakas NA, Fracchia JA. Changing testicular histology in AIDS: its implication for sexual transmission of HIV. Urology 1999; 53: 203–208.

[22] Nicopoullos JD, Almeida P, Vourliotis M, Gilling-Smith C. A decade of the sperm-washing programme: correlation between markers of HIV and seminal parameters. HIV Med 2011; 12: 195–201.

[23] Wanke CA, Silva M, Knox TA, Forrester J, Speigelman D, Gorbach SL. Weight loss and wasting remain common complications in individuals infected with human immunodeficiency virus in the era of highly active antiretroviral therapy. Clin Infect Dis 2000; 31: 803–805.

[24] Dobs AS, Dempsey MA, Ladenson PW, Polk BF. Endocrine disorders in men infected with human immunodeficiency virus. Am J Med 1988; 84: 611–616.

[25] Raffi F, Brisseau JM, Planchon B, Rémi JP, Barrier JH, Grolleau JY. Endocrine function in 98 HIV-infected patients: a prospective study. AIDS 1991; 5: 729–733.

[26] Christeff N, Gharakhanian S, Thobie N, Rozenbaum W, Nunez EA. Evidence for changes in adrenal and testicular steroids during HIV infection. J Acquir Immune Defic Syndr 1992; 5: 841–846.

[27] Dubé MP, Parker RA, Mulligan K, Tebas P, Robbins GK, Roubenoff R, et al. Effects of potent antiretroviral therapy on free testosterone levels and fat-free mass in men in a prospective, randomized trial: A5005s, a substudy of AIDS Clinical Trials Group Study 384. Clin Infect Dis 2007; 45: 120–126.

[28] Klein RS, Lo Y, Santoro N, Dobs AS. Androgen levels in older men who have or who are at risk of acquiring HIV infection. Clin Infect Dis 2005; 41: 1794–1803.

[29] Araujo AB, O'Donnell AB, Brambilla DJ, Simpson WB, Longcope C, Matsumoto AM, et al. Prevalence and incidence of androgen deficiency in middle-aged and older men: estimates from the Massachusetts Male Aging Study. J Clin Endocrinol Metab 2004; 89: 5920–5926.

[30] Grossmann M, Gianatti EJ, Zajac JD. Testosterone and type 2 diabetes. Curr Opin Endocrinol Diabetes Obes 2010; 17: 247–256.

[31] Zitzmann M. Testosterone deficiency, insulin resistance and the metabolic syndrome. Nat Rev Endocrinol 2009; 5: 673–681.

[32] Misra M, Papakostas GI, Klibanski A. Effects of psychiatric disorders and psychotropic medications on prolactin and bone metabolism. J Clin Psychiatry 2004; 65: 1607–1618.

[33] Cooper OB, Brown TT, Dobs AS. Opiate drug use: a potential contributor to the endocrine and metabolic complications in human immunodeficiency virus disease. Clin Infect Dis 2003; 37 Suppl 2: S132–S136.

[34] Bhasin S, Cunningham GR, Hayes FJ, Matsumoto AM, Snyder PJ, Swerdloff RS, et al. Testosterone therapy in men with androgen deficiency syndromes: an Endocrine Society clinical practice guideline. J Clin Endocrinol Metab 2010; 95: 2536–2559.

[35] Bezold G, Politch JA, Kiviat NB, Kuypers JM, Wolff H, Anderson DJ. Prevalence of sexually transmissible pathogens in semen from asymptomatic male infertility patients with and without leukocytospermia. Fertil Steril 2007; 87: 1087–1097.

[36] Ochsendrof FR. Sexually transmitted infections: impact on male fertility. Andrologia 2008; 40: 72–75.

[37] Eggert-Kruse W, Gerhard I, Näher H, Tilgen W, Runnebaum B. Chlamydial infection —a female and/or male infertility factor? Fertil Steril 1990; 53: 1037–1043.

[38] Reichart M, Kahane I, Bartoov B. In vivo and in vitro impairment of human and ram sperm nuclear chromatin integrity by sexually transmitted *Ureaplasma urealyticum* infection. Biol Reprod 2000; 63: 1041–1048.

[39] Svenstrup HF, Fedder J, Abraham-Peskir J, Birkelund S, Christiansen G. *Mycoplasma genitalium* attaches to human spermatozoa. Hum Reprod 2003; 18: 2103–2109.

[40] Michelson HE. Syphilis of the epididymis. JAMA 1919; 73: 1431–1433.

[41] Varma R, Baithun S, Alexander S, Goh BT. Acute syphilitic interstitial orchitis mimicking testicular malignancy in an HIV-1 infected man diagnosed by *Treponema pallidum* polymerase chain reaction. Int J STD AIDS 2009; 20: 65–66.

[42] Garolla A, Pizzol D, Bertoldo A, Menegazzo M, Barzon L, Foresta C. Sperm viral infection and male infertility: focus on HBV, HCV, HIV, HPV, HSV, HCMV, and AAV. J Reprod Immunol 2013; 100: 20–29.

[43] Neofytou E, Sourvinos G, Asmarianaki M, Spandidos DA, Makrigiannakis A. Prevalence of human herpes virus types 1-7 in the semen of men attending an infertility clinic and correlation with semen parameters. Fertil Steril 2009; 91: 2487–2494.

[44] Fichorova RN. Impact of *T. vaginalis* infection on innate immune responses and reproductive outcome. J Reprod Immunol 2009; 83: 185–189.

[45] Brookings C, Goldmeier D, Sadeghi-Nejad H. Sexually transmitted infections and sexual function in relation to male fertility. Korean J Urol 2013; 54: 149–156.

[46] Lewis W, Day BJ, Copeland WC. Mitochondrial toxicity of NRTI antiviral drugs: an integrated cellular perspective. Nat Rev Drug Discov 2003; 2: 812–22.

[47] Pavili L, Daudin M, Moinard N, Walschaerts M, Cuzin L, Massip P, et al. Decrease of mitochondrial DNA level in sperm from patients infected with human immunodeficiency virus-1 linked to nucleoside analogue reverse transcriptase inhibitors. Fertil Steril 2010; 94: 2151–2156.

[48] Lopez S, Coll O, Durban M, Hernandez S, Vidal R, Suy A, et al. Mitochondrial DNA depletion in oocytes of HIV-infected antiretroviral-treated infertile women. Antivir Ther 2008; 13: 833–838.

[49] May-Panloup P, Chretien MF, Jacques C, Vasseur C, Malthiery Y, Reynier P. Low oocyte mitochondrial DNA content in ovarian insufficiency. Hum Reprod 2005; 20: 593–597.

[50] Myer L, Carter RJ, Katyal M, Toro P, El-Sadr WM, Abrams EJ. Impact of antiretroviral therapy on incidence of pregnancy among HIV-infected women in Sub-Saharan Africa: a cohort study. PLoS Med 2010; 7: e1000229.

[51] Toltzis P, Mourton T, Magnuson T. Effect of zidovudine on preimplantation murine embryos. Antimicrob Agents Chemother 1993; 37: 1610–1613.

[52] Toltzis P, Marx CM, Kleinman N, Levine EM, Schmidt EV. Zidovudine-associated embryonic toxicity in mice. J Infect Dis 1991; 163: 1212–1218.

[53] Gerschenson M, Nguyen V, Ewings EL, Ceresa A, Shaw JA, St Claire MC, et al. Mitochondrial toxicity in fetal *Erythrocebus patas* monkeys exposed transplacentally to zidovudine plus lamivudine. AIDS Res Hum Retroviruses 2004; 20: 91–100.

[54] Delvaux T, Nöstlinger C. Reproductive choice for women and men living with HIV: contraception, abortion and fertility. Reprod Health Matters 2007; 15: 46–66.

[55] Agboghoroma CO, Giwa-Osagie OF. Management of infertility in HIV infected couples: a review. Afr J Reprod Health 2012; 16: 13–20.

[56] Stephenson JM, Griffioen A. The effect of HIV diagnosis on reproductive experience. Study Group for the Medical Research Council Collaborative Study of Women with HIV. AIDS 1996; 10: 1683–1687.

[57] Thackway SV, Furner V, Mijch A, Cooper DA, Holland D, Martinez P, et al. Fertility and reproductive choice in women with HIV-1 infection. AIDS 1997; 11: 663–667.

[58] Wilson TE, Massad LS, Riester KA, Barkan S, Richardson J, Young M, et al. Sexual, contraceptive, and drug use behaviors of women with HIV and those at high risk for infection: results from the Women's Interagency HIV Study. AIDS 1999; 13: 591–598.

[59] Floridia M, Tamburrini E, Tibaldi C, Anzidei G, Muggiasca ML, Meloni A, et al. Voluntary pregnancy termination among women with HIV in the HAART era (2002–2008): a case series from a national study. AIDS Care 2010; 22: 50–53.

[60] Townsend CL, Cortina-Borja M, Peckham CS, Tookey PA. Trends in management and outcome of pregnancies in HIV-infected women in the UK and Ireland, 1990–2006. BJOG 2008; 115: 1078–1086.

[61] Bongain A, Berrebi A, Mariné-Barjoan E, Dunais B, Thene M, Pradier C, et al. Changing trends in pregnancy outcome among HIV-infected women between 1985 and 1997 in two southern French university hospitals. Eur J Obstet Gynecol Reprod Biol 2002; 104: 124–128.

[62] Finocchario-Kessler S, Sweat MD, Dariotis JK, Anderson JR, Jennings JM, Keller JM, et al. Childbearing motivations, pregnancy desires, and perceived partner response to a pregnancy among urban female youth: does HIV-infection status make a difference? AIDS Care 2012; 24: 1–11.

[63] Craft SM, Delaney RO, Bautista DT, Serovich JM. Pregnancy decisions among women with HIV. AIDS Behav 2007; 11: 927–935.

[64] Nattabi B, Li J, Thompson SC, Orach CG, Earnest J. A systematic review of factors influencing fertility desires and intentions among people living with HIV/AIDS: implications for policy and service delivery. AIDS Behav 2009; 13: 949–968.

[65] Squires KE, Hodder SL, Feinberg J, Bridge DA, Abrams S, Storfer SP, et al. Health needs of HIV-infected women in the United States: insights from the women living positive survey. AIDS Patient Care STDS 2011; 25: 279–285.

[66] Ethics Committee of the American Society for Reproductive Medicine. Human immunodeficiency virus and infertility treatment. Fertil Steril 2010; 94: 11–15.

[67] Department of Health and Human Services. Guidelines for the use of antiretroviral agents in HIV-1-infected adults and adolescents. Available at: http://aidsinfo.nih.gov/guidelines. Accessed 3 January 2016.

[68] Lundgren JD, Babiker AG, Gordin F, Emery S, Grund B, Sharma S, et al. Initiation of antiretroviral therapy in early asymptomatic HIV infection. N Engl J Med 2015; 373: 795–807.

[69] European AIDS Clinical Society. The European Guidelines for treatment of HIV-infected adults in Europe. Available at: www.eacsociety.org/guidelines/eacs-guidelines/eacs-guidelines.html. Accessed 3 January 2016.

[70] World Health Organization. Consolidated guidelines on the use of antiretroviral drugs for treating and preventing HIV infection. Available at: www.who.int/hiv/pub/guidelines/arv2013/download/en/. Accessed 3 January 2016.

[71] Basaria S, Coviello AD, Travison TG, Storer TW, Farwell WR, Jette AM, et al. Adverse events associated with testosterone administration. N Engl J Med 2010; 363: 109–122.

[72] Kaida A, Lima VD, Andia I, Kabakyenga J, Mbabazi P, Emenyonu N, et al. The WHOMEN's Scale (Women's HAART Optimism Monitoring and EvaluatioN Scale v. 1) and the association with fertility intentions and sexual behaviours among HIV-positive women in Uganda. AIDS Behav 2009; 13: S72–S81.

[73] Galvin SR, Cohen MS. The role of sexually transmitted diseases in HIV transmission. Nat Rev Microbiol 2004; 2: 33–42.

[74] Laga M, Nzila N, Goeman J. The interrelationship of sexually transmitted diseases and HIV infection: implications for the control of both epidemics in Africa. AIDS 1991; 5: S55–S63.

[75] Otten RA, Smith DK, Adams DR, Pullium JK, Jackson E, Kim CN, et al. Efficacy of postexposure prophylaxis after intravaginal exposure of pig-tailed macaques to a human-derived retrovirus (human immunodeficiency virus type 2). J Virol 2000; 74: 9771–9775.

[76] Cardo DM, Culver DH, Ciesielski CA, Srivastava PU, Marcus R, Abiteboul D, et al. A case-control study of HIV seroconversion in healthcare workers after percutaneous exposure. Centers for Disease Control and Prevention Needlestick Surveillance Group. N Engl J Med 1997; 337: 1485–1490.

[77] Kuhar DT, Henderson DK, Struble KA, Heneine W, Thomas V, Cheever LW, et al. Updated US Public Health Service guidelines for the management of occupational exposures to human immunodeficiency virus and recommendations for postexposure prophylaxis. Infect Control Hosp Epidemiol 2013; 34: 875–892.

[78] Abdool Karim Q, Abdool Karim SS, Frohlich JA, Grobler AC, Baxter C, Mansoor LE, et al. Effectiveness and safety of tenofovir gel, an antiretroviral microbicide, for the prevention of HIV infection in women. Science 2010; 329: 1168–1174.

[79] Grant RM, Lama JR, Anderson PL, McMahan V, Liu AY, Vargas L et al. Preexposure chemoprophylaxis for HIV prevention in men who have sex with men. N Engl J Med 2010; 363: 2587–2599.

[80] Baeten JM, Donnell D, Ndase P, Mugo NR, Campbell JD, Wangisi J et al. Antiretroviral prophylaxis for HIV prevention in heterosexual men and women. N Engl J Med 2012; 367: 399–410.

[81] Thigpen MC, Kebaabetswe PM, Paxton LA, Smith DK, Rose CE, Segolodi TM, et al. Antiretroviral preexposure prophylaxis for heterosexual HIV transmission in Botswana. N Engl J Med 2012; 367: 423–434.

[82] Ethics Committee of American Society for Reproductive Medicine. Human immunodeficiency virus (HIV) and infertility treatment: a committee opinion. Fertil Steril 2015; 104: e1–e8.

[83] Mandelbrot L, Heard I, Henrion-Geeant E, Henrion R. Natural conception in HIV-negative women with HIV-infected partners. Lancet 1997; 349: 850–851.

[84] Vernazza PL, Graf I, Sonnenberg-Schwan U, Geit M, Meurer A. Preexposure prophylaxis and timed intercourse for HIV-discordant couples willing to conceive a child. AIDS 2011; 25: 2005–2008.

[85] Semprini AE, Levi-Setti P, Ravizza M, Pardi G. Assisted conception to reduce the risk of male-to-female sexual transfer of HIV in serodiscordant couples: an update [abstract]. Presented at the 1998 Symposium on AIDS in Women, Sao Paulo, Brazil, September 14–15, 1998.

[86] Bujan L, Hollander L, Coudert M, Gilling-Smith C, Vucetich A, Guibert J, et al. Safety and efficacy of sperm washing in HIV-1 serodiscordant couples where the male is infected: results from the European CREAThE network. AIDS 2007; 21: 1909–1914.

[87] Kambin S, Batzer F. Assisted reproductive technology in HIV serodiscordant couples. Sex Reprod Menopause 2004; 2: 92–100.

[88] Sauer MV, Wang JG, Douglas NC, Nakhuda GS, Vardhana P, Jovanovic V, et al. Providing fertility care to men seropositive for human immunodeficiency virus: reviewing 10 years of experience and 420 consecutive cycles of in vitro fertilization and intracytoplasmic sperm injection. Fertil Steril 2009; 91: 2455–2460.

[89] Smith DM, Richman DD, Little SJ. HIV superinfection. J Infect Dis 2005; 192: 438–444.

7

Communicable Diseases Among Refugees with a Focus on the Middle East

Inaya Hajj Hussein, Ibrahim Mortada,
Alice Gerges Geagea and Abdo Jurjus

Abstract

During the past few years, millions of refugees from the Middle East and North Africa fled their countries to almost everywhere in the globe. Civil wars and acts of violence are the main reasons behind the exodus of populations seeking a better life and more secure living conditions. In fact, the current conflict in Syria and Iraq led to massive influx of refugees worldwide and in particular to neighboring countries of the Middle East. This refugee situation is unparalleled since the end of World War II. Besides the individual tragedies of refugees, a public health disaster is being witnessed in the countries of origin which, in many instances, affect the hosting countries as well. Many of these hosting countries witnessed a re-emergence of numerous communicable diseases as a result of the influx of refugees; they were unprepared, and their health sectors did not deliver the adequate response. In this chapter, we review major sexually transmitted diseases in refugees, with a focus on the Middle East. We also discuss the major actions taken in response to the ongoing displacement of refugees by the Government of Lebanon and suggest solutions and recommendations to the Lebanese public health system which is facing new urgent challenges.

Keywords: STIs, refugees' health, communicable diseases, Middle East, Lebanon, Syrian refugees

1. Introduction

During the past decade, millions of refugees worldwide, in particular from the Middle East, fled their home country. The United Nations reported that at the end of 2010, there were over 43 million people in the world displaced because of conflict or persecution [1]. The latest counts conducted by the United Nations High Commissioner for Refugees (UNHCR) revealed that there have been 16,121,427 refugees by the end of 2015 [2]. Over half of the refugees worldwide came from Syria, Iraq, Afghanistan and Somalia and the top hosting countries were Turkey (2.5 millions), Pakistan (1.6 million), Lebanon (1.1 million) and Jordan (0.5 million) [3]. Refugees face multiple barriers in accessing healthcare and maintaining proper follow-ups, including lack of resources needed to cover expenses, cultural differences and lack of health care facilities in the regions of residence.

The purpose of this chapter is to shed light on the reproductive health of displaced people in the Middle East, including sexually transmitted diseases.

2. Health of refugees at the international level

In the United States of America, 18,007 Syrian refugees were resettled between October 1, 2011 and December 31, 2016. Despite the huge resources in the United States of America, the establishment of Medicaid was not sufficient to assure that all refugees have been adequately screened for diseases and have access to proper medical care. In many states, it was difficult to find health clinics that were willing to provide regular appointments to refugees on Medicaid, especially since the services needed to encompass primary care and include specialty clinics and surgery [4].

Europe is experiencing one of the most significant influxes of migrants and refugees in its history. European countries received over 2 million asylum applications in 2015, which represent around a three-fold increase to the number of applications received in 2014 (709,757). Most applications were from Syria (675,668), Afghanistan (406,300) and Iraq (253,558). Around 60% of these applications (1.2 million) were received by European Union member states with Germany and Sweden receiving almost half of the total applications. The number of refugees entering Europe passed the 1 million mark in 2015, a long expected and symbolically significant capstone to a year in which displaced persons flocked to the continent in historic proportions [5].

History is rife with examples of infectious diseases that have been linked to human mobility and migration. Diseases and epidemics often accompanied commercial traders, sailors, pilgrims and other migrants to thrive in new and foreign environments [6]. One particularly famous example is the re-emergence of tuberculosis (TB) in Europe. While once considered a disease of the past, new cases of TB in Europe and the West are frequently attributed to the migration of people from endemic countries, such as Africa and India [7]. In some refugee settings, women and children are believed to comprise about 80% of the population, and they are the most vulnerable to the consequences of displacement, including rape, infectious diseases, and, in particular, sexually transmitted infections (STIs) [8]. In addition, sexual violence and poverty were highlighted as leading to an increase in the transmission of STIs, HIV/AIDS and unwanted and/or high-risk pregnancies. Many become disconnected from their relatives and from their traditional cultural and legal supports. Such issues also impact their reproductive health status. If the hosting countries do not provide adequate reproductive health care services, this could aggravate the situation through unwanted pregnancy and unsafe abortion. In addition, such refugees carry an important disease burden due to disease prevalence in their country of origin, disruption of immunization programs, or even exposure during migration [9].

3. Health of refugees at the regional and national levels

In the Middle East and North Africa, increasing numbers of refugees are being noted as a result of complex political conflicts. Millions of Syrian and Iraqi refugees fled to neighbouring countries or to Europe, the United States of America and other countries. The UNHCR Syria End of Year Report 2015 estimated that 4.2 million of the Syrian populations were refugees, and the average life expectancy of Syrians has fallen by 20 years since the onset of the crisis [10]. Such groups are diverse and require different health and humanitarian interventions, particularly in the reproductive health needs as well as infectious diseases like TB and hepatitis and, in particular, sexually transmitted infections including HIV/AIDS. The UNHCR as well as hosting countries and humanitarian relief organizations agree that reproductive health care should be a priority during such an emergency situation. Several challenges exist to face the situation, and activities must be strengthened in some key areas, such as adolescents' health, in particular HIV and STI prevention and care and an adequate response to sexual and gender-based violence [10].

Lebanon is a country in the Middle East with a population of 4.2 million [11]. Since the 1970s, the Lebanese healthcare system has had to face many challenges due to multiple reasons including wars, political instability, economic difficulties and massive influx of refugees with about 500,000 Palestinian refugees since 1948 [12]. However, the most pressing challenge facing Lebanon is the Syrian refugee crisis. Following the start of the acts of violence in Syria in 2011, there have been an increasing number of Syrian refugees coming to Lebanon. By the end of 2015, their numbers had reached 1.5 million, in addition to 53,000 Palestinians returning from Syria and about 50,000 Iraqis [13]. The new refugees represent more than a 30% increase in Lebanon's pre-crisis population, resulting in the highest refugee density of any country worldwide since 1980 [14]. The refugees from Syria have not been placed in formal camps but are dispersed across Lebanon in houses among the Lebanese population, while about 17% are residing in informal tented settlements [15]. The unprecedented influx of refugees has put a heavy burden on the Lebanese government, society and economy, which is facing many other challenges. The refugee crisis threatens the ability of the government to provide adequate and sustained health services which puts thousands of individuals at risk of acquiring and spreading different infectious diseases. It is estimated that, on average, there are about 50,000–55,000 new deliveries per year among the Syrians in Lebanon. In addition, there are reported cases of HIV infections as well as other sexually transmitted infections.

Previous research by the International Rescue Committee and the Resource Center for Gender Equality ABAAD conducted in Lebanon in August 2012 highlighted that some refugee women and girls in Lebanon have resorted to prostitution as a means to generate an income and meet basic needs. The research noted that 'survival sex' is a type of violence that Syrian women are frequently subjected to [16].

4. Sexually transmitted infections

In this chapter, the discussion will cover the most important sexually transmitted infections among refugee populations, including hepatitis B, hepatitis C, chlamydia/gonorrhea, HIV/AIDS and tuberculosis.

4.1. Hepatitis B

Hepatitis B is a viral infection that is potentially life-threatening and is a major common global health concern. Infection with hepatitis B virus is prevalent among all refugee groups. Screening for hepatitis B identifies susceptible individuals who can be offered vaccine and infected individuals who are eligible for treatment. Most screening protocols test for hepatitis B surface antigen (HBsAg) and its antibody (HBsAb). Refugees identified as HBsAg positive will need further testing to identify the stage of the disease and need for treatment. Understanding beliefs about hepatitis B in refugee populations is important when discussing the implications of test results and will facilitate compliance with prevention strategies and management of the disease. A cross-sectional study among 2769 Tibetan refugees residing in India reported HbsAg seropositivity in 247 (8.9%) individuals of which 60.7% were positive for hepatitis B e antigen, indicating higher infectivity and chances of transmission [17]. In Lebanon, among the Syrian refugees, a rise in hepatitis B incidence was noted from a total of 8 cases in 2013 to 48 cases in 2016 [18]. This shows a trend that is supported by clinical observations. However, a more reliable house-to-house survey could be considered.

4.2. Hepatitis C

Hepatitis C is a contagious blood-borne viral infection caused by the hepatitis C virus (HCV), leading to both acute and chronic hepatitis infection. In a study looking at the prevalence of active hepatitis C virus infections among refugees in the United States of America from various countries in Africa and Asia, it was reported that 63 out of a total of 4890 (1.1%) were positive for HCV RNA. The refugees from Thailand had greater numbers of HCV-positive samples than refugees from other countries [19]. In Lebanon, among the Syrian refugees, the number of reported cases of Hepatitis C doubled from a total of four cases in 2013 to eight cases in 2016 [18], a trend similar to hepatitis B.

4.3. Chlamydia/gonorrhea

Chlamydia and gonorrhea are a major cause of acute disease, infertility and perinatal morbidity and mortality worldwide. It is well known that refugees are at an increased risk of these infections because of many factors associated with civil disruption and displacement, including poor sanitation and/or socioeconomic status resulting in vulnerability to sexual exploitation, sexual violence and abuse and lack of access to prevention and educational efforts. The current CDC guidelines recommend annual screening for chlamydia in sexually active females > 25 years of age with risk factors (e.g., new sex partner or multiple sex partners). Testing is also recommended in those with signs or symptoms of infection or when infection is suspected, usually through medical history and physical examination. In such cases, the use of urine ligase chain reaction to detect gonorrhea and chlamydia infection is most appropriate. Moreover, cervical cancer is the second-most common cause of female cancer mortality worldwide, accounting for approximately 274,000 deaths annually [20]. 70% of cervical cancers are due to high-risk human papillomavirus (HPV) types 16 and 18. The majority of female refugees are from countries where cytologic screening and HPV testing are limited or absent, which leaves this population at a much more increased risk of developing cervical cancer later on in their life. Therefore, cervical cancer screening should be prioritized at the level of other early resettlement issues, such as infectious disease screening and treatment. Results from a screening medical examination of 25,779 refugees arriving to Minnesota during 2003–2010 showed that a total of 18,516 (72%) refugees tested positive for at least one sexually transmitted infection: 183 (1.1%) of 17,235 were seropositive for syphilis, 15 (0.6%) of 2512 were positive for chlamydia, 5 (0.2%) of 2403 were positive for gonorrhea and 136 (2.0%) of 6765 were positive for human immunodeficiency virus [21]. In Lebanon, data are not available concerning such disease entities among refugees. However, clinical observations indicate a rise in their prevalence.

4.4. HIV/AIDS

HIV/AIDS is another commonly seen viral infection caused by the human immunodeficiency virus that still has cure, and currently up to 36.7 million people are living with HIV, with almost half only being treated. This contagious viral infection is spread through bodily fluids attacking the body's immune system mainly the CD4+ cells or T cells, leading to opportunistic infections which are behind the detrimental effects of HIV or the acquired immunodeficiency syndrome [22].

With the extremely high number of people living with HIV, the greatest toll is in sub-Saharan Africa which also accounts for three-quarters of the global death count. The epidemiological impact of HIV has also consequences on the society's development since most of the affected people are young and in their most productive years; there is a negative relationship between the rise of HIV prevalence and the growth of gross domestic product [23]. The only currently available treatment for HIV is through antiretroviral therapy which limits the infections and AIDS; this therapy is also used in pre- and post-exposure prophylaxis treatments in high-risk populations [22].

In Lebanon, a study was conducted exploring the socio-demographic correlates of condom use and HIV testing among men who have sex with men refugees, by surveying and testing 150 participants. Results revealed that a total of four (2.7%) participants tested positive for HIV [24]. The National AIDS Program at the Lebanese Ministry of Public Health (MOPH) reveals a slight increase in the number of newly reported cases of HIV/AIDS from 93 in 2010 to 109 in 2014 with a few being refugees, about 10 cases being reported [25]. All patients have free access to a comprehensive management protocol according to the World Health Organization criteria.

4.5. Tuberculosis

Most cases of TB in immigrants are due to the reactivation of infection with *Mycobacterium tuberculosis*. As refugees often arrive from parts of the world where TB is more common, it is not unusual to identify cases of latent TB infection in these individuals. All refugees must have a physical and mental examination conducted by an approved physician; this medical screening includes a physical examination, including a chest X-ray, and an evaluation for tuberculosis. Any refugee with a chest X-ray suggestive of a current or past TB disease must undergo additional stringent laboratory testing. If laboratory tests are positive for an active TB disease, treatment is required for at least 6 months. Among 11,773 newly arrived asylum seekers in Germany, 16 X-ray investigations gave the suspicion of active tuberculosis, thereof 11 cases could be verified by culture and thereof 9 cases were classified as microscopically positive [26]. In Turkey, the prevalence of TB among 10,689 Syrian refugees was found to be 18.7/100,000. However, the actual prevalence may be even more since many refugees are not in camps and many are homeless in big cities and are therefore at high risk of getting infected with TB. In Jordan, the incidence of TB increased by 40% between 2013 (56 cases/16 months) and 2014 (74 cases/12 months) [27]. In Lebanon, there has been a 27% increase in TB cases since 2011 [28]; the government provides free medical care including the drugs for 6 months to all those living in the country including refugees from various places.

5. Discussion

Since the beginning of the refugee influx to Lebanon, a highly indebted middle-income country with a history of political strife, presence of other vulnerable displaced populations and weak government capacities [29], the conflict brought increasing hardships to both populations. Lebanese and Syrians share economic difficulties and security impacts that are increasing the tensions between the formerly harmonious neighbors [30]. The Regional Refugee and Resilience Plan 2015–2016, including the Lebanese Crisis Response Plan (LCRP), is one of the response plans put in place in an effort to enable the country to cope with the many emerging needs imposed by the refugee crisis. The LCRP is managed by the UNHCR and the United Nations Development Project. It attempts to raise US$2.14 billion to provide protection and humanitarian assistance to 2.2 million de facto Syrian refugees who are highly vulnerable and have acute needs and invest in institutions, services and economies to reach 2.9 million vulnerable people. The LCRP has three strategic priorities or response areas which address the capacities of affected communities, national government and Lebanese. The three response strategies work on nine sectors including basic assistance; food security; shelter; education; water, hygiene, and sanitation (WASH); livelihoods; health; social stability and protection [31].

Moreover, a mapping of ongoing reproductive health (RH) activities was conducted in October 2014, in collaboration with 17 health actors. Results of this mapping revealed that nearly 90% of actors offer RH education through health centers and mobile medical units, 80% implement RH education at community level through outreach and 6% provide RH education through campaigns. The north region is covered by 31% of actors, Beirut and Mount Lebanon regions by 56%, Bekaa region by 50% and the south region by 31%. 90% of health education projects cover family planning, whereas pregnancy and breastfeeding are covered by 80% of projects. Reproductive tract infections and sexually transmitted infections are covered among 68% of the projects and 56% cover prenatal and postnatal care. The age group targeted through RH activities is mostly 14–60 years old, including youth. Women are reached within most of the health education activities, but there are 4 out of 16 actors also reaching men. RH consultation counts revealed around 28,372 pregnant woman and 18,243 family planning visits. All RH education projects target Syrian refugees, whereas 44% target also Lebanese and 12% Palestinians [32].

6. Recommendations

Based on the reviewed data, the authors who are basically partially involved in this field recommend that

1. It is urgent to adopt a new strategy and an innovative approach to support the Lebanese public health system in providing good quality of care to the Syrian and Iraqi refugees while fulfilling their mission to be at the service of the hosting Lebanese citizens and the populations residing in Lebanon.
2. It is imperative to implement pre-departure screening programs at the countries of origin in order to detect and possibly start treatment of communicable diseases as early as possible. This will also limit the risks of spreading any of these diseases among the population of the hosting country. A study assessing the health status of newly arrived refugees in Toronto, Canada, revealed considerably higher rates of various infectious diseases such as HIV and hepatitis B among refugees compared to the Canadian-born population, highlighting the importance of early screening and providing timely preventive and curative care [33].
3. To improve refugees knowledge of available health services, intensifying awareness on the location of the network of health services where support is available is important. This should especially address the subsidies for primary healthcare services and the availability of free vaccines, screening campaigns, essential and chronic medicines and family planning services at facilities in the MoPH network. Awareness-raising should continue through UNHCR reception centers, community centers, outreach workers, municipalities, NGO partners and mass information campaigns.
4. Humanitarian organizations need to promote gender equality. Sex- and age-disaggregated data should be collected, analyzed and used in planning and implementation of aid projects.
5. It is also crucial to draw attention to the situation of women who are forced to engage in paid sex in order to earn an income or women who face exploitation or gender-based violence.
6. Efforts need to be placed on building the capacity of care providers on clinical care for sexual assault survivors, gender-based violence case management and caring for child survivors as well as facilitating access to counseling services for men, women, boys and girls, including mental health services targeted at men, such as anger and stress-management workshops.

7. Conclusion

It should be understood that there is a need to place social suffering on an ease-disease continuum because it connects health to indicators of well-being, quality of life, insecurity and distress, among other manifestations of the ill health including reproductive health and STIs accompanying the traumas of war. Survivors of war oscillate back and forth on this continuum, depending on degree, severity and chronicity of violation as well as the resources available to assist them to recover—health, wealth, strength, cultural stability and social support, among others.

Author details

Inaya Hajj Hussein[1]*, Ibrahim Mortada[2], Alice Gerges Geagea[3] and Abdo Jurjus[4]

*Address all correspondence to: hajjhuss@oakland.edu

1 Oakland University William Beaumont School of Medicine, Rochester, MI, The United States of America

2 Faculty of Medicine, American University of Beirut Medical Center, Beirut, Lebanon

3 Department of Experimental Biomedicine and Clinical Neuroscience, Section of Human Anatomy, (BIONEC), University of Palermo, Italy

4 Department of Anatomy, Cell Biology and Physiological Sciences, Faculty of Medicine, American University of Beirut, Beirut, Lebanon

References

[1] UNHCR. UNHCR Global Trends 2010: 60 Years and Still Counting. Available from: http://www.unhcr.org/4dfa11499.pdf [Accessed: 20-01-2017]

[2] UNHCR. UNHCR Population Statistics. Available from: http://popstats.unhcr.org/en/overview [Accessed: 05-02-2017]

[3] UNHCR. Figures at a Glance. Available from: http://www.unhcr.org/figures-at-a-glance.html [Accessed: 01-02-2017]

[4] Migration Policy Institute (MPI) Tabulation of Data from the U.S. Department of State Refugee Processing Center, "Admissions & Arrivals" Database. Available from: http://ireports.wrapsnet.org/ [Accessed: 04-01-2017]

[5] UNHCR. UNHCR Global Report 2015—Europe Regional Summary. Available from: http://www.unhcr.org/publications/fundraising/574ed7b24/unhcr-global-report-2015-europe-regional-summary.html [Accessed: 02-02-2017]

[6] Gensini GF, Yacoub MH, Conti AA. The concept of quarantine in history: From plague to SARS. Journal of Infection. 2004;**49**(4):257-261

[7] Pareek M, et al. The impact of migration on tuberculosis epidemiology and control in high-income countries: A review. BMC Medicine. 2016;**14**:48

[8] Carballo M, Simic S, Zeric D. Health in countries torn by conflict: Lessons from Sarajevo. Lancet. 1996;**348**(9031):872-874

[9] Barnett ED. Infectious disease screening for refugees resettled in the United States. Clinical Infectious Diseases. 2004;**39**(6):833-841

[10] UNHCR. Protecting and Supporting the Displaced in Syria. UNHCR Syria End of Year Report 2015. 2016. Available from: http://www.unhcr.org/news/editorial/2016/2/56cad5a99/unhcr-syria-2015-end-of-year-report.html?query=syria [Accessed: 09-09-2016]

[11] Ministry of Public Health Lebanon. Statistical Bulletins of the Ministry of Public Health 2006-2013. 2014. Available from: http://www.moph.gov.lb/en/Pages/8/327/statistical-bulletins [Accessed: 15-12-2016]

[12] Ammar W, Kdouh O, Hammoud R, et al. Health system resilience: Lebanon and the Syrian refugee crisis. Journal of Global Health. 2016;**6**(2):020704. DOI: 10.7189/jogh.06.020704

[13] United Nations. Syria Regional Response plan—Midyear Update 2014, Lebanon. 2014. Available from: http://www.unhcr.org/syriarrp6/midyear/ [Accessed: 09-09-2014]

[14] UNCHR. Regional Public Health and Nutrition Strategy for Syrian Refugees Egypt, Iraq, Jordan, Lebanon and Turkey 2014-2015. 2014. Available from: http://reliefweb.int/report/syrian–arab–republic/regional–public–health–and–nutrition–strategy–syrian–refugees–egypt–iraq [Accessed: 01-12-2016]

[15] Government of Lebanon. United Nations. Lebanon. Lebanon Crisis Response Plan 2015-2016. 2014. Available from: http://reliefweb.int/report/lebanon/lebanon–crisis–response–plan–2015-2016 [Accessed: 15-01-2017]

[16] A Gender-Based Violence Rapid Assessment Syrian Refugee Populations, Lebanon. 2012. Available from: https://data.unhcr.org/syrianrefugees/download.php?id=900 [Accessed: 05-02-2017]

[17] Stevens K, Palmo T, Wangchuk T, Solomon S, Dierberg K, Hoffmann CJ. Hepatitis B prevalence and treatment needs among Tibetan refugees residing in India. Journal of Medical Virology. 2016;**88**:1357-1363

[18] Lebanese Ministry of Public Health Epidemiologic Surveillance Department. 2014. Available from: http://www.moph.gov.lb/Prevention/Surveillance/Pages/PastYears.aspx [Accessed: 17-02-2017]

[19] Mixson-Hayden T, Lee D, Ganova-Raeva L, et al. Hepatitis B virus and hepatitis C virus infections in United States-bound refugees from Asia and Africa. The American Journal of Tropical Medicine and Hygiene. 2014;**90**(6):1014-1020. DOI: 10.4269/ajtmh.14-0068

[20] World Health Organization. Cervical Cancer Screening in Developing Countries: Report of a WHO Consultation. 2002. Available from: http://screening.iarc.fr/doc/cervical_cancer_screening_in_dev_countries.pdf [Accessed: 07-02-2017]

[21] Stauffer WM, et al. Sexually transmitted infections in newly arrived refugees: Is routine screening for *Neisseria gonorrheae* and *Chlamydia trachomatis* infection indicated? The American Journal of Tropical Medicine and Hygiene. 2012;**86**(2):292-295

[22] HIV/AIDS | CDC. Cdcgov. 2016. Available from: http://www.cdc.gov/hiv/ [Accessed: 08-02-2017]

[23] Piot P, Bartos M, Ghys P, Walker N, Schwartländer B. The global impact of HIV/AIDS. Nature. 2001;**410**(6831):968-973. DOI: 10.1038/35073639

[24] Wagner GJ, Tohme J, Hoover M, et al. HIV prevalence and demographic determinants of unprotected anal sex and HIV testing among men who have sex with men in Beirut, Lebanon. Archives of Sexual Behavior. 2014;**43**(4):779-788. DOI: 10.1007/s10508-014-0303-5

[25] HIV/AIDS Estimated Incidence in Lebanon. 2014. Available from: http://www.moph.gov.lb/en/DynamicPages/download_file/1516 [Accessed: 12-02-2017]

[26] Meier V, et al. Tuberculosis in newly arrived asylum seekers: A prospective 12 month surveillance study at Friedland, Germany. International Journal of Hygiene and Environmental Health. 2016;**219**(8):811-815

[27] Van Loenhout-Rooyackers JH. Risk of tuberculosis in the inadequate handling of refugees seeking asylum. Nederlands Tijdschrift voor Geneeskunde. 1994;**138**(50):2496-2500

[28] Lebanon Millennium Development Goals Report 2013-2014. Available from: http://www.undp.org/content/dam/undp/library/MDG/english/MDG%20Country%20Reports/Lebanon/MDG%20English%20Final.pdf [Accessed: 26-02-2016]

[29] World Health Organization. Country Cooperation Strategy for WHO and Lebanon 2010-2015. Country Cooperation Strategy. Cairo: World Health Organization; 2010. pp. 15-18

[30] Cherri Z, González PA, Delgado RC. The Lebanese–Syrian crisis: Impact of influx of Syrian refugees to an already weak state. Risk Management and Healthcare Policy. 2016;**9**:165

[31] United Nations. Lebanon Crisis Response Plan 2015-2016. 2014. Available from: https://data.unhcr.org/syrianrefugees/download.php?id=7723 [Accessed: 21-11-2016]

[32] World Health Organization. UNFPA Reproductive Health Education Activities Mapping Report. Lebanon: World Health Organization; September-October 2014

[33] Redditt VJ, et al. Health status of newly arrived refugees in Toronto, Ont Part 1: Infectious diseases. Canadian Family Physician. 2015;**61**(7):e303–e309

8

Circumcision and Sexually Transmitted Disease Prevention: Evidence and Reticence

Marco Vella, Alberto Abrate, Antonina Argo and Alchiede Simonato

Abstract

Circumcision is one of the oldest surgical procedures and the most common surgical procedure performed on males. It is practiced for three main reasons: ritual or religious meanings, prophylactic hygienic purposes, and therapeutic indications. Male circumcision is advocated as an efficacious prevention strategy against sexually transmitted diseases. One of the main biological mechanisms responsible for the lower human immunodeficiency virus (HIV) infection rate in heterosexual circumcised men is the protective effect of keratinization of the glans. Moreover, male circumcision removes the inner part of the prepuce containing Langerhans cells that are targeted by HIV. Several observational studies showed a protective effect of male circumcision regarding the HIV acquisition in heterosexual men, in women with circumcised partners, and in men who have sex with men with an insertive anal role. Circumcision reduced the infection rate of other sexually transmitted diseases like human papillomavirus (HPV), mycoplasma, and genital ulcer disease. It seems now evident that circumcision has no negative effects on sexual function, sensitivity, sexual sensation, and satisfaction. When performed freely after informed consent, male circumcision is a lawful practice in adults. In children, the lack of an informed consent is overcome by the favorable risk/benefit ratio and the decision whether to circumcise or not pertains to the parents.

Keywords: circumcision, HIV, sexually transmitted diseases, sexual function, ethics

1. Introduction

Male circumcision is advocated as an efficacious prevention strategy against sexually transmitted diseases (STDs), other than scaling-up testing and counseling services, campaigns with messages about abstinence, condom use and reducing multiple partners, and universal human immunodeficiency virus (HIV) testing with immediate initiation of antiretroviral therapy. Many controversies exist around male circumcision. In fact, if the procedure can bring benefits in relation to the prevention of several STDs, short-term surgical complications and suspected long-term harms, in relation to sexual dysfunction, have been also advocated by those opponents to the procedure.

2. Circumcision

2.1. Circumcision in the history

Circumcision is practiced for three main reasons. First, it can be performed for ritual or religious meanings (e.g., Jews circumcise children after 8 days of life, while Muslims between 4 and 13 years of age). Second, it can be done for a prophylactic purpose to guarantee a correct hygiene. Third, especially in western countries, it has also a therapeutic indication to treat many diseases of the foreskin, the most common of which is phimosis.

The technique of circumcision is very old and the first documented evidences of this practice are dated as early as the third millennium BC. In the ancient Egypt, circumcision was made for hygienic reasons and documented evidences have been found to date to sixth dynasty tomb (2345–2181 BC). The reasons for circumcision between the different cultural people were different: religious, hygienic, rites of passage, and a way to differentiate cultural groups.

According to Jewish religion (Genesis 17:10-14), God commanded Abraham to be circumcised, an act to be followed by his descendants. Male circumcision is performed by a circumciser (mohel) during a ceremony (covenant of circumcision called "brit milah") on the eighth day of a male infant life.

"Khitan" is the term for male circumcision carried out by Muslims as an Islamic rite. Although the Quran itself does not mention circumcision (and in fact some Quranists are against circumcision adducing that Quran forbids to alter one's body), male circumcision is widely practiced among Muslims like a rite to symbolize their inclusion into the Islamic community. It is considered obligatory in Shia tradition and not obligatory but highly recommended among the Sunni Islam. There is no fixed time for circumcision. The parents should circumcise their children before the age of 10. The preferred age is seven although some Muslims are circumcised as early as on the seventh day after birth (like Jewish people) and as late as at the puberty.

During the nineteenth century in western countries, especially in the United States and Britain, male circumcision has been largely medically adopted like a method to discourage masturbation and became the most common surgical intervention against masturbation.

2.2. Anatomy and functions of the prepuce

The penis is the male reproductive organ. It is located above and in front of the scrotum, below and in front of the pubic symphysis. Its root is in the perineum, attached to the ischio-pubic branches and the suspensor ligament of the penis. The body of the penis has a flattened cylindrical shape, formed by the two corpora cavernosa and corpus spongiosum of the urethra. The corona separates the base of the glans from the shaft of the penis. The glans is formed by the swelling of the corpus spongiosum of the urethra in the shape of a cone.

The skin that covers the penis noticeably moves on the layers below. Its blood supply is independent of the erectile bodies and is derived from the external pudendal branches of the femoral vessels. The skin that covers the glans like a hood is called prepuce or foreskin. The prepuce is a fold, half skin and half mucosa that continues in the mucosa of the glans at the balanopreputial sulcus. So the outer surface is continuous with the skin of the penis, while the inner surface is modeled on the glans adhering only at the level of the balanopreputial sulcus and the frenulum. The frenulum is a triangular mucosal fold that tends from the inner surface of the foreskin to the underside of the glans 8–10 mm behind the external urethral meatus. A short frenulum can prevent complete retraction of the foreskin and can make painful erection and tear.

The virtual cavity of the prepuce is lubricated by the smegma secreted from Tyson's glands. In case of poor hygiene, the smegma can accumulate and become infected generating balanoposthitis. Repeated balanoposthitis may form adhesions between the inner surface of the foreskin and the mucosa of the glans. In most cases, the preputial orifice is quite wide and weak to be freely retracted over the glans, and allows the glans discovering during erection. The restriction of the preputial ring, preventing the glans to escape from the preputial cavity either at rest or during erection, is called phimosis. Phimosis can be congenital or acquired, and can cause disturbances to urination and erection, and facilitate the appearance of inflammation and infection. In the newborn boy in the first months of life, the prepuce is contracted around the glans. The retraction of the foreskin is possible in the 50% of cases after 1 year of life, and in the 89% at 3 years of age [1]. Phimosis is then present in the 8% of 6–7-year-old children and in only 1% of 16–18-year-old males [2]. In some cases, the glans can go out the foreskin but then cannot be able to reenter generating a swelling accompanied by pain or ulceration; this process is called paraphimosis and requires an immediate manual reduction maneuver.

2.3. Surgical techniques

Literally from Latin, circumcision means "to cut around." The procedure aims to expose the glans sufficiently to prevent phimosis or paraphimosis (**Figure 1**). It is one of the oldest surgical procedures, performed since the age of the Egyptians. It is surely the most common surgical procedure performed on males. Over the world, it is estimated that 30% of males are circumcised. In the US, an average of a million newborn males is circumcised yearly. Circumcision rate in US is as high as 70%, while in Britain it is 6%.

Absolute indications for medical circumcision are secondary phimosis at any age, primary phimosis with recurrent balanoposthitis and urinary tract infection, and sexual discomfort. The European Association of Urology (EAU) does not recommend routine neonatal circumcision to prevent penile cancer as a recent meta-analysis could not find any risk in uncircumcised patients without a history of phimosis [1]. On the other hand, contraindications for

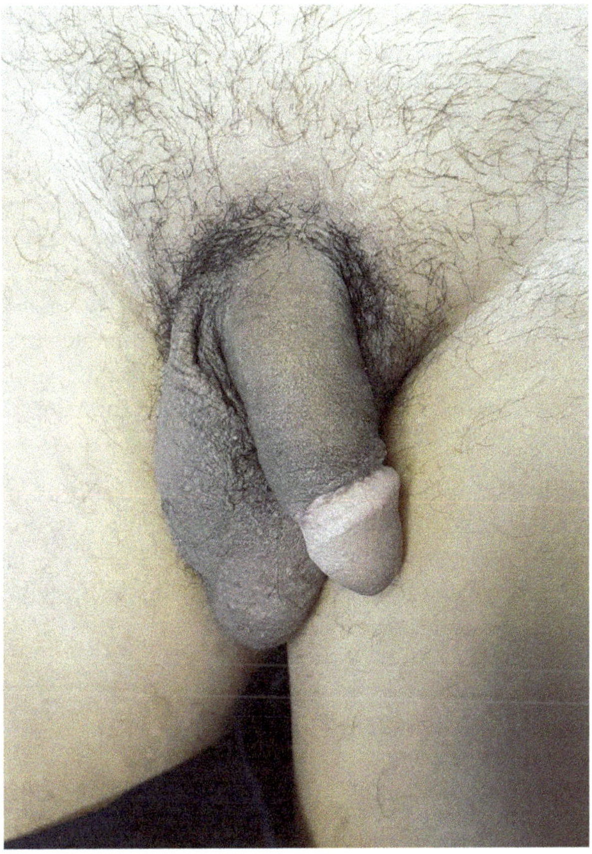

Figure 1. Short-term aesthetic result after circumcision in an adult patient.

circumcision are acute local infection and congenital anomalies of the penis (e.g., hypospadias or buried penis, in which the foreskin may be required for a reconstructive procedure). Asepsis, adequate excision of the outer and inner preputial skin layers, hemostasis, protection of the glans and urethra, and cosmetics are the principles of circumcision.

Circumcision is generally performed under local anesthesia (topical anesthetic cream or anesthetic infiltration at the base of the penis). Different techniques were described depending on the age of the patient and the surgeon's experience. There are device methods and free-hand techniques.

In pediatric settings, the device methods are favored. In this case, the Gomco clamp and its variations, like the Plastibell, are suture-less techniques that use devices that protect the glans, resect the prepuce, and provide hemostasis. The Gomco clamp uses a metal bell placed over the glans after the prepuce is fully retracted. The prepuce is then replaced over it. This is sometimes facilitated by a dorsal slit. A metal plate is placed over the bell and thus the prepuce lies between the two parts. The device is then tensioned to trap the foreskin in position to be adequately removed after a scalpel incision. The Plastibell is a plastic device with a groove on its back that has to be slipped between the glans and the prepuce. In this case, suture material is looped around in the groove and tied tightly. The foreskin withers and drops off in 7–10 days as the suture cuts off the blood supply distally to the groove.

In adulthood, the Sleeve technique or the dorsal slit technique is preferred. In the first case, the prepuce is retracted over the glans penis and a circumferential incision is made around the shaft, usually distal to the corona. The prepuce is returned to cover the glans and another circumferential incision is made around the shaft at the same position as the first one. The strip of the skin is then removed and the free edges are sutured. When the foreskin cannot be retracted over the glans, a dorsal slit may be suggested. The prepuce is freed from the glans of adhesions and with the aid of forceps, and then a longitudinal incision of both layers of the prepuce is done to some millimeter of the corona. It is cosmetically unacceptable to carry out a dorsal slit alone without excising the prepuce.

Male circumcision has low complication rates when properly performed. The most common complications are bleeding, incomplete removal of the foreskin, infection, urethral meatitis, inclusion cyst, excessive removal of the skin that can lead to severe cosmetic consequences, and functional problems. Injury of the glans, severe scarring, and urethra-cutaneous fistula are major although rare complications of the procedure.

3. Circumcision and HIV infection

3.1. Biological evidence of reduced HIV transmission in circumcised men

Between 75 and 85% of cases of HIV infection worldwide have probably occurred during sexual activity. Two main biological mechanisms are thought to be responsible of the lower HIV infection rate in heterosexual circumcised men [3].

The first is the protective effect of keratinization of the glans and the sulcus following the procedure. Thereafter, male circumcision removes the inner part of the prepuce that is more susceptible to HIV infection. In fact, the inner surface of the foreskin contains Langerhans' cells (LCs) exposing HIV receptors. LCs are antigen-presenting cells (APCs) and are likely to be the primary point of viral entry into the penis of an uncircumcised man [4].

HIV binds to the CD4 and CCR5 receptors on antigen-presenting cells—which include Langerhans' cells and dendritic cells—in the genital and rectal mucosa [5].

A keratinized, squamous epithelium covers the penile shaft and outer surface of the foreskin providing a protective barrier against HIV infection. By contrast, the inner mucosal surface of the foreskin is not keratinized and is rich in LCs making it particularly susceptible to the virus.

A widely accepted model for the sexual transmission of HIV is based on infection of the genital tract of rhesus macaques with Simian immunodeficiency virus (SIV). The same sequence of cellular events involving the infection of LCs has been sperimentally shown in male macaques following the SIV inoculation into the penile urethra or onto the foreskin [6]. Once infected, LCs fuse with adjacent CD4 lymphocytes and migrate to deeper tissues. Within 2 days of infection, the virus can be detected in the internal iliac lymph nodes and shortly thereafter in systemic lymph nodes.

Other mechanisms of increased incidence of HIV infection in uncircumcised men are the ulcerative and inflammatory lesions of the foreskin, and frenulum or glans caused by other STDs. In uncircumcised males, the highly vascular frenulum is particularly susceptible to trauma during intercourse, and ulcerative lesions produced by other STDs increase the ability of HIV to enter in the submucosal layer and link to APCs and CD4 cells. So that circumcision further reduces the risk of infection by lowering the synergy that normally exists between HIV and other STDs.

3.2. Male circumcision and HIV infection

Several observational studies showed a protective effect of male circumcision regarding the human immunodeficiency virus acquisition in heterosexual men (**Table 1**).

In 2000s, three large randomized trials specifically designed to evaluate the effect of male circumcision on the risk of HIV infections were performed in South Africa, in Uganda, and in Kenya [7–9] for a total of more than 11,000 subjects enrolled. Male circumcision showed a

<20% circumcised	Seroprevalence	>80% circumcised	Seroprevalence
(A) Sub-Saharan Africa			
Zimbabwe	25.84	Kenya	11.64
Botswana	25.10	Congo	7.64
Namibia	19.94	Cameroon	4.89
Zambia	19.07	Nigeria	4.12
Swaziland	18.50	Gabon	4.25
Malawi	14.92	Liberia	3.65
Mozambique	14.17	Sierra Leone	3.17
Rwanda	12.75	Ghana	2.38
(B) South/southeast Asia			
Cambodia	2.40	Pakistan	0.09
Thailand	2.23	Philippines	0.06
Myanmar	1.79	Indonesia	0.05
India	0.82	Bangladesh	0.03

Table 1. HIV-1 seroprevalence in relation to circumcision status in some high-incidence areas (A) and low-risk areas (B): June 1998 UNAIDS/WHO percentage estimates.

protective effect with a relative risk (RR) reduction of acquiring HIV infection of 50% after 12 months and 54% after 24 months. All the studies were stopped early due to these significant findings. The results have also been confirmed by a meta-analysis of the studies [10]. The number needed to treat was 56; it means that circumcision prevented 17 HIV infections per 1000 men at 2 years.

According to some mathematical models, the full coverage of male circumcision in those countries at high rate of HIV incidence, like sub-Saharan Africa, could avert 0.3 million deaths in the first 10 years and a further 2.7 million in the next 10 years [11].

The evidences of male circumcision benefits have also been shown from observational studies conducted in the USA and Israel [12], where the HIV burden is lower than Africa, and in low-incidence countries like India [13].

A consultation in Montreux (Switzerland) held on 28 March 2007 and sponsored by the World Health Organization (WHO) and the Joint United Nations Program on HIV/AIDS (UNAIDS) resulted in the recommendation of circumcision as a strategy for the prevention of heterosexually acquired HIV infection in men.

3.3. Effect of male circumcision on the risk of women HIV acquisition

An earlier observational study in Rakai, Uganda, found a relative male-to-female HIV transmission rate ratio of 0.41 (confidence interval (CI): 0.10–1.14) in couples with circumcised versus uncircumcised HIV-infected men. In the same study, for all HIV-positive male partners with viral loads of less than 50,000 copies/ml, no transmissions were observed in circumcised men, compared with a transmission rate of 9.6 per 100 patients (CI: 6.1–13.1, $p = 0.02$) in uncircumcised men [14].

In particular, it was estimated that circumcision may confer a 46% reduction in the rate of HIV transmission from circumcised men to their female partners [15].

Assuming a reduction in male-to-female transmission, the projected impact of circumcision on HIV spread is substantially enhanced, especially for women. Although male circumcision is an intervention applied to men, it brings substantial benefits for women as well.

An increase in the risk of acquisition and transmission of HIV during circumcision wound-healing period is an admitted possibility [16], but it is unlikely to have a major effect on the population. Premature resumption of sexual activity before the wound is healed or "compensatory" increase in risk following circumcision are both unlikely to substantively undermine the benefits of male circumcision on HIV incidence among women or men.

3.4. Infection of men who have sex with men

A Cochrane systematic review and meta-analysis including more than 65,000 participants showed that circumcision may reduce HIV acquisition among men who have sex with men having an insertive anal role but probably have no role among those having a receptive role [17].

4. Male circumcision and other sexually transmitted infections

4.1. Human papillomavirus

Circumcision was shown to decrease human papillomavirus (HPV) infection rates among both HIV-negative and HIV-positive heterosexual men included in a randomized controlled trial (RCT) performed in Uganda (RR 0.40, 95% CI: 0.19–0.84), control event rate 24.7% [18]. Male circumcision decreases also HPV infection rates in female partners especially of circumcised HIV-negative males [19, 20]. It is important to note that female partners of circumcised males have a lower risk of cervical cancer [21].

4.2. Mycoplasma

Circumcision was found to nearly halve the odds of Mycoplasma infection of the genitalia in circumcised men (odds ratio (OR) 0.54; 95% CI: 0.29–0.99) [22]. On the contrary, genital Mycoplasma is not reduced in female partners of circumcised men [23].

4.3. Genital ulcer disease

Two large RCTs showed that male circumcision reduce genital ulcer disease (GUD) incidence with a risk ratio of 0.51 and 0.52 [24]. The risk for GUD is also decreased in female partners of circumcised males as for Chlamydia trachomatis infection [25], bacterial vaginosis, and trichomonas infection [26].

4.4. Syphilis

The relation between male circumcision and new acquisition of syphilis is not clear. In fact, one large RCT showed no significant difference between circumcised and uncircumcised men (adjusted hazard ratio 1.10, 95% CI: 0.75–1.65, $p = 0.44$) [27]. However, another large RCT showed that circumcision was associated with a 42% reduction in the incidence of syphilis (adjusted hazard ratio 0.58, 95% CI: 0.37–0.91). In particular, a 62% reduction of syphilis among HIV-infected men was noted, whereas a nonsignificant reduction in the incidence of syphilis was observed among men without HIV [28].

4.5. Herpes simplex virus

A discrepancy of results exists between the trials conducted in order to evaluate the association of male circumcision and herpes simplex virus (HSV) prevalence. The reason for such a discrepancy is due to the nonunivocal use of the test employed for HSV detection and because of nonhomogeneous characteristics of the subjects and their sexual life.

In fact, two RCTs from Uganda [27] and South Africa [29] showed a significant reduction in HSV infection rates after circumcision. Two other trials conducted in Kenya failed to show such a reduction [24, 30].

4.6. Gonorrhea and Chlamydia

Male circumcision probably does not interfere with gonorrhea incidence. In fact, both observational [31] and randomized [32] did not show a risk reduction of gonococcus infection after circumcision.

Similarly, there is no association between Chlamydia infection and circumcision status [32].

5. Circumcision and sexual function

The possible implication of circumcision on sex needs more thorough discussion. The dorsal nerves provide sensory innervation to the penis. These nerves follow the course of the dorsal arteries and richly supply the glans. The prepuce is also a primary sensory part of the penis. In fact, it contains a high concentration of Meissner's corpuscles and sensory cells, which make it a specialized sensory mucosa. The effect of circumcision on sexual sensation is widely discussed and contradictory results have been shown. Some authors reported that the foreskin is important for normal sexual activity and affirm that circumcision removes the most sensitive parts of the penis. In addition to this, the glans of circumcised penis was found to be less sensitive compared to the glans of uncircumcised men, probably due to the subsequent thickening of the glans epithelia. Conversely, other authors showed that there is no substantial difference in sexual pleasure in circumcised and uncircumcised males, but an increased penile sensitivity. The same contradictory results were reported for women partners. In fact, the gliding mechanism, which makes the penis shaft to glide in its own skin covering during intercourse, was thought to add to the comfort of both partners in theory.

However, although one trial conducted in Denmark [33] reported a reduction in sexual satisfaction, more orgasm difficulties, and higher rate of dyspareunia among women partners of circumcised men, the most part of the studies supported the thesis that circumcision does not change or even improve sexual pleasure of women partners.

Krieger et al. [34] assessed, in a randomized trial, the effect of adult male circumcision on men sexual function and pleasure concluding that the procedure did not cause sexual dysfunction. Moreover, using the Brief Male Sexual Function Inventory (BMFSI) and the Intravaginal Ejaculation Latency Time (IELT), after an observational 12-week study, Senkul et al. [35] noted a prolonged mean ejaculatory latency time, which may be considered an advantage, and no substantial differences in the mean BMSFI (**Table 2**).

To analogous conclusions arrived, the studies of Kigozi et al. [36] and Collins et al. [37] use, respectively, the International Index of Erectile Function (IIEF) and the Brief Male Sexual Function Inventory (BMFSI).

On the contrary, the World Health Organization in 2007 [38] stated that there was little evidence to support a negative effect of male circumcision on sexual pleasure.

Author	Study	Sexual assessment	Outcome
Senkul et al. [35]	Observational	BMFI	Increase IELT and no change
Kigozi et al. [36]	Randomized	IIEF	No difference between groups
Collins et al. [37]	Observational	BMFSI	No change
Krieger et al. [34]	Observational	Non-validated questionnaire	No difference (very satisfied)
Frisch et al. [33]	Case-control	Survey	More orgasm difficulties

Table 2. Effects of male circumcision on sexual function.

However, a recent systematic review analyzing the highest quality studies, conducted by Morris and Krieger [39], concluded that male circumcision has no negative effects on sexual function, sensitivity, sexual sensation, or satisfaction.

6. Ethical and legal arguments of male circumcision

6.1. Adults

An ethical argumentation regarding male circumcision should focus on four bioethical principles: autonomy, dignity, integrity, and vulnerability, which are to be understood without giving priority to one principle over another, but according to their mutual connections [40]. Bodily integrity is not a value worthy of respect in his own meaning (per se), unless related to dignity and values of a human person under all circumstances concerning health. Integrity, as mentioned in the Barcelona Declaration (1998), is not limited to the body, conversely it concerns the whole life of every person, in its physical, mental, and narrative dimension [41]. Dignity is considered a property of every human being who has dignity if it is the expression of his/her autonomy, at a given moment of his/her life. Strongly related to the notion of autonomy is the obligation of informed consent during the course of health care, with the focus on self-determination [40]. By applying the principle of autonomy in medical ethics, one could even justify the refusal of medical and surgical treatment deemed necessary or, on the contrary, admit the possibility that a competent adult person consent to medical treatment, in spite of the possibility of unwanted negative effects and outcomes. In fact, since last century, patient's informed consent was considered the expression of a wiliness permitting to attempt patient physical integrity and, if it had been missed, any medical act could be understood as "violence."

Some authors opposing to male medical circumcision, skeptical about the Center for Disease Control and Prevention (CDC) guidelines, argued about supposed health benefits of female "circumcision," some forms of which may be even considered as less invasive than male circumcision, trying to balance similarities [42]. This argument is strongly denied by medical classification of the WHO that named "mutilation" as all forms of female circumcision and consequently no far similarities must be drawn between two practices. Thus, the practices banned by the WHO, as female genital mutilations, even with patient consent, could not be considered lawful [43].

On the point of view of health professionals and physicians duties, by applying the "beneficence" ethical principle, benefits must "simply" exceed predictable risks and complications, all evaluated in the light of scientific evidence principles. Values of integrity and honesty of health professionals are moral aptitudes worldwide mentioned, which must contribute to reach a convinced opinion of the patient [44], with a proper illustration of pros and cons attributable to each medical practice, taking into account all aspects worthy of consideration in patient's perspective [45–48]. The ratio between risks and benefits, in the case of adult patient, may justify the proposal and adoption of male circumcision, within updated medical guidelines evidence, provided it does not impose to anyone an also minimal genital surgery, even in consideration of absolutely rare frequency of risks and complications related to this practice.

6.2. Children

With regard to health-care decisions for young children, it is generally assumed that their parents should make these. Only when parents make decisions that are very clearly against the interest of their children, an external imposition could be assumed. It is also worthy of consideration for the family that have to live with the results of health decision, and every family has its own set of values; the basis for decision making is related to the model of "surrogate decision-making standard" or, alternatively, the "best interest" standard. Disagreement between the parents' decision and the health-care professionals involved in the care and the treatment sometime should require legal evaluation in Court.

Criticism related to the Guidelines of the American Academy of Pediatrics (AAP) 2012 policy statement and technical report is yet reported and debated in scientific literature [41]. Basically, this matter regards prophylactic infant male circumcision and parents' consent, in the view of the best child's interest and future consequences related to circumcision. One position concludes that, before an age of consent, circumcision is not a desirable health-promotion strategy, given more effective and less ethically problematic alternatives [42]. On the contrary, from a scientific point of view, like infant vaccinations, the benefits of male circumcision exceed risks by a large margin; following these clinical and epidemiological indications, the pro-male circumcision arguments include also legal arguments [49]. Within this favorable approach, parents must make many decisions on behalf of their children. The decision whether to circumcise or not, as for some not obligatory vaccination, is one of those pertaining to parents.

7. Conclusions and key messages on male circumcision

- Male circumcision is effective to reduce HIV infection in heterosexual men, especially in areas at high incidence of the disease.
- Male circumcision should be provided freely after informed consent, ensuring surgical safety and quality.

- Male circumcision is an addition to, not a substitute for, other proven methods for preventing HIV infection, as it provides only partial protection.
- Male circumcision is a preventive measure with an optimal cost/benefit ratio.
- Sex should be resumed at least 6 weeks after circumcision and after a medical examination confirming that the healing process is complete.
- Male circumcision seems to confer protection against HIV infection also in women assuming that sexual intercourses are avoided during the wound-healing period.
- Male circumcision reduces HIV acquisition among men who have sex with men having an insertive anal role.
- Male circumcision reduces the incidence of HPV infection in males and of cervical cancer in women.
- Male circumcision has a protective effect regarding Mycoplasma genitalia infection and genital ulcer disease.
- Conflicting data are available about the benefits of circumcision over the transmission of other sexually transmitted diseases.
- There is no substantial difference in sexual pleasure between circumcised and uncircumcised men.
- Male circumcision is generally well accepted by female partners.
- Several surgical techniques are available, but none has demonstrated superiority over the others.
- Surgical complications are rare in hospital settings.
- When performed freely after informed consent, male circumcision is a lawful practice in adult.
- In children, the lack of an informed consent is overcome by the favorable risk/benefit ratio and the decision whether to circumcise or not pertains to the parents.
- Male circumcision and female genital mutilation are very different things.

Author details

Marco Vella[1*], Alberto Abrate[1], Antonina Argo[2] and Alchiede Simonato[1]

*Address all correspondence to: marco.vella@unipa.it

1 Urological Section, Department of Surgical, Oncological and Stomatological Science, University of Palermo, Palermo, Italy

2 Medico-Legal Section, Department for Health Promotion, Maternal and Child Care, University of Palermo, Palermo, Italy

References

[1] Tekgül S, Dogan HS, Hoebeke P, Kocvara R, Nijman JM, Radmayr C, Stein R. EAU Guidelines on Paediatric Urology: European Association of Urology. 2016. Available from: http://www.uroweb.org/guideline/paediatric-urology/

[2] Gairdner D. The fate of the foreskin, a study of circumcision. British Medical Journal. 1949;**2**:1433-1437, illust

[3] Szabo R, Short RV. How does male circumcision protect against HIV infection? British Medical Journal. 2000;**320**:1592-1594

[4] McCoombe SG, Short RV. Potential HIV-1 target cells in the human penis. AIDS. 2006;**20**:1491-1495. DOI: 10.1097/01.aids.0000237364.11123.98

[5] Hussain LA, Lehner T. Comparative investigation of Langerhans' cells and potential receptors for HIV in oral, genitourinary and rectal epithelia. Immunology. 1995;**85**:475-484

[6] Miller CJ. Localization of Simian immunodeficiency virus-infected cells in the genital tract of male and female Rhesus macaques. Journal of Reproductive Immunology. 1998;**41**:331-339

[7] Auvert B, Taljaard D, Lagarde E, Sobngwi-Tambekou J, Sitta R, Puren A. Randomized, controlled intervention trial of male circumcision for reduction of HIV infection risk: The ANRS 1265 Trial. PLoS Medicine. 2005;**2**:e298. DOI: 10.1371/journal.pmed.0020298

[8] Bailey RC, Moses S, Parker CB, Agot K, Maclean I, Krieger JN, Williams CF, Campbell RT, Ndinya-Achola JO. Male circumcision for HIV prevention in young men in Kisumu, Kenya: A randomised controlled trial. Lancet. 2007;**369**:643-656. DOI: 10.1016/S0140-6736(07)60312-2

[9] Gray RH, Kigozi G, Serwadda D, Makumbi F, Watya S, Nalugoda F, Kiwanuka N, Moulton LH, Chaudhary MA, Chen MZ, Sewankambo NK, Wabwire-Mangen F, Bacon MC, Williams CF, Opendi P, Reynolds SJ, Laeyendecker O, Quinn TC, Wawer MJ. Male circumcision for HIV prevention in men in Rakai, Uganda: A randomised trial. Lancet. 2007;**369**:657-666. DOI: 10.1016/S0140-6736(07)60313-4

[10] Siegfried N, Muller M, Deeks JJ, Volmink J. Male circumcision for prevention of heterosexual acquisition of HIV in men. Cochrane Database Systemic Revision. 2009:CD003362. DOI: 10.1002/14651858.CD003362.pub2

[11] Williams BG, Lloyd-Smith JO, Gouws E, Hankins C, Getz WM, Hargrove J, de Zoysa I, Dye C, Auvert B. The potential impact of male circumcision on HIV in Sub-Saharan Africa. PLoS Medicine. 2006;**3**:e262. DOI: 10.1371/journal.pmed.0030262

[12] Chemtob D, Op de Coul E, van Sighem A, Mor Z, Cazein F, Semaille C. Impact of male circumcision among heterosexual HIV cases: Comparisons between three low HIV prevalence countries. Israel Journal of Health Policy Research. 2015;**4**:36. DOI: 10.1186/s13584-015-0033-8

[13] Arora P, Nagelkerke NJ, Jha P. A systematic review and meta-analysis of risk factors for sexual transmission of HIV in India. PLoS One. 2012;**7**:e44094. DOI: 10.1371/journal.pone.0044094

[14] Gray RH, Kiwanuka N, Quinn TC, Sewankambo NK, Serwadda D, Mangen FW, Lutalo T, Nalugoda F, Kelly R, Meehan M, Chen MZ, Li C, Wawer MJ. Male circumcision and HIV acquisition and transmission: Cohort studies in Rakai, Uganda. Rakai Project Team. AIDS. 2000;**14**:2371-2381

[15] Hallett TB, Alsallaq RA, Baeten JM, Weiss H, Celum C, Gray R, Abu-Raddad L. Will circumcision provide even more protection from HIV to women and men? New estimates of the population impact of circumcision interventions. Sexually Transmitted Infections. 2011;**87**:88-93. DOI: 10.1136/sti.2010.043372

[16] Wawer MJ, Makumbi F, Kigozi G, Serwadda D, Watya S, Nalugoda F, Buwembo D, Ssempijja V, Kiwanuka N, Moulton LH, Sewankambo NK, Reynolds SJ, Quinn TC, Opendi P, Iga B, Ridzon R, Laeyendecker O, Gray RH. Circumcision in HIV-infected men and its effect on HIV transmission to female partners in Rakai, Uganda: A randomised controlled trial. Lancet. 2009;**374**:229-237. DOI: 10.1016/S0140-6736(09)60998-3

[17] Wiysonge CS, Kongnyuy EJ, Shey M, Muula AS, Navti OB, Akl EA, Lo YR. Male circumcision for prevention of homosexual acquisition of HIV in men. Cochrane Database Systemic Revision. 2011; Issue 6: CD007496. DOI: 10.1002/14651858.CD007496.pub2

[18] Serwadda D, Wawer MJ, Makumbi F, Kong X, Kigozi G, Gravitt P, Watya S, Nalugoda F, Ssempijja V, Tobian AA, Kiwanuka N, Moulton LH, Sewankambo NK, Reynolds SJ, Quinn TC, Oliver AE, Iga B, Laeyendecker O, Gray RH. Circumcision of HIV-infected men: Effects on high-risk human papillomavirus infections in a randomized trial in Rakai, Uganda. Journal of Infectious Disease. 2010;**201**:1463-1469. DOI: 10.1086/652185

[19] Wawer MJ, Tobian AA, Kigozi G, Kong X, Gravitt PE, Serwadda D, Nalugoda F, Makumbi F, Ssempiija V, Sewankambo N, Watya S, Eaton KP, Oliver AE, Chen MZ, Reynolds SJ, Quinn TC, Gray RH. Effect of circumcision of HIV-negative men on transmission of human papillomavirus to HIV-negative women: A randomised trial in Rakai, Uganda. Lancet. 2011;**377**:209-218. DOI: 10.1016/S0140-6736(10)61967-8

[20] Davis MA, Gray RH, Grabowski MK, Serwadda D, Kigozi G, Gravitt PE, Nalugoda F, Watya S, Wawer MJ, Quinn TC, Tobian AA. Male circumcision decreases high-risk human papillomavirus viral load in female partners: A randomized trial in Rakai, Uganda. International Journal of Cancer. 2013;**133**:1247-1252. DOI: 10.1002/ijc.28100

[21] Castellsague X, Bosch FX, Munoz N, Meijer CJ, Shah KV, de Sanjose S, Eluf-Neto J, Ngelangel CA, Chichareon S, Smith JS, Herrero R, Moreno V, Franceschi S. Male circumcision, penile human papillomavirus infection, and cervical cancer in female partners. New England Journal of Medicine. 2002;**346**:1105-1112. DOI: 10.1056/NEJMoa011688

[22] Mehta SD, Gaydos C, Maclean I, Odoyo-June E, Moses S, Agunda L, Quinn N, Bailey RC. The effect of medical male circumcision on urogenital Mycoplasma genitalium among men in Kisumu, Kenya. Sexually Transmitted Disease. 2012;**39**:276-280. DOI: 10.1097/OLQ.0b013e318240189c

[23] Tobian AA, Gaydos C, Gray RH, Kigozi G, Serwadda D, Quinn N, Grabowski MK, Musoke R, Ndyanabo A, Nalugoda F, Wawer MJ, Quinn TC. Male circumcision and Mycoplasma genitalium infection in female partners: A randomised trial in Rakai, Uganda. Sexually Transmitted Infections. 2014;**90**:150-154. DOI: 10.1136/sextrans-2013-051293

[24] Mehta SD, Moses S, Parker CB, Agot K, Maclean I, Bailey RC. Circumcision status and incident herpes simplex virus type 2 infection, genital ulcer disease, and HIV infection. AIDS. 2012;**26**:1141-1149. DOI: 10.1097/QAD.0b013e328352d116

[25] Castellsague X, Peeling RW, Franceschi S, de Sanjose S, Smith JS, Albero G, Diaz M, Herrero R, Munoz N, Bosch FX. Chlamydia trachomatis infection in female partners of circumcised and uncircumcised adult men. American Journal of Epidemiology. 2005;**162**:907-916. DOI: 10.1093/aje/kwi284

[26] Gray RH, Kigozi G, Serwadda D, Makumbi F, Nalugoda F, Watya S, Moulton L, Chen MZ, Sewankambo NK, Kiwanuka N, Sempijja V, Lutalo T, Kagayii J, Wabwire-Mangen F, Ridzon R, Bacon M, Wawer MJ. The effects of male circumcision on female partners' genital tract symptoms and vaginal infections in a randomized trial in Rakai, Uganda. American Journal of Obstetrics & Gynecology. 2009;**200**:42 e1-7. DOI: 10.1016/j.ajog.2008.07.069

[27] Tobian AA, Serwadda D, Quinn TC, Kigozi G, Gravitt PE, Laeyendecker O, Charvat B, Ssempijja V, Riedesel M, Oliver AE, Nowak RG, Moulton LH, Chen MZ, Reynolds SJ, Wawer MJ, Gray RH. Male circumcision for the prevention of HSV-2 and HPV infections and syphilis. New England Journal of Medicine. 2009;**360**:1298-1309. DOI: 10.1056/NEJMoa0802556

[28] Gray RH, Serwadda D, Tobian AA, Chen MZ, Makumbi F, Suntoke T, Kigozi G, Nalugoda F, Iga B, Quinn TC, Moulton LH, Laeyendecker O, Reynolds SJ, Kong X, Wawer MJ. Effects of genital ulcer disease and herpes simplex virus type 2 on the efficacy of male circumcision for HIV prevention: Analyses from the Rakai trials. PLoS Medicine. 2009;**6**:e1000187. DOI: 10.1371/journal.pmed.1000187

[29] Sobngwi-Tambekou J, Taljaard D, Lissouba P, Zarca K, Puren A, Lagarde E, Auvert B. Effect of HSV-2 serostatus on acquisition of HIV by young men: Results of a longitudinal study in Orange Farm, South Africa. Journal of Infectious Disease. 2009;**199**:958-964. DOI: 10.1086/597208

[30] Mehta SD, Moses S, Agot K, Maclean I, Odoyo-June E, Li H, Bailey RC. Medical male circumcision and herpes simplex virus 2 acquisition: Posttrial surveillance in Kisumu, Kenya. Journal of Infectious Disease. 2013;**208**:1869-1876. DOI: 10.1093/infdis/jit371

[31] Sobngwi-Tambekou J, Taljaard D, Nieuwoudt M, Lissouba P, Puren A, Auvert B. Male circumcision and Neisseria gonorrhoeae, Chlamydia trachomatis and Trichomonas vaginalis: Observations after a randomised controlled trial for HIV prevention. Sexually Transmitted Infections. 2009;**85**:116-120. DOI: 10.1136/sti.2008.032334

[32] Mehta SD, Moses S, Agot K, Parker C, Ndinya-Achola JO, Maclean I, Bailey RC. Adult male circumcision does not reduce the risk of incident Neisseria gonorrhoeae, Chlamydia trachomatis, or Trichomonas vaginalis infection: Results from a randomized, controlled trial in Kenya. Journal of Infectious Disease. 2009;**200**:370-378. DOI: 10.1086/600074

[33] Frisch M, Lindholm M, Gronbaek M. Male circumcision and sexual function in men and women: A survey-based, cross-sectional study in Denmark. International Journal of Epidemiology. 2011;**40**:1367-1381. DOI: 10.1093/ije/dyr104

[34] Krieger JN, Mehta SD, Bailey RC, Agot K, Ndinya-Achola JO, Parker C, Moses S. Adult male circumcision: Effects on sexual function and sexual satisfaction in Kisumu, Kenya. Journal of Sexual Medicine. 2008;**5**:2610-2622. DOI: 10.1111/j.1743-6109.2008.00979.x

[35] Senkul T, Iser IC, Sen B, Karademir K, Saracoglu F, Erden D. Circumcision in adults: Effect on sexual function. Urology. 2004;**63**:155-158

[36] Kigozi G, Watya S, Polis CB, Buwembo D, Kiggundu V, Wawer MJ, Serwadda D, Nalugoda F, Kiwanuka N, Bacon MC, Ssempijja V, Makumbi F, Gray RH. The effect of male circumcision on sexual satisfaction and function, results from a randomized trial of male circumcision for human immunodeficiency virus prevention, Rakai, Uganda. BJU International. 2008;**101**:65-70. DOI: 10.1111/j.1464-410X.2007.07369.x

[37] Collins S, Upshaw J, Rutchik S, Ohannessian C, Ortenberg J, Albertsen P. Effects of circumcision on male sexual function: Debunking a myth? Journal of Urology. 2002;**167**: 2111-2112

[38] World Health Organization. Male Circumcision: Global Trends and Determinants of Prevalence, Safety and Acceptability. 2007. Available from: http://whqlibdoc.who.int/publications/2007/9789241596169_eng.pdf

[39] Morris BJ, Krieger JN. Does male circumcision affect sexual function, sensitivity, or satisfaction?--A systematic review. Journal of Sexual Medicine. 2013;**10**:2644-2657. DOI: 10.1111/jsm.12293

[40] Pegoraro R, Putoto G, Wray E, editors. Hospital Based Bioethics. A European Perspective. Padova: Piccin; 2007. p. 198

[41] Kemp P, Rendtorff JD. The Barcelona Declaration. Towards an integrated approach to basic ethical principles. Synthesis Philosophica. 2008;**46**:239-251

[42] Earp BD. Do the benefits of male circumcision outweigh the risks? A critique of the proposed CDC guidelines. Frontiers in Pediatrics. 2015;**3**:18. DOI: 10.3389/fped.2015.00018

[43] Vella M, Argo A, Costanzo A, Tarantino L, Milone L, Pavone C. Female genital mutilations: Genito-urinary complications and ethical-legal aspects. Urologia. 2015;**82**:151-159. DOI: 10.5301/uro.5000115

[44] Argo A, Zerbo S, Triolo V, Averna L, D'Anna T, Nicosia A, Procaccianti P. Legal aspects of sexually transmitted diseases: Abuse, partner notification and prosecution. Giornale Italiano di Dermatologia e Venereologia. 2012;**147**:357-371

[45] Friedman B, Khoury J, Petersiel N, Yahalomi T, Paul M, Neuberger A. Pros and cons of circumcision: An evidence-based overview. Clinical Microbiology and Infection. 2016;**22**:768-774. DOI: 10.1016/j.cmi.2016.07.030

[46] Homfray V, Tanton C, Miller RF, Beddows S, Field N, Sonnenberg P, Wellings K, Panwar K, Johnson AM, Mercer CH. Male circumcision and STI acquisition in Britain: Evidence from a national probability sample survey. PLoS One. 2015;**10**:e0130396. DOI: 10.1371/journal.pone.0130396

[47] Jiang J, Su J, Yang X, Huang M, Deng W, Huang J, Liang B, Qin B, Upur H, Zhong C, Wang Q, Ruan Y, Ye L, Liang H. Acceptability of male circumcision among college students in medical universities in Western China: A cross-sectional study. PLoS One. 2015;**10**:e0135706. DOI: 10.1371/journal.pone.0135706

[48] Westercamp M, Bailey RC, Bukusi EA, Montandon M, Kwena Z, Cohen CR. Male circumcision in the general population of Kisumu, Kenya: Beliefs about protection, risk behaviors, HIV, and STIs. PLoS One. 2010;**5**:e15552. DOI: 10.1371/journal.pone.0015552

[49] Morris BJ, Bailey RC, Klausner JD, Leibowitz A, Wamai RG, Waskett JH, Banerjee J, Halperin DT, Zoloth L, Weiss HA, Hankins CA. Review: A critical evaluation of arguments opposing male circumcision for HIV prevention in developed countries. AIDS Care. 2012;**24**: 1565-1575. DOI: 10.1080/09540121.2012.661836

9

Cervical Cancer, a Sequela of a Sexually Transmitted Infection: The Human Papillomavirus Infection

Tamunomie K Nyengidiki, Goddy Bassey and Ikechukwu Durugbo

Abstract

Cervical cancer has contributed to a large number of gynecologically related oncologic deaths in most developing countries. Almost all cases of cervical cancer are related to the presence of persistent strains of sexually transmitted oncogenic strains of human papillomavirus infection (HPV). Steps taken to decrease infection rate will reduce the long-term sequelae of cervical cancer globally.

Keywords: cervical cancer, sexually transmitted disease, HPV

1. Introduction

Cervical cancer is a malignant lesion of the cervix. The squamous cell carcinoma consists of about 90–95% of the cases while adenocarcinoma makes up about 5–10% [1]. Other histological variants do exist such as adenosquamous, sarcomas, lymphomas, carcinomas, etc. Cervical cancer arises either from the ectocervix or from the endocervix. The site of the growth bears no relationship to the histological type as some squamous carcinoma are found in the endocervical canal [1]. Worldwide, every 2 min, a woman dies of cervical cancer, and it is the leading cause of cancer deaths in women of the developing countries as about 85% of the women dying from cervical cancer reside in the developing countries [2].

Currently, about 200 different strains or genotypes of human papillomavirus infection (HPV) have been isolated. Thirty of these have a predilection for the epithelium of the genital tract of which 15 strains are regarded as oncogenic and are responsible for virtually all cases of cervical cancer worldwide. Oncogenic strains or high-risk genotypes which include serotypes 16,

18, 31, 35 and 45 are responsible for most cases of cervical cancer, although multiple infections with a combination of genotypes have been isolated in 6% of cases. It is estimated that only 20% of women will escape HPV infection in their lifetime and this underscores the importance of this infection [2, 3].

Human papillomavirus, a non-envelop double-stranded DNA virus, measures about 55 nm in diameter and consist of a genome that encodes for early and late proteins. It causes both benign and malignant conditions of the skin, cervix, vagina, vulva and anus. The main routes of transmission are through sexual intercourse and skin-skin contact; it is projected that about half of all sexually active adolescent will acquire the infection; however, the infection is usually self-limiting and harmless depending on the host immunity among other factors. Failure of the host immunity to clear the infection is responsible for persistence of the infection and eventual development of cervical cancer [3–5]. This chapter exploits cervical cancer as sexually transmitted infection sequelae with the human papillomavirus virus, largely the causative agent.

1.1. Epidemiology of cervical cancer

Worldwide, about 500,000 new cases of cervical cancer are diagnosed annually and there are about 300,000 associated deaths per year. Most of the new cases of cervical cancer and the associated cancer deaths occur in the less developed regions of the world [6]. Projections indicate that more than one million new cases of cervical cancer will occur each year by 2050 [7].

Every year, across Africa about 79,000 women are diagnosed with cervical cancer [6]. The epidemiology of cervical cancer is different in North and sub-Saharan Africa, due to differences in cervical screening, cultural differences and human immunodeficiency virus (HIV) prevalence. Organized cervical screening is limited or absent in several African countries [6].

Yearly across Africa, about 62,000 women die from cervical cancer with a similar distribution of mortality rates to incidence rates. High incidence and mortality rates occur in sub-Saharan Africa while lower rates occur in North Africa [6]. In Nigeria, cervical cancer age standard incidence rate at the Ibadan population-based cancer registry was 36.0 per 100,000 and 30.3 per 100,000 at Abuja population-based cancer registry [8].

In Europe and North America, the incidence of cervical cancer is about 60,000 and 14,000, respectively, with a lower annual mortality rate of about 30,000 and 5000, respectively [6, 9]. The low incidence and mortality may reflect the availability of well-established screening program in developed countries [7, 9].

1.2. Burden of HPV infection and regional variation of genotypes

Human papillomavirus virus is a relatively small sexually transmitted virus containing circular double-stranded DNA with affinity to cutaneous and mucosal epithelium resulting in cytopathic changes. It is the most common sexually acquired infection in the world with more than half in young, sexually active adolescents. The persistence of the oncogenic HPV types causes cervical cancer in women. Several studies have been done on the prevalence of HPV genotypes in women with different genotypes implicated in different histological types of cervical cancer.

Cervical cancers constitute two-thirds of all genital cancers in developing countries like Nigeria with most of the patients presenting with clinical stage III or IV disease [4, 10]. Therefore, the main burden of cervical cancers is in the developing world where it contributes significantly to maternal death. This is contrary to the developed countries where there is decreasing incidence of cervical cancer. This is due to the establishment of effective cervical cancer screening protocol, education and access to good medical care [10, 11]. In the UK, screening has prevented up to 70% of cervical cancer death since its inception in 1988 [12].

Worldwide, an estimated 291 million women are harboring HPV DNA at any point in time and 23% of these infections are related to HPV 16 while 8.5% are related to HPV 18 [13]. The adjusted global prevalence has been reported to be 10.41% [14]. The oncogenic HPV incidence is highest in young women and the risk of infection remains throughout life [15]. There are regional differences in the prevalence of the oncogenic HPV infection [16].

A study done in Benin, West Africa, showed an overall prevalence of 32.2% [17]. High-risk types were involved in 88% of the infection, most notably HPV 16, 18, 35, 45, 58 and 59. Another study done in Mexico for a prevalence of HPV genotypes in women from a rural region of Puebla revealed the prevalence of 25.4% [18]. The study also revealed two peaks of higher HPV prevalence in those aged 18–24 and 55–64 years. The individual genotypes in the study were 9.6% HPV 6, 4.6% HPV 11, 54.2% HPV 16, 37.3% HPV 18 and 9.6% HPV 31. HPV 16 was the most common type found in all the cervical lesions.

A study on the prevalence of HPV and its genotypes done in Ibadan, Nigeria, showed that the overall prevalence of HPV was 26.3% in women with cervical cancer and 24.8% in the women without cervical lesions [4]. It also revealed that the high-risk HPV was predominant (19.7%) and was mostly due to viral types 16, 31, 35 and 58. The low-risk HPV were found in 6.6% and mixed infections of more than one HPV type occurred in 33.5% of HPV-positive cases. A similar incidence of 21.6% was found in Okene, north-central Nigeria with the high-risk HPV prevalence of 16.6 and 3.5% having mixed infections [19].

In immunocompromised patients, the genotypic distribution also differs as observed in a cross-sectional prospective study conducted out in LUTH, Lagos which determined the prevalence of high-risk HPV among HIV-positive and HIV-negative women in 2012 [20]. The study revealed that the prevalence of HPV among the HIV-positive women was 44.9% with the prevalence of the high-risk types constituting 37.5%. The most common high-risk types seen were types 31, 52, 53 and 35. It also showed that the prevalence of HPV among the HIV-negative women was 11% while the most common high-risk types seen in them were types 18, 16, 52 and 56. Similar study for the prevalence of HPV genotypes enrolled HIV-positive and HIV-negative women presenting for cancer screening program [21]. Among the HIV-positive women, HPV 35 (8.7%) and HPV 56 (7.4%) were the most prevalent high-risk HPV while HPV 52 and HPV 68 (2.8% each) were the most prevalent among HIV-negative women. The study suggested that the oncogenic HPV types 35, 52, 56 and 68 may be more important risk factors for cervical pre-cancers among African women hence polyvalent high-risk HPV vaccines meant for African populations should protect against HPV types other than 16 and 18.

A cross-sectional epidemiological study that assessed HPV prevalence and type distribution in women with invasive cervical cancer in Ghana, Nigeria and South Africa revealed that the most commonly detected HPV types were HPV 16 (51.2%), HPV 18 (17.2%), HPV 35 (8.7%), HPV 45 (7.4%), HPV 33 (4.0%) and HPV 52 (2.2%). The prevalence of single and multiple HPV infections seemed higher among the HIV-positive women. Therefore, HPV 16, 18, 45 and 35 were the most common HPV types in sub-Saharan African women [22]. Another study in Abuja showed HPV types 18 and 16 to be the most predominant in the metropolis [23].

2. HPV genotypes and distribution in cervical cancer

The most common oncogenic HPV genotypes are 16, 18, 45, 31, 33 and 51 [24]. Others are 52, 56, 58, 59 and 68. HPV genotypes 16, 18, 45, 33 and 31 are usually associated with squamous cell carcinoma while types 16, 18, 45, 31 and 51 are usually associated with adenocarcinoma [24]. These oncogenic strains are those linked to cervical cancer.

Globally, HPV types 16 and 18 together account for more than 70% of the cervical cancer cases while the next most common oncogenic HPV types are 45, 31 and 33 and together account for about an additional 10% [16, 25]. HPV 18 is more prevalent in adenocarcinoma than the squamous cell carcinoma while HPV 16 in more prevalent in squamous cell carcinoma [16]. The non-oncogenic genotypes are 6, 11, 44, 43, 44, 54 and 55 and are associated with benign genital warts. HPV types 6 is most commonly detected in the benign genital lesions (about 90% of warts) and followed by HPV 11 (10–30% of genital warts) [26].

2.1. HPV and other cancers

Despite its contribution to the development of cervical cancer, HPV is also associated with oropharyngeal, vaginal, vulva and anal cancers [26, 27]. About 12% of cancers of the oropharynx and 3% of cancers of the mouth are attributed to HPV infection [26]. However, the major risk factors for these cancers are tobacco use and alcohol consumption. The effects of these two risk factors are multiplicative [26, 27].

The HPV infection results in about 90% of anal cancers [27]. The other risk factors to the development of anal cancers are HIV infection, cigarette smoking, anal intercourse and multiple sexual partners [27]. The HPV infection and pathologies are both increased in HIV-positive individuals [2]. The mechanism of interaction of HIV and HPV is not known but it may involve immune suppression rather than direct interaction [2].

The vaginal intraepithelial neoplasia, which is a preinvasive disease of the vagina, has been associated with HPV infection [28]. The vagina lacks a transformation zone, whereas in the cervix immature epithelial cells are infected with HPV [28]. It has been theorized that the HPV entry mechanism involves abrasions from coitus and the use of tampons. The HPV may begin its growth in a healing abrasion in a similar fashion as in the transformation zone. The upper third of the vagina is vulnerable to the development of dysplasia and carcinoma *in situ* whether or not hysterectomy has been performed previously for intraepithelial neoplasia [28]. Each of these entities has a potential for progression to invasive cancer. For this reason, women who have had a hysterectomy with a history of HPV or intraepithelial neoplasia should continue to have periodic cytologic screening of the vaginal apex [28].

The HPV infection is strongly associated in younger women with vulvar cancer. This is preceded with high-grade vulvar intraepithelial neoplasia which is commonly associated with high oncogenic type 16 and to a lesser extent type 18 [25]. Although the incidence of vulvar intraepithelial neoplasia and HPV has increased over the past decade, the incidence of vulvar cancer has remained relatively constant [25].

2.2. HPV and non-oncogenic conditions

The non-oncogenic or low-risk HPV types can cause benign condyloma acuminata (genital warts) [22]. The low-risk HPV types 6 and 11 are found in most of the genital warts [26, 29]. The HPV type 6 is most commonly detected in genital warts (about 90% of warts) followed by HPV type 11 (10–30% of warts) [30, 31]. The low-risk HPV types are rarely associated with dysplasia or cervical cancer [26]. Clinically apparent genital warts affect 1% of the sexually active population (15–49 years) in the USA [26, 29]. In the UK, genital warts were the second most commonly diagnosed sexually transmitted infection (after chlamydia) among young people (16–24 years) in a genitourinary medicine clinic [32].

3. Anatomy of the cervix in relation to HPV infection

Generally, HPV requires epithelial tissue for the completion of its viral cycle and the rich epithelial network of the cervix makes it susceptible to colonization by HPV. The epithelium of the cervix is divided into mature and differentiated cells which constitute the parabasal and basal layers adjacent to the basement membrane and the end-stage fully differentiated cells of the superficial layer [33]. The anatomical placement of the cervix in the vagina exposes it to the seminal fluid which harbor the HPV virus which usually has a predilection to the transformation zone, which has the most actively dividing cells.

3.1. Human papillomavirus, life cycle and invasion

The human papillomavirus measures about 55 nm in diameter and its viral genome is divided into three regions: the upstream regulatory region (URR), the early region (E1–E7) and the late region (L1 and L2) [34]. The genes in the early region dictate the production of copies of viral DNA, development of new messenger RNAs (mRNA) and eventual transformation of the host genome. In addition, E6 and E7 encode for the major transforming proteins which are capable of inducing cell proliferation and immortalization. The genes in the late region are responsible for the development of the viral coat. HPVs are epitheliotropic viruses and are responsible for several mucous and skin lesions. Infection is initiated when the virus gains entry into the basal cells of the epithelium.

The HPV life cycle is restricted to the cervical epithelium as shown in **Figure 1** [35]. The virus is thought to infect the basal cell layer of the epithelium via micro-abrasions and then uses the host cell machinery to replicate viral DNA and express virally encoded oncogenes [36]. The HPV has several mechanisms for avoiding the immune system. This includes the restriction of its life cycle to the epithelial cells that have short lifespan and therefore has no replication in the blood (no viraemia) and the infection is not spread systematically [35]. As a result, HPV does not need to destroy the host cell, and in the absence of cell death or a danger signal, HPV fails to trigger inflammation and an immune response [35, 36].

In addition, HPV down-regulates the expression of interferon genes. Type 1 interferon is a cytokine that has antiviral and antiproliferative properties. The HPV oncoproteins E6 and E7 can directly inhibit these antiviral pathways in the cell [35]. Then, the new viral particles are assembled in the upper layers of the epithelium. The virus will be released with the cells as they are shed from the epithelial surface. HPV immune evasive mechanisms enable the infection to persist [35].

3.2. HPV transmission

The majority of the anogenital HPV is sexually transmitted. If one partner has HPV, the other partner's chance of being infected with the same HPV type increases by >50 times [37]. Sexual intercourse and/or genital skin-to-skin contact are the primary routes of anogenital HPV transmission [38]. Condom use does not provide complete protection from HPV transmission and self-inoculation is possible [39]. Infection is thought to occur through microscopic tears or abrasions in the epithelium. Transmission by non-sexual routes is thought to be uncommon, but the possible routes include transmission from mother to newborn [40].

Other non-sexual routes of transmission are through finger-to-genital contact and transmission through fomites and environmental surfaces [41]. Vertical transmission together with other non-sexual routes may contribute to anogenital HPV infections in children [42].

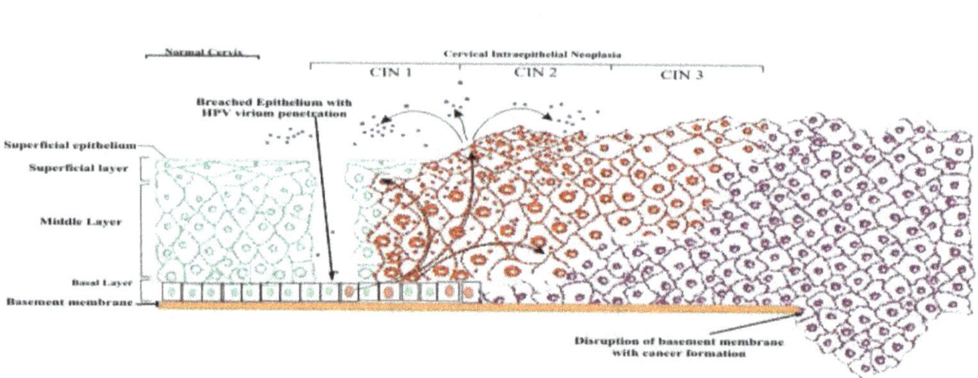

Figure 1. Diagram indicating the life cycle from HPV infection to frank carcinoma (adapted from Nature Rev Cancer, 2007).

In children, prior to any sexual activity, anogenital HPV DNA detection rates range between 3 and 55% and this variation is likely to be caused by different sample collection and HPV detection methods.

4. Risk of HPV infection

Every sexually active woman is at risk of acquiring an oncogenic HPV infection which may cause cervical cancer [43]. The risk of acquiring oncogenic HPV infection is high even after first intercourse and continues throughout a woman's sexually active lifetime [44]. HPV infections are very common with up to 80% of women acquiring HPV infection in their lifetime [26, 44]. While most HPV infections resolve naturally, there is currently no way of predicting which infection will persist [26]. The cumulative risk of acquiring cervical HPV infection in women with only one sexual partner is 46% (3 years after first sexual encounter) [45]. New HPV infections can be acquired at any age [46, 47] and the prevalence of infection is greatest (approximately 20%) in women less than 25 years of age [14]. The incidence of oncogenic HPV infection is around 5% in women 25–55 years of age [48]. Although new infections decrease with age, the risk of persistence of infection increases with age [15].

4.1. Co-factors that increase the risk of progress to cervical cancer

The persistence of HPV infection with the oncogenic HPV types is necessary but insufficient alone to cause cervical cancer [49]. Approximately 70% of cervical cancers worldwide is associated with HPV types 16 and 18 [25]. The HPV types 16 and 18 persist longer than low-risk HPV types [50]. Several other factors are associated with the development of cervical cancer following oncogenic HPV infection [26, 51]. These factors include environmental factors like smoking, sexual exposure especially for early onset of sex (coitarche) and high parity [46]. The other factors are hormonal, like in long-term use of oral contraceptives and immunosuppressive factors such as HIV, transplant recipients and long-term systemic steroid use [36, 39].

4.2. Pathway of HPV infection to cervical cancer

The progression of HPV infection to cervical cancer is a multi-step process. The initial infection of the cervix with HPV leads to viral entry into target basal epithelial cells. HPV oncogenes (E6 and E7) will be expressed and they modulate the effect of the tumor suppressor proteins p53 and Rb [34]. The HPV genome integrates into the host genome and this results in cytogenetic instability. These genetic changes allow for uncontrolled cell growth (immortalization) [34]. The final stage involves malignant transformation to invasive cervical cancer.

After the cervix is infected with HPV, the infection may cause mild Papanicolaou abnormalities and/or mild cervical intraepithelial neoplasia (CIN), which usually clear spontaneously [49, 52]. Studies have demonstrated that the persistence of high-risk HPV is a key factor in the progression to precancerous lesions or high-grade dysplasia (CIN 2/3), which has a greater likelihood of progression to invasive cancer [49].

It has also been shown that for every one million women infected with HPV about 100,000 will develop precancerous changes, about 8000 will develop carcinoma *in situ* while about 1600 will develop invasive cervical cancer if precancerous changes and CIS are not detected or treated [38]. Cervical cancer is an outcome of the oncogenic HPV infection. However, over 80% of HPV infection are asymptomatic, transient and resolve spontaneously [49, 52, 53]. This progression of HPV infection from precancerous conditions to cervical cancer is unpredictable and may take up to 20 years to complete [48].

5. Diagnosis

The aim of HPV testing is to determine the presence of high-risk HPV which can persist and result in a premalignant lesion of the cervix and subsequently cervical cancer [52]. The HPV test checks for the genetic material (DNA) of the HPV. The HPV test is done on a sample of cells from cervical smears collected with cytobrush among other methods of collection. The multiplex polymerase chain reaction (PCR) kits are used in determining the specific HPV genotypes while the real-time PCR kits are used in quantifying the HPV genotypes.

HPV genotypes are determined by polymerase chain reaction (PCR) and hybrid capture 2 (HC2). In determining the genotype by PCR, the process by hybridization using type-specific probes is utilized. The sequencing or restriction fragment length of the viral genome is determined in the process. Among various PCR methods, one of the most useful PCR methods for genotyping of HPV is the non-radioactive reverse line blot (RLB). In 37 mucotropic HPV types, the late region (L1) of the HPV genome is amplified using the general primers GP5+/GP6+ [50, 51, 54].

Another method of HPV DNA testing/genotyping is the digene which is a hybrid capture 2 (HC2). Hybrid capture 2 is a commercially available standardized kit that uses RNA probes to detect DNA from the oncogenic HPV types. The DNA of interest is merged with a specific HPV RNA probe cocktail. The combination created is fixed on a microplate coated with antibodies specific for the hybrid created and detected by a chemiluminescent substrate. The ability to detect low-risk or high-risk genotypes are determined by the RNA probe pool used during the process. RNA probe A when used is able to detect low-risk genotypes while RNA probe B identifies oncogenic genotypes. If an HPV test shows that high-risk types of HPV are present, further investigations such as a colposcopy and/or cervical biopsy may be recommended.

5.1. Treatment and prevention of HPV infection

The prevention of HPV infection is very important if the associated disease conditions are to be reduced. Abstinence and HPV vaccines are the two most important ways of preventing HPV infection. However, there are other ways of reducing the risk of transmission of the virus. Not having genital intercourse is an important way of avoiding the HPV infection but this is not realistic for most adults hence the need for other methods of prevention. For the sexually active women, the use of barrier methods such as condom during intercourse and dental dams for mouth-to-genital contact can help to reduce the transmission of HPV [50].

To be most effective, these barrier methods should be used with every sex act, from start to finish. The HPV can infect the areas that are not covered by a condom, so condoms may not fully protect against HPV infection. The other methods of reducing the risk of HPV infection are by having a faithful relationship with one partner, limiting the number of sexual partners and being with a partner who has had no or fewer prior sex partners [50]. But even people with only one lifetime sex partner can get infected with human papillomavirus [55, 56].

5.1.1. HPV vaccines

The HPV vaccines generate neutralizing antibodies which prevent the HPV infection. The induction of high and sustained levels of the neutralizing antibodies is a key mechanism of vaccine-induced protection. The neutralizing antibodies bind the HPV's outer shell (capsid) and prevent infection of the host cell [57]. Therefore, the neutralizing antibodies are likely the mediator of the protection [57, 58]. Currently, there are two vaccines administered for the prevention of HPV. They are the Cervarix and the Gardasil as illustrated in **Table 1**. The Cervarix contains antigens of virus-like particles of HPV 16 and 18 while the Gardasil contains those of HPV 16, 18, 6 and 11. The Cervarix protects against HPV 16 and 18 while the Gardasil protects against HPV 16, 18, 6 and 11. Therefore, the Gardasil protects against cervical cancer like the Cervarix and also protects against genital warts [59]. The vaccines are most effective if given before the female becomes sexually active. It is recommended that they are administered at the age of 11 or 12 years although a 9-year-old child can receive the vaccines (before the age of sexual debut) [59].

Catch-up vaccines could be given to girls and women between the ages of 13 and 26. This is for those who did not get any or all of the doses when they were younger. The vaccines are safe and effective and given in 3 doses over 6 months [60]. Boys and men can also get the HPV vaccines to prevent the HPV infection and the associated conditions such as genital warts and anal cancers. In addition, the male vaccination is recommended in order to reduce the reservoir

Vaccine	Target population	Serotypes	Disease targets	Dose schedules
Cervarix (Glaxosmithkline)	Girls and women aged 9–26 years	16 and 18	Prevention of cervical cancer caused by the 16 and 18 genotypes	Dose: 0.5 ml IM Schedule: 0, 1 and 6 months
Gardasil (MSD)	Girls and women aged 10–26 years	6, 11, 16 and18 (1° Gardasil) inclusive of HPV types 31, 33, 45, 52 and 58 (Gardasil 9)	Prevention of cervical cancer of listed serotypes and genital warts	Dose: 0.5 ml IM Schedule: 0, 2 and 6 months

Table 1. Vaccines against the human papillomavirus infection in prevention of cervical cancer [59].

load of the HPV in the males and hence reduce its transmission to the female partners. Neither Gardasil nor Cervarix can provide complete protection against the persistent infection with other HPV types, some of which also cause cervical cancer [61]. Therefore, about 30% of cervical cancers and 10% of genital warts will not be prevented by these vaccines. Despite the two vaccines, there are debates and researches on the need for booster doses [62–64]. In December 2014, Food and Drug Administration in the USA approved a nine-valent Gardasil-based vaccine called Gardasil-9. Gardasil-9 protects against infection with the four strains of HPV covered by the first generation of Gardasil as well as other strains responsible for 20% of cervical cancers (HPV types 31, 33, 45, 52 and 58) [65].

5.1.2. Booster vaccines for HPV

Vaccinations raise antibody levels to HPV, then antibody levels wane. The immune correlate of protection for HPV vaccination remains unknown [61]. Additional vaccine dose will boost immune memory in vaccinated women but recall of vaccine-induced immune memory by natural HPV exposure is unproven [62, 63]. The pace of HPV pathogenesis is uncertain, therefore, the requirement for booster vaccination is currently unknown [61].

Author details

Tamunomie K Nyengidiki*, Goddy Bassey and Ikechukwu Durugbo

*Address all correspondence to: tammynyengs@yahoo.com

Gynaecological Oncology Unit, Department of Obstetrics and Gynaecology, University of Port Harcourt Teaching Hospital, Port Harcourt, Rivers State, Nigeria

References

[1] Anorlu RI. Tumours of the cervix uteri. In: Agboola A, editor. Textbook of Obsterics and Gynaecology for Medical Students. 2nd ed. Ibadan: Heinemann Educational Books; 2006. pp. 167-182

[2] Parkin DM, Bray F. The burden of HPV-related cancers. Vaccine. 2006;**24**(suppl 3):S11–S25

[3] Hernandez BU, Wikens LR, Zhu X. Transmission of HPV in heterosexual couples. Emerging Infectious Diseases. 2008;**14**:888-894

[4] Thomas JO, Herrero R, Omigbodun AA, Oje-makinde K, Ajayi OI, et al. Prevalence of Papillomavirus infection in women in Ibadan, Nigeria: A population-based study. British Journal of Cancer. 2004;**90**(3):638-645

[5] Chinchai Y, Chansaenroj J, Swangvarees, Junyagdkul P, Poovorawan Y. Prevalence of HPV genotypes in cervical cancer. International Journal of Gynecological Cancer. 2012;**22**(6):1063-1068

[6] Ferlay J. GLOBOCAN 2002 Cancer Incidence, Mortality and Prevalence Worldwide. Lyon: IARC Cancer Base; 2004

[7] Parkin DM, Bray Fl, Devesas S. Cancer burden the year 2000. The global picture. European Journal of Cancer. 2001;**37**(suppl 8):S4–S66

[8] Jedy- Agba E, Girado MP, Ogunbiyi O, Oga E, Fabowale T, et al. cancer incidence in Nigeria; A report from population based cancer registries. Cancer Epidemiology. 2012;**36**(5):e271–e278

[9] Ferlay J, Shin HR, Bray F. GLOBOCAN: 2008 v 1.2 Cancer Incidence and Mortality Worldwide: IARC CancerBase No10 [Internet]. Lyon, France: International Agency for Research in cancer; 2010. Available from: http: globocan; iarc.fr

[10] Tabone T, Garland SM, Mola G, O'Connor M, Danielewski J, Tabrizi SN. Prevalence of HPV in women with cervical cancer in Papua New Guinea. International Journal of Gynecology & Obstetrics. 2012;**117**(1):30-302

[11] Tabrizi SN, Law I, Buadromo E, Steven MP, Fong J et al. Prevalence of HPV genotype in cervical biopsies from women diagnosed with cervical intra-epithelial neoplasia or cervical cancer in Fiji. Sex Health. 2011;**8**(3):338-42.

[12] The Ten Teachers. Malignant diseases of the uterus and cervix. In: Monga A, Dobbs S, editors. Gynaecology by Ten Teachers. 19th ed. London Book Power; 2011. pp. 52-53

[13] De Sanjose A, Qiunt WG. Worldwide prevalence and genotype distribution of cervical HPV DNA in women with normal cytology: A meta-analysis. Lancet Infectious Diseases. 2007;**7**(7):453-459

[14] Borchell AN, Winer RL, De Sanjose S, Franco EL. Epidemiology and transmission dynamics of genital HPV infection. Vaccine. 2006;**24**(suppl 3):L52–L61

[15] Castle PE, Schiffman M, Hererro R. A prospective study of age trends in cervical HPV acquisition and persistence in Guamacaste, Costa Rica. Journal of Infectious Diseases. 2005;**191**:1808-1816

[16] Bosch FX. Epidemiology and natural history of HPV infections and type-specific implications in cervical neoplasia. Vaccine. 2008;**26**(suppl 10):K1–K16

[17] Franco P, Michela P, Antonella DM, Ahissou RF, Luigi M. prevalence of HPV infection in women in Benin, West Africa. Journal of Virology. 2011;**8**:514

[18] Noe-velazque M, Maria A. Prevalence of HPV genotypes in women from the rural region of Puebla, Mexico. International Journal of Infectious Diseases. 2008;**13**(6):690-695

[19] Schnatz PF, Markelova NV, Holmes D. The prevalence of cervical HPV and cytological abnormalities in association with reproductive factors of rural Nigerian women. Journal of Women's Health. 2008;**17**:279-284

[20] Nweke IG, Baryor AF, Abdulkareem FB, Nwadike VU. Prevalence of HPV DNA in HIV positive women in LUTH, Lagos. British Microbiology Research Journal. 2013;**3**(3): 400-413.

[21] Akarolo- Anthony SN, Ogbonna CC, Famooto OA, Dareng EO et al. HIV associated high risk HPV infection among Nigerian women. Biomed Central Infect Dis.2013;**31**(13):521-27

[22] Denny L, Ademole I, Anorlu R. HPV prevalence and type distribution in invasive cervical cancer in Sub-saharan Africa. International Journal of Cancer. 2014;**134**(6):1389-1398

[23] Ajobiewe OJ, Isu NR, Agwale S, Ajobiewe HF, Dagana A. Epidemiology of subtypes of HPV in Abuja Metropolis. Nigerian Journal of General Practice.2012;**10**(1):1-8

[24] Smith JS. HPV type distribution in invasive cervical cancer and high-grade cervical lesions: A meta- analysis update. International Journal of Cancer. 2007;**121**:621-632

[25] Munoz N, Bosch FX, De Sanjose S. Epidemiologic classification of HPV types associated with cervical cancer. New England Journal of Medicine. 2003;**348**:518-527

[26] Baseman JG, Koutsky. The epidemiological HPV infections. Journal of Clinical Virology. 2005;**32**:S16–S25

[27] Hillemans P. The most common sexual transmitted infections worldwide. BMC Infectious Diseases. 2008;**8**:76-85

[28] Cameron JE, Hargensee ME. HPV infection and disease in HIV individuals. Cancer Treatment and Research. 2007;**133**:185-213

[29] Markowitz LE, Dunne EF, Saraiya M, Lawson HW. CDC Advisory Committee on Immunization Practices (ACIP). Quadrivalent HPV vaccine: Recommendations of ACIP. MMWR Recommendations and Reports. 2007;**56**:1-24

[30] Gall S. Female genital warts; Global trends and treatment. Infectious Diseases in Obstetrics and Gynecology. 2001;**9**(3):149-154

[31] Greer CE, Wheeler CM, Ladner MB. HPV type particles in patients with genital warts. Journal of Clinical Microbiology. 1995;**33**:2058

[32] Brown DR, Schroeder JM, Bryan JT. Detection of multiple HPV types in condyloma acuminata lesions from otherwise healthy and immunosuppressed patients. Journal of Clinical Microbiology. 1999;**37**:3316-3322

[33] Martins AW, Erin M, Elizabeth RU. Human papillomavirus and molecular considerations for cancer risk. Cancer. 2008;**113**(10):2981-2994

[34] Kwawukume EY, Srofenyoh EK. Premalignant Lesions of the Female Genital Tract. Comprehensive Gynaecology in the Tropics. 1st ed. Accra: Graphic packaging Ltd; 2005. pp. 396-411

[35] Frazer IH. Prevention of cervical cancer through papilloma virus vaccination. Nature Reviews Immunology. 2004;**4**:46-54

[36] Burd EM. Human papilloma virus and cervical cancer. Clinical Microbiology Reviews. 2003;**16**:1-17

[37] Burchell AN, Tellier PP, Hanler J. Coutlee F, Franco EL. Influence of partners infection status on prevalent of HPV among persons with new sex partner. Sexually Transmitted Diseases. 2010;**37**:34-40

[38] McIntosh N. Frequently asked question on vaccines and immunization practices. JHPIEGO. 2008; Strategy paper 8.16-18

[39] Schiffman M, Kjaer SK. Natural history of anogenital HPV infection and neoplasia. Journal of the National Cancer Institute Monographs. 2003;**31**:14-19

[40] Smith EM, Ritche JM, Yankowitz J, Swarnavel S. Hangen TH. HPV prevalence and types in newborns and parents: Concordance and modes of transmission. Sexually Transmitted Diseases. 2004;**31**:57-62

[41] Strauss S. Sastry P, Soenex C, Edwards S, Gray J. Contamination of environmental surfaces by genital HPV. Sexually Transmitted Infections. 2002;**28**:135-138

[42] Doerfler D, Bernhaus A, Kottmel A, Christine S. HPV infection prior to coitarche. American Journal of Obstetrics & Gynecology. 2009;**200**:479.el–487.e5

[43] Gravitte PE, Jamshidi R. Diagnosis and management of oncogenic cervical HPV infection. Infectious Disease Clinics of North America. 2005;**19**:439-458

[44] Brown DR, Shew ML, Qudari B. A Longitudinal study of genital HPV infection in a cohort of closely followed adolescent women. Journal of Infectious Diseases. 2005;**191**:182-192

[45] Collins S, Mazloamzadeh S, Winter H. High incidence of cervical HPV infection in women during the first sexual relationship. British Journal of Obstetrics and Gynaecology. 2002;**109**:96-98

[46] Grainge MJ, Seth R, Guo L. Cervical HPV screening among older women. Emerging Infectious Diseases. 2005;**11**:1680-1685

[47] Franco EL, Harper DM. Vaccination against HPV infection. A new paradigm in cervical cancer control. Vaccine. 2005;**23**:2388-2394

[48] Munoz N, Mendez F, Posso H. Incidence, duration, and determinants of cervical HPV infection in a cohort of Colombian women with normal cytological results. Journal of Infectious Diseases. 2004;**190**:2077-2087

[49] Bosch FX, Lorincz A, Munoz N, Meijer CJ, Shan KV. The causal relation between HPV and cervical cancer. Journal of Clinical Pathology. 2002;**55**(4):244-265

[50] Schmitt M, Dondog B, Waterboer T, Pawlita M. Homogenous amplification of genital HPV by PCR using novel broad spectrum GP5+ and GP6+ primers. Journal of Clinical Microbiology. 2008;**46**:1050-1059

[51] Lee JK. Kim MK, Song SH, Hong JH, Min KJ. Comparison of HPV and typing by hybrid capture 2, linear array, DNA chip and cycle sequencing in cervical swabs. International Journal of Gynecological Cancer. 2009;**19**(2):266-272

[52] Moscicki AB, Shiboski S, Broering J. The natural history of HPV infection as measured by repeated DNA testing in adolescent and young women. Journal of Paediatrics. 1998;**132**:277-284

[53] Guiliano AR, Papenfuss MR, Dewman CA, Hunter JB. HPV prevalence at the USA-Mexico border among women 40 years of age and older. International Journal of STD & AIDS. 2005;**16**:247-251

[54] Schmitt M, Dondog B, Waterboer T, Pawlita M, Tommasino M. Abundance of multiple high-risk HPV infections found in cervical cells analyzed by use of ultrasensitive HPV genotyping assay. Journal of Clinical Microbiology. 2010;**48**:143-149

[55] Human Papillomavirus. In Centre for Disease Control and prevention, Epidemiology and Prevention of Vaccines Preventable Diseases. Hamborsky J, Kroger A, Wolfe S edns. 13th edition, Washington DC. Public Health Foundation Publishers. 2015;175-178.

[56] The Health Protection Agency (HPA). Centre for Infection Annual Data UK. London: National Press Release; 2010

[57] Stanley M, Lowy DR, Frazer I. Prophylactic HPV vaccine: Underlying mechanism. Vaccine. 2006;**24**(Suppl 3):S106–S113

[58] HPV WHO position paper. Weekly Epidemiological Record. 2009;**84**:118-131

[59] Brown DR, Kjaer SK, Sigurdsson K, Iversen OE. The impact of quadrivalent HPV vaccine on infection and disease due to oncogenic non-vaccine HPV types in generally HPV-naïve women aged 16-26. Journal of Infectious Diseases. 2009;**199**:926-934

[60] Slade BA, Leidel L, Vellozi C, Woo EJ. Post licensure safety surveillance for quadrivalent HPV recombinant vaccine. Journal of the American Medical Association. 2009;**302**:750-757

[61] Paavonen J, Naud P, Salmeron J, Wheeler CM. Efficacy of HPV vaccine against cervical infection and precancer caused by oncogenic HPV types (PATRICIA): Final analysis of double-blind randomized study in young women. Lancet. 2009;**374**:302-314

[62] Pichichero ME. Booster vaccinations: Can immunologic memory outpace disease pathologenesis? Paediatrics. 2009;**124**:1633-1641

[63] Olsson SE, Vlla LL, Costa RL, Petta CA. Induction of immune memory following administration of a prophylactic quadrivalent HPV types 6/11/16/18 virus-like particle vaccine. Vaccine. 2007;**25**:4931-4939

[64] Einstein MH. Acquired immune response to oncogenic HPV associated with prophylactic cervical cancer vaccines. Cancer Immunology Immunotherapy. 2008;**57**:443-451

[65] FDA Approves Gardasil-9 for Prevention of Certain Cancers Caused by Additional Types of HPV. Press release of 10 December 2014 [Internet]. 2017. Available from: www.fda.gov/news events/newsroom @13.00hrs [Accessed 20th February]

10

Bacterial Vaginosis and Sexually Transmitted Diseases: Relationship and Management

Marco Bertini

Abstract

In the last few decades, bacterial vaginosis (BV) has become an emerging pathology; its relationship with pregnancy, pelvic inflammatory disease (PID), infertility, preterm delivery, and neonatal small for gestational age are well established. BV substantially changes vaginal microbiome and these modifications could facilitate sexually transmitted infections (STIs). Several studies have reported an association between abnormal vaginal microbiota, in particular, BV and depletion of lactobacilli species, and increased risk of sexually transmitted infections (STIs) acquisition. Immunologic, enzymatic, and metabolic mechanisms could operate independently or in combination to enhance STIs' transmission. Several studies have pointed out this association: vaginal microbiome modifications in BV could predispose to sexually transmitted diseases (STDs). Considering the high social impact of BV together with its relationship with STDs, it seems to be "crucial" to restore vaginal microbiome in childbearing age women in order to reduce STIs acquisition. Some experimental clinical data seem to confirm this observation: vaginal microbiome restoration by probiotics/synbiotics seems to improve not only STIs' acquisition but also STDs' pathology progression. Restoring vaginal microbiome could represent an international, innovative, and less-expensive gold standard to counteract STDs' spread and acquisition.

Keywords: bacterial vaginosis (BV), sexually transmitted diseases (STDs), vaginal microbiome, probiotics/synbiotics, *Lactobacillus*

1. Introduction

The infections of the human reproductive system include sexually transmitted diseases (STDs) that are defined as "infection that spreads primarily through person-to-person," and non-STDs that are "endogenous infections of the genital organs such as "bacterial vaginosis" (BV) [1].

Both STDs and non-STDs are a major concern for public health system worldwide [1].

Sexually transmitted diseases (STDs) are the most frequently "unrelieved" diseases in the United States [2]; its prevalence is high all over the world, especially in the United States where about 12 million new cases occur each year [2].

Surprisingly, STDs represent a public health problem also in the developing countries, being the second cause of health loss in childbearing women [2].

STDs have a lot of health-related consequences between women, adolescent, and children, particularly in ethnic/racial minority group: In U.S. a lot of women (more than a million) experienced an episode of pelvic inflammatory disease (PID) per year: considering that PID represents an important health consequences of STDs and that 15% of the infertile U.S. women experienced a tubal inflammation related to PID, it seems obvious to ascribe to STDs as playing a leading role in women health [2].

Also, the relationship between untreated STDs and pregnancy are well known: neonatal pneumonia, neonatal ophthalmia, mental and physical developmental disabilities, and fetal death related to syphilis are the more impacting consequences of untreated STDs [2].

Unprotected sexual encounters and having multiple sexual partners, together with higher biologic aptness, are the leading causes of STDs in adolescents between 10 and 19 years, which seems to be the higher risk category among all age groups [2].

Bacterial vaginosis (BV) is a clinical syndrome resulting from the replacement of normal hydrogen peroxide-producing lactobacillus species in the vagina with high concentration of anaerobic bacteria such as *Gardnerella vaginalis* and *Mycoplasma hominis* [3].

BV is the most prevalent form of vaginal infection among women of reproductive age, affecting 8–23%, and is the most common etiology of vaginal symptoms prompting women to seek medical care [4].

It does not appear to be a sexually transmitted disease, although it has been associated with having multiple sex partners [3].

It is the most common cause of vaginal discharge or malodor and is commonly encountered in the context of STDs [3].

Since the relationship between BV and STDs is not well established, the aim of this chapter will be to describe the role of BV in determining STDs and to point out how BV management could improve STDs' epidemiology and prevalence.

2. Vaginal microbiome

There are approximately 10 times as many microbes associated with a human as there are human cells in the body [4]: despite recognition of the importance of the interactions between the host human body and the bacteria it supports, there remain many unanswered questions regarding how the microbial environment varies with and among individuals in healthy and diseased states [5, 6].

Historically, bacteria have been identified using Gram stain or culture-based techniques but, unfortunately, as few as 20% of bacteria closely associated with the human body can be cultivated via culture-based techniques [6].

Culture-based methods may therefore underestimate the diversity of microbiome [5, 6].

During the past decade there has been an explosion of interest in molecular-based, culture-independent techniques to study the microbiome [7–14].

Molecular-based techniques involve analysis of 16S ribosomal RNA (rRNA), DNA hybridization, or fingerprinting and next-generation sequencing [7–14].

The National Institute of Health, recognizing the potential of molecular techniques to further understand human bacterial communities, initiated the Human Microbiome Project (HMP) in 2007 [15].

The HMP targeted the genitourinary system because it has been well established for more than a century that bacteria are present within the vagina and that an imbalance within this microbial environment may be associated with disease [16–19].

Research has demonstrated that alterations in the vaginal microbiome affect susceptibility to gynecologic infections, including cervicovaginitis, postoperative infections, and human immunodeficiency virus (HIV) infection, but also that many of the differences in the vaginal microbiome may represent normal variation and may not necessarily indicate disease [20–24].

However, despite evidence from both culture-dependent and independent methods supporting the dynamic nature of the vaginal microbiome, both methods suggest that the microbiome is relatively stable through periods of hormonal fluctuation, such as puberty or the menstrual cycle [20–24].

It can be partially confirmed by the old statement of Albert Doderlein (1892): by using culture method he found that vaginal microbiome of healthy women possess a predominance of Gram-positive rods named "Doderlein lactobacillus" from his name [25].

More than 120 years later, it is universally accepted that lactobacilli are the predominant species of the human microbioma and that they have a key role in maintaining an acidic environment able to protect women against virus and bacteria responsible for opportunistic infections and STDs [26].

It was remarkable to observe that humans species are the only one with this relative abundance of lactobacilli in vagina (more than 70%), while other mammals present not more than 1% of lactobacilli in the vaginal microbiota [26] (**Figure 1**).

To date, most comparative studies in mammals find that hosts with similar lifestyles and evolutionary histories harbor similar microbiomes at a given body site, both in the bacteria taxa they contain and the functions they provide to hosts [27, 28].

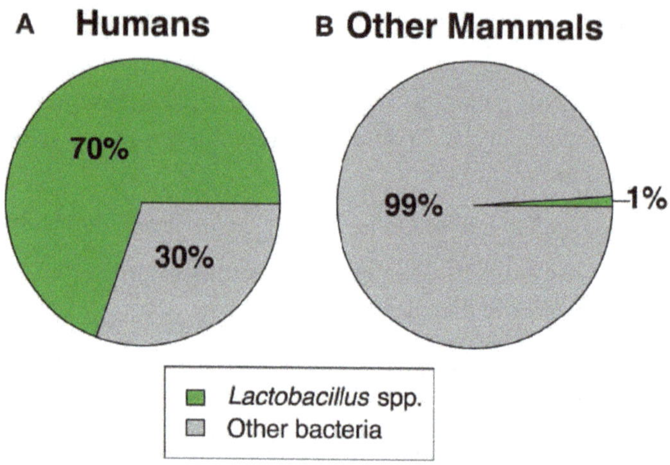

Figure 1. Mean vaginal relative abundance of *Lactobacillus* spp. vs other bacteria in humans (A) and nonhumans (B) [26].

One important exception to this pattern is the vaginal microbiome, where humans exhibit striking differences in community composition compared to other mammals; specifically, the human vaginal microbiome is dominated by *Lactobacillus* spp. [29, 30].

These lactobacilli process glycogen and it breaks down products to produce lactic acid, leading to an exceptional low vaginal pH of < 4.5 [26].

Lactobacilli dominance and low pH of the human vaginal microbiome are hypothesized to benefit women by reducing disease risk [31].

Furthermore, the loss of lactobacilli dominance is linked to bacterial vaginosis (BV), which is associated with an overgrowth of anaerobic bacteria, relatively high vaginal pH (>4.5) infertility, preterm birth, maternal infections, and increased risk of STDs [21, 30–33].

To date, four hypotheses have been proposed to explain the uniqueness of the human vaginal microbiome relative to other mammals: two mechanistic explanation and two evolutionary explanation: the first "mechanistic hypothesis" considers that the differences in vaginal microbioma between human and nonhuman mammals are related to the differences in reproductive physiology: a typical 28 days ovarian cycle of the humans is quite different from other mammals [34].

This 28 days ovarian cycle in reproductive women is orchestrated by steroids and lactobacilli abundance is strictly linked to estrogen levels [35].

The second "mechanistic hypothesis," the common function hypothesis, proposes that in nonhuman mammals, other bacteria may protect hosts via mechanisms other than lactic acid and low vaginal pH so that the presence of lactobacilli may not be a requirement for a healthy vaginal environment [34, 35].

In addition to these mechanistic hypothesis, two evolutionary explanation have been proposed, the first, referred to as the "disease risk hypothesis," proposes that humans have higher STDs risk than nonhuman mammals because species with promiscuous mating strategies are predicted to have higher STD risk than those with only single, brief reproductive episode per breeding season [36, 37].

The last evolutionary explanation, the "obstetric protection hypothesis" suggests that selection for lactobacilli in the human vagina is due to the high risk of microbial complications associated with pregnancy and childbirth, thus lactobacilli and low vaginal pH may serve as a protective function during human birth, and these traits are unnecessary in mammals with less pregnancies and birth risks [38, 39].

An understanding of the diversity of the vaginal microbial environment during states of health and disease is essential for the identification of risk factors for disease and the development of appropriate treatment [26].

2.1. Vaginal microbiome in the healthy state

Nowadays, it is well established that the normal vaginal microbiome is dominated by lactobacilli species [16, 40, 41].

Years of research have clearly demonstrated that the vaginal microbiota represents the first barrier against obligatory or facultative pathogens in the female reproductive tract [43].

It is well known that women with low lactobacillus species in vaginal microbioma are at high risk for urogenital infective diseases and adverse pregnancy outcomes [42].

Lactobacilli help to prevent vaginal infection by producing lactic acid, hydrogen peroxide, bacteriocins, or through competitive exclusion of other bacteria [43–46].

Studies utilizing 16S rRNA PCR have demonstrated that the vaginal microbial environment is usually dominated by one or two lactobacilli species, most frequently *Lactobacillus iners*, *Lactobacillus crispatus*, *Lactobacillus gasseri*, or *Lactobacilli jensenii* [9, 47].

Of the 73% of women with lactobacilli-dominant environment, the most frequently detected organism was *L. iners*, which was the predominant organism in 34% of women sampled [9].

The second most common Lactobacilli-dominant environment was *L. crispatus* (26.2% of women) [9].

The identification of an *L. iners*-dominant microbial environment was in contrast to findings from early molecular-based and culture-dependent studies which suggested other dominant *Lactobacilli* spp, including *Lactobacillus acidophilus*, *L. crispatus*, and *L. jensenii* [48, 49].

It seems that the species of lactobacilli that dominate the vaginal environment may have implications for gynecologic health: different species may differentially predispose to dysbiosis [50, 51].

For example, it has been suggested that an *L. crispatus* vaginal microbiome is more stable and less likely to transition to bacterial vaginosis (BV) than *L. iners* or mixed lactobacilli environment [52, 53].

Culture-dependent and microscopy methods demonstrated that the composition of normal vaginal flora may also fluctuate within an individual woman: this "fluctuation" is related to the menstrual cycle or as result of sexual activities [54, 55].

During menses there is a decrease in lactobacilli and a relative increase in the proportion of bacteria associated with higher Nugent Scores [54, 55].

Recent sexual activity may also affects the microbial composition of the vagina by decreasing the proportion of the lactobacilli species present, which may predispose to dysbiosis with the loss of the protective effects of lactobacilli [53, 56].

Decreased of lactobacilli have also been observed in postmenopausal women, specifically those with vaginal dryness or atrophy [57–59].

The observed fluctuation throughout the menstrual cycle may be explained by evidence that high levels of E2 may favor a lactobacilli-dominant environment [53, 60, 61].

Evidence from culture-dependent and independent methods supported the dynamic nature of the vaginal microbiome [62–64].

A lot of studies have evaluated the vaginal microbiota in tandem by both culture-based and molecular techniques: the results demonstrate a moderate level of concordance providing similar but not identical vaginal microbiome profiles [62–64].

Also interesting is the fact that the quantity and proportion of specific microorganisms in the vagina may vary between women of different ethnic origins: African-American women may have an increased *L. iners* and decreased *L. crispatus* levels compared with Caucasian or Asian women [53].

This distinction is important because *L. iners* dominated flora may predispose to BV [53].

Molecular studies have also demonstrated that African-American and Hispanic women are more likely to harbor a vaginal microbiome dominated by bacteria other than lactobacilli species compared with Caucasian women [9, 66, 67].

These studies suggest that African-American women may have higher levels of *Gardnerella, Atopobium, Clostridiales,* and BV-associated bacterial species or be more likely to harbor a polymicrobial environment compared with Caucasian women [9, 65, 66].

Taken together, these data suggest that the differences in the microbiome between women of various races may alter woman's predisposition to infection and may at least in part explain the racial disparities in the incidence of BV and STDs [67, 68].

Concluding, vaginal microbiome in healthy women is a lactobacilli-dominated environment in which pH (under 4.5), lactic acid, hydrogen peroxide, bacteriocins, biosurfactants and co-aggregant activities counteract the growth of Gram-negative anaerobes bacteria such as *G. vaginalis*, Bacteroides, Mobiluncus spp, E. coli: when this equilibrium is broken (decreased of lactobacilli and increased of Gram-negative bacteria) vaginal pH increases and BV was detected.

2.2. Vaginal microbiome in pathologic state

2.2.1. Vaginal microbiome in bacterial vaginosis

From the beginning of 1900, the medical community accepted that a shift in the microbial environment of the vagina, specifically a decrease in "Doderlein's rods" (later identified as lactobacilli) can lead to symptomatic vaginitis with vaginal discharge [16, 40].

Subsequent studies by Gardner and Dukes demonstrated that nonspecific vaginitis (the old name of BV) was associated with a relative increase in rod-shaped bacteria on Gram stain, later identified as *G. vaginalis* [17, 69, 70].

These studies also described the "clue-cells" as characteristic of BV, resulting from vaginal epithelial cells with grainy cell borders [17, 69].

In order to implement standardized diagnostic criteria, researchers pointed out diagnostic clinical criteria (Amsel's criteria) and Gram stain criteria (Nugent scores): Amsel's criteria requires almost three of four "clinical conditions" to be present: (1) thin, white, vaginal discharge; (2) vaginal pH > 4.5; (3) "clue cells" on microscopy evaluation; (4) positive "whiff test" (10% KOH addition to sample produces fishy odor) [19, 71].

Are Amsel's criteria "Clinical Criteria"? Are we sure that pH values or clue cells or whiff test evaluation are "Clinical Criteria"?

The only "real" clinical criteria for women is "vaginal discharge" but, only taking into account TV and media campaigns for the use of panty-liners in women, it is easy to understand "the reason why" BV is underdiagnosed by gynecologists; on one side, the women feel their "vaginal discharge" like "physiological," and on the other side, vaginal symptoms are not "so urgent" for gynecological consultation.

This is the reason why BV is "a very dangerous pathology": the time from the beginning of the BV and the diagnosis is too much and, during this time, the local defense of the vagina disappeared leading, in the meanwhile, to more susceptibility to STDs and the bacteria facultative pathogen of vagina such as *Mobiluncus, Prevotella,* and *Escherichia coli* could determine an ascending pelvic inflammatory disease (PID) with subsequent infertility.

The Nugent score is evaluated by calculating the proportion of large, Gram-positive rods (*Lactobacilli*), small, Gram-variable rods (*Gardnerella*), and curved, Gram-variable rods (*Mobiluncus* species) on Gram stain [71].

The sensitivity and specificity of Amsel's criteria was estimated to be around 70% and 94%, respectively, and of the Nugent score were 89 and 83%, respectively [72].

Culture-dependent studies of BV demonstrate increased diversity of vaginal bacteria (including an increase in facultative anaerobes as *Gardnerella, Mycoplasma,* and *Prevotella*), with a simultaneous decrease of lactobacilli [73].

With an increasing use of molecular-based techniques to study the vaginal microbiome, bacteria that seemingly evaded detection using culture-based methods have now been associated with BV, including *Atopobium vaginae, Clostridiales,* and *Megasphaera* species [47, 66, 74, 75].

2.2.2. *Vaginal microbiome in sexually transmitted infection*

It seems universally accepted that increased bacterial diversity, as in BV, with the well-known vaginal ecosystem modifications, could be associated with gynecological infections, such as *Chlamydia trachomatis, Neisseria gonorrhoeae, Trichomonas vaginalis,* human papilloma virus (HPV), and herpes simplex virus (HSV) 2 infections [21, 76–78].

It is unclear whether it is the altered levels of bacteria themselves that predispose to infection or whether the altered vaginal microbiome leads to BV, which predispose to these pathologies owing, for example, to altered pH (leading to less efficient neutralization of pathogen, decreased of immune response, loss of hydrogen peroxide activity).

Numerous studies have demonstrated the association between BV and an increased risk of HIV acquisition: hydrogen peroxide produced by lactobacilli is known to have viricidal activities and, consequently, the relative decrease in lactobacilli in BV women may increase susceptibility to HIV infection [23, 24, 39, 79].

A prospective cohort study evaluating the relationship between the vaginal microbial environment and infection risk, the absence of lactobacilli on culture, and the presence of abnormal vaginal flora on Gram stain were associated with an increased risk of HIV acquisition, even after controlling for risk factors [22].

Nevertheless, molecular-based techniques and culture methods confirmed that vaginal microbiome in STDs is usually modified and different from women in healthy status and that the absence of lactobacilli on culture and the presence of abnormal vaginal flora on Gram stain were associated with an increased risk of STDs.

2.2.3. *Vaginal microbiome in upper genital tract infection*

The vaginal microbiome modifications affect vaginal health, and pathology may also predispose to upper genital tract infection, such as pelvic inflammatory disease (PID) [79].

Subclinical PID (histological evidence of endometritis) was detected in 15% of women with BV diagnosed by clinical and Gram stain criteria [79].

Women with vaginal samples (Gram stain and culture) positive for "BV-associated bacteria (BVAB)" (*Gardnerella, Mycoplasma,* anaerobic Gram-negative rods, and Ureaplasma urealyticum) were at increased risk for PID [80].

Since isolation of BV-associated bacteria in the vagina has been demonstrated to increase the risk of sexually transmitted infection acquisition, the correlation of BV with PID may be related to altered vaginal flora that predisposes to STIs and subsequent ascending infection [76, 77].

Available data from upper genital tract structures confirm that BV-associated bacteria can be isolated from upper genital tract.

In a study on 89 women affected by acute salpingitis (45 with pathology and 44 as control group) 16SrDNA detected bacteria in the fallopian tubes of 24% of cases and none of controls [81].

There was a statistically significant difference in the proportion of upper genital tract microbiome based on race: African-American and Hispanic women were more likely to harbor an upper genital tract microbiome dominated by a nonlactobacilli species compared with Caucasian, and this is in contrast with those of vaginal microbiome.

The reasons of this "discrepancy" are not clear and, probably, future acquisitions on molecular-based techniques may facilitate to better understand these differences.

3. Bacterial vaginosis

Bacterial vaginosis is a polymicrobial clinical syndrome resulting from replacement of the normal hydrogen peroxide producing Lactobacillus spp in the vagina with high concentration of anaerobic bacteria (e.g., *Prevotella* sp, *Mobiluncus* sp, *G. vaginalis, Ureaplasma,* and *Mycoplasma*) [10].

BV is a common vaginal condition among U.S. women and also worldwide, especially in childbearing age women [79].

A recent analysis of the National and Nutrition Examinations Surveys demonstrated that almost one-third of women were positive for BV [80].

BV is almost three times more common among black than white women [12], and it has been correlated with particular sexual behavior such as young age at coitarche, life time number of sex partners, a recent history of multiple sex partners, and a recent history of new sex partner [80–83].

The reason for the higher prevalence of BV among black women is unknown but the relationship between BV and race is remarked also from the number of the percentage of black infants born preterm in U.S. (17.5%) vs 10.2% of white infants [82].

BV could account for as much as 30% of the racial difference in premature birth and infant mortality [82].

Other risk factors for BV seem to be "vaginal douching" and use of intrauterine device (IUD) for birth control so that these practices must be limited in women of childbearing age [83].

BV seems not to be a self-limiting pathology since it has been consider a predisponent factor for PID, infertility, PPROM, preterm delivery, and neonatal small for gestational age [82, 83].

Since a lot of cross-sectional and prospective cohort studies have found that BV is associated with acquisition of both HIV and sexually transmitted infections, it seems to be almost interesting to fully understand this vaginal pathology to better clarify its role in determining STDs.

One of the most important "practical problems" of BV is that it is a "silent vaginitis" from a symptomatic point of view.

Comparing BV with specific vaginitis (e.g., vaginal infections clearly referred to vaginal obligatory pathogen such as *Candida vaginalis* or *T. vaginalis*), it is easy to understand why BV diagnosis is underestimated by gynecologists [84] (**Table 1**).

Approximately 50% of the women affected by BV are asymptomatic [82, 83].

In addition, also considering the standard clinical criteria for the diagnosis of BV (Amsel's criteria): almost three of four "clinical conditions" are to be present: (1) thin, white, vaginal discharge; (2) vaginal pH > 4.5; (3) "clue cells" on microscopy evaluation; and (4) positive "whiff test" (10% KOH addition to sample produces fishy odor) [19]. It seems to be obvious that the only real clinical condition is the vaginal discharge that can often be perceived by women like "a kind of physiologic condition."

	Bacterial vaginosis	Candidiasis	Trichomoniasis
Symptoms	Approx. 50% asymptomatic	10–20% asymptomatic	10–50% asymptomatic
	Offensive fishy smelling discharge	Vulval itching	Offensive vaginal discharge
		Vulval soreness	Vulval itching/irritation
		Vaginal discharge (nonoffensive)	Dysuria
		Superficial dyspareunia	Rarely low abdominal discomfort
Clinical signs	Thin white homogenous discharge, coating walls of vagina, and vestibule	Vulval erythema	Vulval erythema
	Absence of vaginitis	Vulval fissuring	Vaginitis
		Vaginal discharge may be curdy (nonoffensive)	Vaginal dsicharge in up to 70% frothy and yellow in 10–30%
		Satellite skin lesions	Approx. 2% "strawberry" cervix visible to naked eye
		Vulval oedema	5–15% no abnormal signs

Table 1. Symptoms and clinical signs of bacterial vaginosis, candidiasis, and trichomoniasis (adapted from) [85].

This means that the rupture of vaginal microbiome equilibrium determining BV could frequently happened without a real alarm in women and, consequently, this long-lasting vaginal imbalance in "apparently healthy women" could bring to invalidate ascending pathologies such as PID or STDs.

- Why the presence of BV could lead to such as improving urogenital pathologies?
- Why the "natural vaginal microbiome" of healthy people could protect against vaginal infections?
- Why the presence of lactobacilli seems to be pivotal in women health?

These Gram-positive bacteria possess a lot of activities that could be useful to counteract vaginal facultative and obligatory pathogen.

It is well known that the term lactobacilli means bacteria that are able to hydrolyze sugars (especially glycogen in the vagina) producing lactic acid and other acids (e.g., pyroglutamic acid): this happened because they try to conserve the optimal vaginal pH for their survival.

Vaginal pH < 4.5 is the optimal condition for their life but it is detrimental for other bacteria such as a lot of anaerobes Gram-facultative bacteria that are commonly present in vagina, also in the healthy women, but with low vaginal concentration: once that lactobacilli decrease, we assist to an increase in vaginal pH with a consequent increase in anaerobes facultative bacteria [82–84].

Low vaginal pH seems to possess also direct antiviral and antimicotic activities related to unfavorable vaginal condition for these infective agents [82–84].

Lactic acid is a potent broad-spectrum bactericide and virucide [83].

During the process of glycogen metabolism in the vagina, hydrogen peroxynitrite is produced: this molecule possesses antiviral, antibacterial, and antimicotic properties [82–84].

In addition, lactobacilli produced a lot of bacteriocins, substances that locally possess antibacterial activities [82–84].

Lactobacilli have demonstrated to possess some cosurfactant and antiaggregant activities that could be useful in controlling vaginal anaerobes growing-up [82–87].

Last but not the least, the ability of a lactobacilli predominants spp. to modulate local immunosystem [86, 87].

Genital epithelial cells and human microbiota seems to regulate the innate immune response: so that genital tract immune response plays a key role in the etiopathogenesis and pathophysiology of BV [87].

It has been demonstrated that the derangement of vaginal microbiota modifies pathogen's susceptibility encouraging HIV shedding/replication in women genital tract and consequently leading to an increase in the transmission of HIV from female to male [86–88].

It seems that activation of Toll-like receptors (TLRs) could lead to BV-associated inflammation [87].

Recurrence of BV in HIV-infected people seems to be associated with agenetic variation in TLR4, TLR9, and TLR2 in African-American adolescents [89].

BV has also been associated with a polymorphism in TLR2 suggesting that different BV-associated bacteria (BVAB) were able to control cytokines secretion and that activation of immunity in differentiate vaginal epithelial cells was related to different bacteria: an increase in proinflammatory cytokines and in epithelial cells has been associated with the presence of *A. vaginae* while *L. iners* seems to activate receptor signaling activity: on the contrary, *Prevotella bivia* and *L. crispatus* do not possess these effects [89].

BVAB infections could result in a proinflammatory immune response that disrupts barrier functions where other microbes could elicit different responses [90].

Recently, the pivotal role of Gamma Delta (GD) cells in the innate and adaptive immune system has been demonstrated: these cells are well represented in the female reproductive tract and seems to play a key role in the vaginal epithelial barrier against pathogens [91].

The decrease in cervical GD1 cells and increase in GD2 cells among women with abnormal vaginal flora predisposes women with BV to HIV acquisition [91].

Considering the high rate of correlation between these parameters, the authors proposed to use GDT cells as markers of female genital tract vulnerability to HIV [91].

GD1 cells and GD2 cells substantially differentiates in vaginal localization and functioning: GD1 cells are well represented in mucosal tissue and play a leading role in maintaining mucosal structure, while GD2 cells are well represented in peripheral blood and are important in maintaining humoral immunity and in the development of the immune response to pathogens [91].

Increased cervical vaginal lavages seem to increase sialic acid residues leading to an increase in sialidase levels that are associated with BV [92].

BVBlue System method has been used to measure sialidase levels and to make diagnosis of BV [93].

Mucinases, sialidases, and biofilm production seem to be related with sialidase secretion by *G. vaginalis* and *Bacteroides* spp leading to STDs [94] by disrupting the integrity of the mucosa, facilitating the adhesion of pathogens to mucins, and underlying epithelial cells [95].

The relationship between sialidases and HIV infection has recently been evaluated [95–98], as gp 120 and CD4 seem to carry sialic acid residues: sialidases administration to HIV cells has demonstrated to enhance HIV infection [9, 97] suggesting that sialic acid disruption could help virus-binding and enhanced virus transmission.

In addition, the negatively charged sialic acid molecules at the terminal ends of the O-linked sugar chains determine changes in mucosal viscosity [98, 99].

Concluding, there are a lot of activities related to lactobacilli presence in the vagina that seems to be helpful in counteracting BV and preventing BV-associated pathologies.

Treatment of BV is recommended in order to relieve vaginal symptoms and signs of infection and to reduce the risk of acquiring *C. trachomatis, Neisseria gonorrhea, T. vaginalis*, HIV, and herpes simplex type 2 infections.

Obviously, the treatment is necessary also to avoid risk of PID, infertility, and pregnancy/newborn's complication.

Center for Disease Control's (CDC) recommended regimen for B.V. is [83]:

a. Metronidazole 500 mg orally twice a day for 7 days

OR

b. Metronidazole gel 0–75% one full application (5 g) intravaginally, once a day for 5 days

OR

c. Clindamycin cream 2% one full application (5 g) intravaginally at bedtime for 7 days

Women treated with nitroimidazoles must remember that alcohol consumption should be avoided during treatment [83].

To reduce the possibility of disulfiram-like reaction, abstinence from alcohol use should continue for almost 24 hours after completion of metronidazole [83].

We also have to remember that clindamycin cream is oil-based and consequently might weaken latex condoms and diaphragms for almost 5 days after use; women should be advised to refrain from sexual activities or use condoms consistently and correctly during the treatment regimen [83].

Since no clinical data support the use of vaginal douching for symptoms relief or treatment of BV, and since vaginal douching increases recurrence of BV, this procedure must be avoided by gynecologists [83].

CDC's alternative regimens to treat BV are:

a. Clindamycin 300 mg orally bid for 7 days or

b. Clindamycin vaginal ovules 100 mg once a day (bedtime) for 3 days or

c. Tinidazole 1 g oral route once a day for 7 days or

d. Tinidazole 2 g oral route for 5 days

Also, in this case we have to remember the same disulfiram-like reaction for nitroimidazoles so that alcohol consumption should be avoided during treatment and almost 72 hours after the completion of the tinidazole regimen [83].

For Clindamycin ovules, since an oleaginous base that might weaken latex or rubber products is present (condom and diaphragma), we have to remember to avoid condoms and diaphragms use during treatment and within 72 hours following treatment [83].

Treatment of vaginal infections requires different drugs although the recurrence rate post-treatment remains high due to adverse effects on the beneficial microbiota [86].

Metronidazole and clindamycin treatment do not prevent recurrent BV infections as the lactobacilli population is rarely reconstituted [86].

Thus, there could be clear clinical advantages for the use of biotherapeutic agents (prebiotics and/or probiotics) for treating these infections [84].

Biotherapeutic agents have been defined by McFarland and Elmer in 1995 as living microorganisms that are used to prevent or treat human disease by interacting with natural microbial ecology of the host [84].

Probiotics could though be highly beneficial in modulating the mucosal flora, maintaining the integrity of the epithelial barrier and regulating the immune response [84].

Hydrogen peroxide–producing lactobacilli have been shown to be protective against a number of bacterial infections [84].

Reid et al. observed that a vaginal application of Lactobacillus casei sub-rhamnosus was able to survive in vagina after 7 weeks of exogenous application concluding that "it was surprising and it was the first and unique observation referring to exogenously-applied Lactobacilli vaginal application" [100].

Consistently with this information, a lot of clinical trials have recently been performed by using vaginal commercial probiotics containing selected Lactobacillus rhamnosus spp [100–109].

Since the recurrence rate of BV is higher also after treatment with CDC-recommended protocols, the "probiotic vaginal approach" with *Lactobacillus rhamnosus* BMX 54 has recently been tested in controlled, randomized clinical trial for the prevention of the recurrence rates of BV [100–109].

A review on its long-term use after CDC regimen administration seems to point out on a big sample size of women that its chronic use (almost 6 months) after CDC treatment administration in women affected by BV could significantly decrease the BV recurrence rates when confronted with the simple CDC regimen [104].

Lactobacillus rhamnosus BMX 54 has also recently demonstrated to be able to control HPV infection in women affected by BV [109].

While this "vaginal approach" with selected Lactobacilli spp seems to be encouraging, to lower the recurrence rates of BV, the oral approach with probiotics seems to be ineffective for BV treatment [110].

Considering the relationship between BV and STDs, it could be useful to consider this biotherapeutics approach to prevent and control STDs.

4. Sexually transmitted diseases

The term sexually transmitted diseases (STDs) refers to many diseases and the number keeps expanding with the discovery of new pathogens (e.g., HIV) or a new route of acquisition of a known pathogen (e.g., hepatitis C) [3].

Historically, all the diseases known to be transmitted only by sexual intercourse have been classified as "venereal diseases"; Other terms, such as "sexually transmitted infections" (STIs), "sexually transmitted diseases and infections" and "reproductive tract infections" have been used [3].

All these diseases will be included in this chapter under the term "sexually transmitted diseases."

STDs have complex political, social, and public health implications, in addition to their medical significance [3].

Syphilis continues to remain an important disease in spite of the introduction, more than 60 years ago, of effective treatment such as penicillin; its rate is on the rise in men who have sex with men (MSM) in some areas of U.S. [3].

STDs still remain the most common infectious diseases in developed and developing countries [3].

Considering the availability of effective therapies and that STDs could be prevented by changing one's behavior, it is surprising that these pathologies have been on the rise in developed and developing countries: only the complex nature of these diseases and the complex relationship between public health and social community could explain this continuous rise [3].

In this chapter, we divided the STDs in two main categories: diseases characterized by genital ulcers and diseases characterized by genital discharge; HIV infection will not be discussed in this chapter.

4.1. Sexually transmitted diseases with ulcers

Syphilis, herpes simplex virus (HSV), and chancroid are STDs with ulcer; each of these diseases has been associated with an increased risk of HIV infection [2, 3].

Genital ulcers diseases (GUD) facilitate enhanced HIV transmission among sexual partners. In the presence of genital ulcers, there is a fivefold increase in susceptibility to HIV, and HIV-infected individuals with genital ulcer disease may transmit HIV to their sexual partner more efficiently [2, 3].

A genital ulcer is defined as a breach in the skin or mucosa of the genitalia.

Genital ulcers may be single or multiple and may be associated with inguinal or femoral lymphadenopathy.

HSV is the most common cause of genital ulcers in U.S. among young, sexually active partners, *Treponema pallidum* (syphilis) is the next common cause of GUD, while chancroid, caused by H. ducreyl, has been infrequently associated with cases of GUD in U.S. [2, 3].

In developing countries, the most frequent genital ulcer disease is represented by "chancroid" [2, 3].

Travelers or native in the tropics could present *Lymphogranuloma venereum* (LFG) by *C. trachomatis* and Granuloma inguinale by *Calymmatobacterium granulomatis*: these GUDs are endemic in tropical countries [2, 3].

The relationship between GUD and pathogens are strictly related to patient population and geographic area [2].

There is a considerable overlap in the clinical presentation of herpes, primary syphilis, and chancroid [2].

Genital herpes typically presents with multiple, shallow ulcers and bilateral lymphadenopathy [2].

Primary syphilis can usually been differentiated from genital herpes by the presence of single deep, defined ulcer with induration [2, 3].

Also from chancroids and syphilis, a difference could be done according to the presence of a painful, undetermined ulcer with a purulent base that tender to lymphadenopathy [2, 3].

The cause of genital ulcers cannot be based on clinical findings alone because it possesses only 30–34% of sensitivity: this means that diagnostic testing should be performed [3].

4.2. Sexually transmitted diseases with vaginal discharge

Vaginal discharge is a frequent gynecologic complaint, accounting for more than 10 million office visits annually in U.S. [2, 3].

The three most common causes of vaginal discharge are BV (40–50% of cases), vulvovaginal candidiasis (20–25% of cases), and *T. vaginalis* (15–20% of cases); of these vaginitis, only Trichomoniasis is a STD, while BV is a "borderline" pathology that occurs in women with a high rate of STDs as well as in women who have never been sexually active [3].

Pelvic inflammatory diseases (PIDs), Gonococcal infections (*N. gonorrhea*), and *C. trachomatis* infections are three other STDs with vaginal discharge [2, 3].

Human papilloma virus (HPV) infections are the most common viral STDs worldwide; 1% of the sexually active persons in U.S. between the ages of 15 and 49 years are estimated to have genital warts from HPV [3].

Most genital HPV infections are subclinical and are transmitted primarily through sexual contact. HPV is a double-stranded DNA virus that causes a spectrum of clinical diseases ranging from asymptomatic infection to frank malignancy. External genital warts have various morphological manifestations such as condyloma acuminata, smooth dome-shaped papular warts, keratotic warts, and flat warts [3].

Because of the well-known relationship between HPV and cervical cancer, in June 2006, U.S. Food and Drug Administration approved a quadrivalent vaccine for HPV [2, 3].

Several states have already recommended HPV prevention making HPV vaccination mandatory for middle school girls [2, 3].

5. Bacterial vaginosis and sexually transmitted diseases: relationship

Several prospective studies have reported an association between abnormal vaginal microbiota, in particular BV and depletion of lactobacillus species and increased risk of STIs' acquisition [32, 111–121].

Human papilloma virus (HPV), human immunodeficiency virus (HIV), human herpes simplex virus (HSV), and PID infections/acquisition seem to be more frequent in women affected by BV [32, 111–121].

Also, *T. vaginalis, N. gonorrhea, C. trachomatis* genital infections, and PID seem to be more frequent in women with BV or depletion of vaginal lactobacilli [32].

The vaginal microbiome has been well characterized although cultivation-based and molecular methods and data from epidemiological studies indicate that the vaginal microbiota influences and enhanced STI susceptibility [20, 32, 113, 115, 116].

Immunologic, enzymatic, and metabolic mechanisms could operate independently or in combination to enhance STI acquisition [20, 115].

An increasing number of evidences provide a strong foundation for a biologic relationship between BV and increased STIs susceptibility.

It is well known that vaginal Lactobacilli spp fermented local sugars (e.g., glycogen) producing an acidic vaginal pH that have been associated with decreased *in vitro* activity of *C. trachomatis* and *N. gonorrhea* [32, 118, 119].

This acidic environment seems to be unfavorable also for HPV, HIV, and HPS infections [32].

Hydrogen peroxynitrite produced in vagina by Lactobacilli spp through sugar fermentation seems to be a key point for reducing risk of STIs [32].

Hydrogen peroxynitrite possesses a well-known bactericidal and virucidal activity [32].

Cervical mucus has the ability to trap pathogens but, unfortunately, this mucus barrier may be compromised by mucin-degrading enzymes such as sialidase and mucinase, which are produced by BV-associated bacteria: loss of the protective mucus provides pathogens with unhindered access to target cells, increasing epithelial binding potential [32, 114].

Sialidase also cleaves terminal sialic acids from glycoproteins, exposing other sugar on their carbohydrate side chains, which can be used as energy for bacteria [32, 116].

Several BV-associated bacteria produced indole that is used by *C. trachomatis* to overcome the bactericidal effect of interferon gamma [32].

The relationship between genital epithelial cells in the vagina and vaginal microbiota seems to strongly influence the innate immune response suggesting a pivotal role of the reproductive tract immune response in determining BV and its compliances: vaginal microbiota derangement could decrease local immunity with a consequent increase of STDs risks in the women urogenital tract [87].

Lactobacilli have historically been considered keystone species of vaginal communities in reproductive-age women [32, 87].

Lactobacilli produce bacteriocins (low molecular weight proteins) that can inhibit the growth of a variety of bacteria reinforcing the concept of reducing susceptibility to STDs [32, 87].

BV may predispose to acquisition of STDs upon exposure because local cytokine production associated with BV may facilitate the acquisition of STDs [32].

Finally, lactobacilli exhibit cosurfactant and coaggregant activities that could envelop STDs virus or bacteria so that in BV the absence of these "mechanical inhibition" could facilitate the acquisition of STDs [32] (**Figure 2**).

Concluding, BV, a worldwide common vaginal infection, which is mostly asymptomatic, could be a predisposing factor, also if asymptomatic, to STDs acquisition and then to eradicate this very frequent pathology in developed and developing countries could represent a gold standard for STDs' primary prevention.

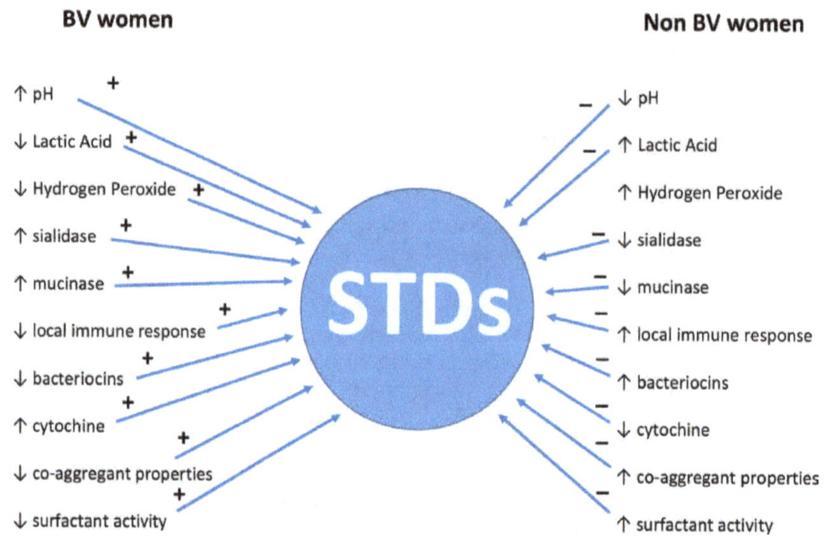

Figure 2. Differences in BV and non-BV in predisposing factors for STDs.

6. Bacterial vaginosis control for sexually transmitted diseases' primary prevention

Since BV is one of the key risk factors for STDs' acquisition, and since asymptomatic and symptomatic BV actually represents the most common vaginal infection worldwide (account for almost one-third of childbearing women), it seems obvious that BV treatment and definitive infection's eradication could be one of the most important plan for STDs' primary prevention.

Considering that BV increases susceptibility to STDs, two limiting factors are associated with BV treatment:

1. The fact that treatment for BV asymptomatic nonpregnant women is not currently recommended [118, 120–122];
2. The urgent need to develop more effective intervention for BV because the recurrence following current treatment is disappointingly high [42].

Women with an abnormal vaginal microbiota were at an increased risk of acquiring STDs compared to women with a normal vaginal microbiota; it seems that the risk of STD acquisition increased with higher Nugent score category [32].

Considering vaginal microbiome modifications as a predisposing factor for STDs acquisition, restoration of vaginal flora seems to be the crucial keystone for long-term BV treatment and, consequently, for STDs primary prevention.

Interventions that decrease the incidence and the recurrence rates of BV and promote a normal vaginal microbiota could potentially contribute to the reduction in STDs' incidence.

Current available and recommended treatment for BV [83] as follows:

CDC's (Center for Disease Control) recommended regimens are:

a. Metronidazole tablet 500 mg oral route bid for 7 days or
b. Metronidazole vaginal gel 0.75% (5 g intravaginally every day for 5 days) or
c. Clindamycin vaginal cream 2% (5 g intravaginally every day at bedtime for 7 days)

CDC's alternative regimens to treat BV are:

a. Clindamycin 300 mg orally bid for 7 days or
b. Clindamycin vaginal ovules 100 mg once a day (bedtime) for 3 days or
c. Tinidazole 1 g oral route once a day for 7 days or
d. Tinidazole 2 g oral route for 5 days

Failure to produce sustained changes in the vaginal microbiota [113, 115, 120] clearly demonstrated that alternative regimens that improve cure rates and produce sustained changes in the vaginal microbiota are needed.

The CDC recommended therapies failed to control relapses of BV (almost 40% of recurrences rate at 3 months and 50% of relapses at 6 months), and this seems to be the most relevant problem in treating BV eradication in order to prevent STDs acquisition [104].

With >500 million new cases of STIs each year, the development of innovative strategies for STIs prevention is a global public health priority [32].

By using only Nugent score to classified and scoring BV, the relationship between BV and STDs seems to be clear: BV microbiota as gauged by Gram stain is associated with a significant elevated risk for acquisition of STDs [32].

Obviously, the Human Microbiome Project (http://nihroadmap.nih.gov/hmp/), providing also the genomic studies of the vagina, is expected to describe the structure of the complex microbial communities and how they contribute to disease susceptibility: when it will be available we will probably add more information to control BV recurrence.

Anyway, only by using Gram stain culture and Amsel's clinical criteria, which is available worldwide today, it is possible to make a BV diagnosis and to have a picture of the women "more susceptible" for STIs acquisition.

From the other side we have to manage the problem related to treatment recommendations that differentiate between women who report symptoms and those who do not; to our knowledge there are no published studies on differences in sequelae between asymptomatic and symptomatic BV [114, 115, 118].

Adverse outcomes linked to BV are probably caused by alterations in the vaginal flora that are seen in both [117, 118].

Screening and treatment for asymptomatic BV women would prevent STDs by restoring optimal vaginal flora, thus reducing susceptibility to STDs as supported by studies demonstrating a clear association between BV and an increase prevalence and incidence of STDs and HIV infection [114–118].

So the first recommendation is:

1. to treat also asymptomatic BV women in order to reduce STDs acquisition susceptibility;

However, recent largest study to evaluate the impact of treatment of BV on STD outcomes demonstrated that treatment of women with oral metronidazole does not affect the incidence of gonorrhea and chlamydia concluding that we are waiting for more effective therapies for BV [113, 119].

Standard of care for BV treatment is effective in the short term, and it is not able to restore vaginal microbiota. So by using this regimen, we obtain a clearance of BV more than a real eradication and, consequently, the long-term effect is detrimental with a high percentage (more than 50%) of recurrence after 6 months.

Nowadays, we could describe BV recurrences as a "drug-free pathology" for which every effort has to be done in order to restore vaginal pH and, obviously, to reduce the acquisition susceptibility of STDs.

If STDs acquisition is related to asymptomatic and symptomatic BV, and if standard of care seems to be unable to modify, almost in long term, STIs' epidemiology, the relationship between vaginal microflora modifications and STIs' susceptibility seem to be a key point to prevent STDs.

So that BV management in terms of restoring vaginal microflora such as in healthy women seems to be pivotal in STDs' primary prevention: taking into account that almost one-third of the women worldwide are affected by asymptomatic and symptomatic BV and that most of them are undiagnosed, untreated, or treated with the only available standard of care, BV management could represent a new/old cost-effective modality to primary prevent STDs.

Since sexual behaviors are changing year by year especially in young population, and since the percentage of sexually active girls/women that could have sexual intercourse with STDs people are increasing, we strongly believe that vaginal microbiota restoration could become the next milestone in STDs prevention.

So, the second recommendation is:

2. to restore vaginal microbiota in every sexually active women of childbearing age in order to reduce STDs acquisition susceptibility;

Since the standard of care (CDC recommended therapy) seems not to be able to restore vaginal microflora and possess a high rate of recurrences, alternative approaches are needed.

Biotherapeutic agents (living microorganism used to prevent or treat human disease by interacting with natural microbial ecology of the host) have been used to treat vaginal infections during the time [84].

Vaginal biotherapeutic agents can be divided in three classes:

1. Prebiotic (carbohydrates that topically stimulated the growth of the body's indigenous lactobacilli) [84];
2. Probiotic (living microorganisms—usually *Lactobacilli*) [84];
3. Synbiotic (a combination of the two concept) [84].

A lot of clinical trials have been done with vaginal probiotics; probiotics such as *Lactobacillus rhamnosus* GR-1, *Lactobacillus rhamnosus* Lcr 35, *Lactobacillus reuteri* RC-14, and *L. crispatus* CTV-05 taken orally or vaginally in various doses can improve vaginal flora without side effects [84].

Other strains such as *Lactobacillus rhamnosus* L60 and *Lactobacillus fermentum* L23 have been considered for probiotic development due to their specific characteristics including the production of bacteriocins, adherence properties, etc. [84].

Vaginal probiotics have been compared with vaginal metronidazole in a randomized clinical trial and the results show the superiority in terms of effectiveness for two intravaginal capsules of probiotic containing Lactobacillus rhamnosus GR-1 and Lactobacillus reuteri RC-14 taken once a day for 5 day vs 0.75% metronidazole vaginal gel applied daily for 5 days; another randomized clinical trial showed that there was no difference in BV treatment of patients administered Lactobacillus acidophilus and 0.03 mg estriol with vaginal metronidazole at 3–7 days [84].

Probiotics can be used as complementary to traditional therapies to improve the treatment of vaginal infections and to reduce recurrences of such episodes [84].

Probiotics can also be prophylactic in healthy subjects with a history of recurrent BV [84].

Unfortunately, a review published on EFSA Journal points out the ineffectiveness of probiotics for oral use in restoring vaginal microbiome [111], and another review published on Cochrane showed that probiotics clinical trials were inconsistent to demonstrate clinical efficacy of this approach in BV women [122].

The reported data on a vaginal tablet synbiotic containing *Lactobacillus rhamnosus* BMX 54 plus lactose seem to be interesting. Clinical data on a sample size of more than 800 women affected by BV and treated with standard of care (metronidazole) followed by a long-term course of this synbiotic clearly demonstrated a significant reduction in the recurrence rate of BV [101–109].

The results obtained in controlled trials [101–109] substantiated the effectiveness of the combination therapy (metronidazole 500 mg twice daily for 1 week followed by a once weekly application of vaginal tablets containing Lactobacillus rhamnosus and lactose for 6 months in preventing BV relapses, not only during the treatment time (6 months) but also during the 6-month follow-up without any treatment) (**Figure 3**).

Another controlled clinical trial performed by using the same synbiotic for 12 weeks once weekly in pregnant women vs no-treatment control group supported its effectiveness in preventing the

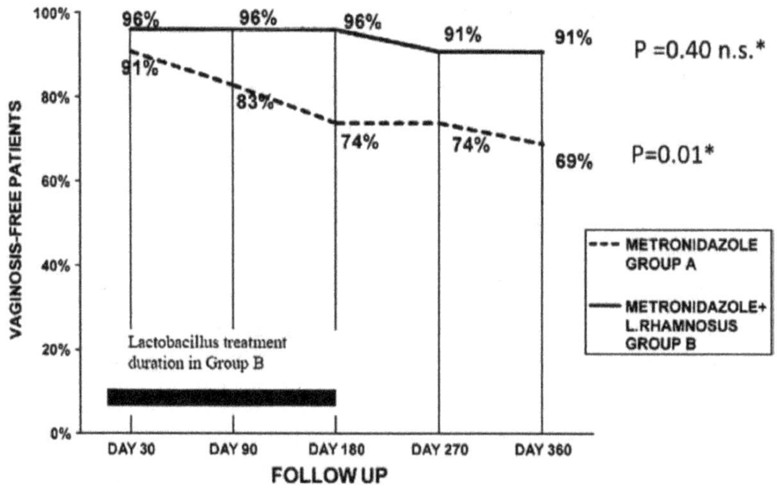

Figure 3. Trend of "vaginosis-free" patients in each group during follow-up. *A p-value for repeated measures in each group was considered to be significant if $p = 0.05$ [107].

development of abnormal vaginal microflora and in control of cervical parameters that could represent risk factors for preterm delivery [108].

A very long-lasting clinical trial (24 months) showed that the same combination between lactose and Lactobacillus rhamnosus BMX 54 via vaginal tablets was able to control vaginal pH in BV during the long-lasting treatment [103].

This "synbiotic vaginal approach" seems to be useful especially if administered for long time course (from 6 months to 3 years) to restore vaginal microflora and to prevent BV recurrences and mutually supported the standard of care for BV.

This probably means that the right Lactobacillus together with the right prebiotic could add complementary effectiveness vs the only therapy with vaginal probiotics resulting in an interesting option to prevent STDs' infections and acquisition.

A recent controlled clinical trial performed on 117 women affected by BV/vaginitis and associated HPV infection showed a significant decrease in HPV-related cytological anomalies (71.9 vs 36.6%: $p = 0.04$) and HPV clearance (33.3 vs 13.3%) in metronidazole or fluconazole plus *Lactobacillus rhamnosus* BMX 54/lactose long-term (8 months) treated group vs metronidazole or fluconazole plus a short-term course (2 months) of vaginal application of the same synbiotic [109].

Synbiotic vaginal tablets were administered after metronidazole or fluconazole treatment with a precise long-term schedule (once a day for 10 days, then every 3 days for a month, then once every 5 days till 2 months, and the last 6 months 1 vaginal tablet once a week) [109].

These results support the evidence from Mitra et al. [123] "there is emerging evidence which leads us to conclude that increased diversity of vaginal microbiota combined with reduced relative abundance of Lactobacillus species is involved in HPV acquisition and persistence and the development of cervical precancer and cancer."

Concluding, considering the lack of short-long term efficacy of standard of care in decreasing BV prevalence and recurrences, it seems that every effort must be done during the next years to control "microbioma modifications related to BV": selected biotherapeutic agents, using for long-term course, could be an interesting and cost-effective treatment to prevent STDs acquisition.

Author details

Marco Bertini

Address all correspondence to: bertini@baldaccilab.com

R&D Department, Laboratori Baldacci SpA, Pisa, Italy

References

[1] Shaskolsky B, Dementieva E, Leinsoo A, Runina A, Vorobyev D, Plakhova X, Kubanov A, Deryabin D, Gryadunov D. Drug resistance mechanism in bacteria causing sexually transmitted disease and associated with vaginosis. Frontiers in Microbiology. 18th May 2016;**7**(7). DOI: 10.3389/fmicb.2016.00747

[2] Bryan C. Infectious Disease. Chapter eight. Sexually Transmitted Diseases. Richard Hunt. editor Microbiology and Immunology on line – Edited by Richard Hunt

[3] Shresta RK, Englund K. Cleveland Clinical Sexually Transmitted Diseases. Published on August 2010 – TeachMeMedicine.org

[4] Gordon JI, Klaenhammer TR. A rendezvous with our microbes. Proceedings of the National Academy of Sciences of the United States of America. 2011;**108**(Suppl 1): 4513-4515

[5] Eckburg PB, Bik EM, Bernstein CN, Purdom E, Dethlefsen L, Sargent M, et al. Diversity of the human intestinal microbial flora. Science. 2005;**308**:1635-1638

[6] Dethlefsen L, McFall-Ngai M, Relman DA. An ecological and evolutionary perspective on human-microbe mutualism and disease. Nature. 2007;**449**:811-818

[7] Spear GT, Sikaroodi M, Zariffard MR, Landay AL, French AL, Gillevet PM. Comparison of the diversity of the vaginal microbiota in HIV-infected and HIV-uninfected women with or without bacterial vaginosis. The Journal of Infectious Diseases. 2008;**198**:1131-1140

[8] Zozaya-Hinchliffe M, Lillis R, Martin DH, Ferris MJ. Quantitative PCR assessments of bacterial species in women with and without bacterial vaginosis. Journal of Clinical Microbiology. 2010;**48**:1812-1819

[9] Ravel J, Gajer P, Abdo Z, Schneider GM, Koenig SS, McCulle SL, et al. Vaginal microbiome of reproductive-age women. Proceedings of the National Academy of Sciences of the United States of America. 2011;**108**(Suppl 1):4680-4687

[10] Spear GT, Gilbert D, Landay AL, Zariffard R, French AL, Patel P, et al. Pyrosequencing of the genital microbiotas of HIV-seropositive and seronegative women reveals *Lactobacillus iners* as the predominant Lactobacillus species. Applied and Environmental Microbiology. 2011;**77**:378-381

[11] Dols JA, Smit PW, Kort R, Reid G, Schuren FH, Tempelman H, et al. Microarray-based identification of clinically relevant vaginal bacteria in relation to bacterial vaginosis. American Journal of Obstetrics & Gynecology. 2011;**204**:305.e1-305.e7

[12] Hugenholtz P, Goebel BM, Pace NR. Impact of culture-independent studies on the emerging phylogenetic view of bacterial diversity. Journal of Bacteriology. 1998;**180**: 4765-4774

[13] Baker GC, Smith JJ, Cowan DA. Review and re-analysis of domain-specific 16S primers. Journal of Microbiological Methods. 2003;**55**:541-555

[14] Weng L, Rubin EM, Bristow J. Application of sequence-based methods in human microbial ecology. Genome Research. 2006;**16**:316-322

[15] Human Microbiome Project Consortium. Structure, function and diversity of the healthy human microbiome. Nature. 2012;**486**:207-214

[16] Doderlein A. Das scheidensekret und seine bedeutung fur puerperalfieber. Bakteriology. 1892;**11**:699

[17] Gardner HL, Dukes CD. *Haemophilus vaginalis* vaginitis: A newly defined specific infection previously classified non-specific vaginitis. American Journal of Obstetrics & Gynecology. 1955;**69**:962-976

[18] Spiegel CA, Amsel R, Ecshenbach D, Sckoenknecht F, Holmes KK. Anaerobic bacteria in nonspecific vaginitis. The New England Journal of Medicine. 1980;**303**:601-607

[19] Amsel R, Totten PA, Spiegel CA, Chen KC, Eschenbach D, Holmes KK. Nonspecific vaginitis. Diagnostic criteria and microbial and epidemiologic associations. American Journal of Medicine. 1983;**74**:14-22

[20] Schwebke JR. Gynecologic consequences of bacterial vaginosis. Obstetrics and Gynecology Clinics of North America. 2003;**30**:685-694

[21] Cherpes TL, Meyn LA, Krohn MA, Lurie JG, Hiller SL. Association between acquisition of herpes simplex virus type 2 in women and bacterial vaginosis. Clinical Infectious Diseases. 2003;**37**:319-325

[22] Martin HL, Richardson BA, Nyange PM, Lacreys L, Hiller SL, Chohan B, et al. Vaginal lactobacilli microbial flora and risk of human immunodeficiency virus type 1 and sexually transmitted disease acquisition. Journal of Infectious Diseases. 1999;**180**:1863-1868

[23] Cu-Uvin S, Hogan JW, Caliendo AM, Harwell J, Mayer KH, Carpenter CC, et al. Association between bacterial vaginosis and expression of human immunodeficiency virus type 1 RNA in the female genital tract. Clinical Infectious Diseases. 2001;**33**: 894-896

[24] Cohen CR, Lingappa JR, Baeten JM, Ngayo MO, Spiegel CA, Hong T, et al. Bacterial vaginosis associated with increased risk of female to male HIV-1 transmission: A prospective cohort analysis among African couples. PLOS Medicine. 2012;**9**:e1001251

[25] Albert DM, Doderlein G. A critical view to the bibliographies of two German professors. Zentralblatt für Gynäkologie. 2006;**128**(2):56-59

[26] Miller EA, Beasley DE, Dunn RR, Archie EA. Lactobacilli dominance and vaginal pH: Why is the human vaginal microbiome unique? Frontiers in Microbiology. 1936–Dec 2016;**7**:article 1936. DOI: 10:3389/fmicb.2016.01936

[27] Delsuc F, Metcalf JL, Wegener Parfrey L, Song SJ, Gonzales A, Knight R. Convergence of gut microbiomes in myrmecophagus mammals. Molecular Ecology. 2014;**23**:1301-1317. DOI: 10.1111/mec.12501

[28] Ley RE, Hamady M, Lozupone C, Turnbaugh PJ, Ramey RR, Biircher JS, et al. Evolution of mammals and their gut microbes. Science. 2008;**320**:1647-1651. DOI: 10.1126/Science.1155725

[29] Graver MA, Wade JJ. The role of acidification in the inhibition of *Neiseria gonorrhea* by vaginal lactobacilli during anaerobic growth. Annals of Clinical Microbiology and Antimicrobials. 2011;**10**:8. DOI: 10.1186/1476-0711-10-8

[30] Brotman RM. Vaginal microbiome and sexually transmitted infections: An epidemiologic perspective. Journal of Clinical Investigation. 2011;**121**:4610-4617. DOI: 10.1172/JCI57172

[31] Adunate M, Srbinovski D, Hearps AC, Latham CF, Ramsland P, Gugasyan R, et al. Antimicrobial and immune modulatory effects of lactic acid and short chain fatty acids produced by vaginal microbiota associated with eubiosis and bacterial vaginosis. Frontiers in Physiology. 2015;**6**:164. DOI: 10.3389/fphys.2015.00164

[32] Atashili J, Poole C, Ndumbe PM, Adimora AA, Smith JS. Bacterial vaginosis and HIV acquisition: A meta-analysis of published studies. AIDS. 2008;**22**:1493-1501. DOI: 10.1097/QAD.0b013e3283021e37

[33] DiGiulio DB, Callahan BJ, McMurdie PJ, Costello EK, Lyell GJ, Robaczeska A, et al. Temporal and spatial variation of the human microbiota during pregnancy. Proceedings of the National Academy of Sciences of the United States of America. 2015;**112**:11060-11065. DOI: 10.1073/pnas. 152875112

[34] Stumpf RM, Wilson BA, Rivera A, Yildirim S, Yeoman CJ, Polk JD, et al. The primate vaginal microbiome: Comparative context and implications for human health and disease. American Journal of Physical Anthropology. 2013;**152**:119-134. DOI: 10.1002/ajpa.22395

[35] Ayre WB. The glycogen-estrogen relationship in the vaginal tract. The Journal of Clinical Endocrinology and Metabolism. 1951;**11**:103-110

[36] Abt MC, Artis D. The dynamic influence of commensal bacteria on the immune response to pathogens. Current Opinion in Microbiology. 2013;**16**:4-9. DOI: 10.1016/J. Mib.2012.12.002

[37] Nunn CL, Gittleman JL, Antonovics J. Promiscuity and the primate immune system. Science. 2000;**290**:1168-1170. DOI: 10.1126/science.290.5494.1168

[38] Ahsel S, Abee CR. A pelvimetry method for predicting perinatal mortality in pregnant squirrel monkeys (Salmiri Scluresus). Laboratory Animal Science. 1983;**33**:156-167

[39] Sheldon IM, Lewis GS, LeBlanc S, Gilbert RG. Defining postpartum uterine disease in cattle. Theriogenology. 2006;**65**:1516-1530. DOI: 10.1016/j.theriogenology.2005.08.021

[40] Thomas S. Doderlein's bacillus: *Lactobacillus acidophilus*. Journal of Infectious Diseases. 1928;**43**:218-227

[41] Redondo-Lopez V, Cook RL, Sobel JD. Emerging role of lactobacilli in the control and maintenance of the vaginal bacterial microflora. Reviews of Infectious Diseases. 1990;**12**:856-872

[42] Ravel J, Brotman R. Translating the vaginal microbiome: Gaps and challenges. Genome Medicine. 2016;**8**:35. DOI: 10.1186/s13073-016-0291-2

[43] O'Hanlon DE, Moench TR, Cone RA. Vaginal pH and microbicidal lactic acid when lactobacilli dominate the microbiota. PLOS One. 2013;**8**:e80074

[44] Eschembach DA, Davick PR, Williams BL, Klebanoff SI, Young-Smith K, Critchlow CM, et al. Prevalence of hydrogen peroxide-producing lactobacillus species in normal women and women with bacterial vaginosis. Journal of Clinical Microbiology. 1989;**27**:251-256

[45] McGroarty JA. Probiotic use of lactobacilli in the human female urogenital tract. FEMS Immunology & Medical Microbiology. 1993;**6**:251-254

[46] Sobel JD, Schneider J, Kaye D, Levison ME. Adherence of bacteria to vaginal epithelial cells at various times in the menstrual cycle. Infection and Immunity. 1981;**32**:194-197

[47] Zhou X, Bent SI, Schneider MG, Davis CC, Islam MR, Forney LI. Characterization of vaginal microbial communities in adult healthy women using cultivation-independent methods. Microbiology. 2004;**150**:2565-2573

[48] Antonio MA, Hawes SE, Hiller SL. The identification of vaginal lactobacillus species and the demographic and microbiologic characteristics of women colonized by these species. Journal of Infectious Diseases. 1999;**180**:1950-1956

[49] Ocana VS, Bru E, De Ruiz Holgado AA, Ndler-Macias ME. Surface characteristics of lactobacilli isolated from human vagina. The Journal of General and Applied Microbiology. 1999;**45**:203-212

[50] Santiago GL, Cools P, Verstraelen H, Verhelst R, Trog M, Missine G, El Aila N, et al. Longitudinal study of the dynamics of vaginal microflora during two consecutive menstrual cycles. PLOS One. 2011;**6**:e28180

[51] Santiago GL, Tency I, Verstraelen H, Verhelst R, Trog M, Tenmerman M, et al. Longitudinal qPCR study of the dynamics of *L. crispatus, L. iners, A. vaginae*, (sialidase positive) *G. vaginalis* and *P. bivia*. Plos One. September 2012;**7**(9):e45281

[52] Castro J, Henriques A, Machado A, Henriques M, Jefferson KK, Cerca N. Reciprocal interference between *Lactobacillus* species and *Gardnerella vaginalis* on initial adherence to epithelial cells. International Journal of Medical Sciences. 2013;**10**:1193-1198

[53] Gajer P, Brotman RM, Bai G, Sakamoto J, Schtte UM, Zhong X, et al. Temporal dynamics of the human vaginal microbiota. Science Translational Medicine. 2012;**4**:132ra52

[54] Schwelbe JR, Richey CM, Weiss HL. Correlation of behaviors with microbiological changes in vaginal flora. Journal of Infectious Diseases. 1999;**180**:1632-1636

[55] Eschenbach DA, Thwin SS, Patton DL, Hooton TM, Stapleton AE, Agnew K, et al. Influence of the normal menstrual cycle on vaginal tissue, discharge, and microflora. Clinical Infectious Diseases. 2000;**30**:901-907

[56] Jespers V, Van De Wijgert J, Cools P, Verhelst R, Verstraelen H, Delany-Moretwe S, et al. The significance of *Lactobacillus crispatus* and *L. vaginalis* for vaginal health and the negative effect of recent sex: A cross-sectional descriptive study across groups of African women. BMC Infectious Diseases. 2015;**15**:115

[57] Petricevic L, Dornig KJ, Nierscher FJ, Sandhofer MJ, Krondorfer I, Kneifel W, et al. Differences in the vaginal lactobacilli of postmenopausal women and influence of rectal lactobacilli. Climacteric. 2013;**16**:356-361

[58] Zhang R, Daroczy K, Xiao B, Yu L, Chen R, Liao Q. Qualitative and semiquantitative analysis of *Lactobacillus* species in the vaginas of healthy fertile and postmenopausal Chinese women. Journal of Medical Microbiology. 2012;**61**:729-739

[59] Van De Wigert JH, Borgdorff H, Verhelst R, Crucitti T, Francis S, Verstraelen H, et al. The vaginal microbiota: What have we learned after a decade of molecular characterization? PLOS One. 2014;**9**:e105998

[60] Jakobsson T, Forsum U. Changes in the predominant human *Lactobacillus* flora during in vitro fertilization. Annals of Clinical Microbiology and Antimicrobials. 2008;**7**:14

[61] Hickey RJ, Abdo Z, Zhou X, Nemeth K, Hansmann M, Osborn TW, et al. Effects of tampons anti menses on the composition and diversity of vaginal microbial communities over time. British Journal of Obstetrics and Gynaecology. 2013;**120**:695-704. discussion 704-6

[62] Hickey RJ, Zhou X, Settles ML, Erb J, Malone K, Hansmann MA, et al. Vaginal microbiota of adolescent girls prior to onset of menarche resemble those of reproductive age women. mBio. 2015;**6**:e00097-15

[63] Chaban B, Links MG, Jayaprakash TP, Wagner EC, Bourque DK, Lohn Z, et al. Characterization of the vaginal microbiota f the healthy Canadian women through the menstrual cycle. Microbiome. 2014;**2**:23

[64] Balkus JE, Mitchelll C, Agnew K, Liu C, Fiedler T, Cohon SE, et al. Detection of hydrogen peroxide-producing *Lactobacillus* species in the vagina: A comparison of culture and quantitative PCR among HIV-1 seropositive women. BMC Infectious Diseases. 2012;**12**:188

[65] Fetweis JM, Brooks JP, Serrano MG, Sheth NU, Girerd PH, Edwards DJ, et al. Differences in vaginal microbiome in African American women versus women of European ancestry. Microbiology. 2014;**160**:2272-2282

[66] Zhou X, Brown CJ, Abdo Z, Davis CC, Hansmann MA, Joyce P, et al. Differences in the composition of vaginal microbial communities found in healthy Caucasian and black woman. The ISME Journal. 2007;**1**:121-133

[67] Koumans EH, Sternberg M, Bruce C, McQuillan G, Kendrick J, Sutton M, et al. The prevalence of bacterial vaginosis in the United States, 2001-2004, associations with symptoms, sexual behaviors, and reproductive health. Sexually Transmitted Infections. 2007;**34**:864-869

[68] Ness RB, Hiller S, Ritcher HE, Soper DE, Stamm C, Bass DC, et al. Can known risk factors explain racial differences in the occurrence of bacterial vaginosis? Journal of the National Medical Association. 2003;**95**:201-212

[69] Gardner HL, Dukes CD. New etiologic agent in nonspecific bacterial vaginitis. Science. 1954;**120**:853

[70] Piot P, Van Dick E, Goodfellow M, Falkow SA. A taxonomic study of *Gardnerella vaginalis* (*Haemophilus vaginalis*): Gradner and Dukes (1955). Journal of General and Applied Microbiology. 1980;**119**:373-396

[71] Nugent RP, Krohn MA, Hiller SL. Reliability of diagnosing bacterial vaginosis is improved by standardized method of gram stain interpretation. Journal of Clinical Microbiology. 1991;**29**:297-301

[72] Schwebke JR, Hiller SL, Sobel JD, MaGregor JA, Sweet RL. Validity of the vaginal gram stain for the diagnosis of bacterial vaginosis. Obstetrics and Gynecology. 1996;**88**:573-576

[73] Hiller D, Holmes K, Marrazzo J. Bacterial vaginosis. In: Holmes KK, Sparling PF, Mardhet PA, editors Sexually Transmitted Diseases. 4th ed. New York: McGraw-Hill, Health Profession Division; 2008. pp. 737-768

[74] Mendes-Soares H, Krishan V, Settles ML, Ravel J, Brown CJ, Forney LJ. Fine scale analysis of 16S rRNA sequences reveals a high level of taxonomic diversity among vaginal Atrobium spp. Pathogens and Diseases. 2015. **73**. Doi.org/10.1093/ferrspd/fdv020

[75] Fredricks DN, Fiedler TL, Marrazzo JM. Molecular identification of bacteria associated with bacterial vaginosis. New England Journal of Medicine. 2005;**353**:1899-1911

[76] Wiesenfeld HC, Hiller SL, Krohn MA, Landers DV, Sweet RL. Bacterial vaginosis is a strong predictor of *Neisseria gonorrhea* and *Chlamydia trachomatis* infection. Clinical Infectious Diseases. 2003;**36**:663-668

[77] Dareng EO, Ma B, Famooto AO, Akarolo-Anthony SN, Offiong RA, Olaniyan O, et al. Prevalent high risk HPV infection and vaginal microbiota in Nigerian women. Epidemiology and Infection. 2015;**144**:1-15. doi.org/10.1017/S0950268815000965

[78] Brotman RM, Klebanoff MA, Nansel TR, Yu KF, Andrews WW, Zhang J, et al. Bacterial vaginosis assessed by gram stain and diminished colonization resistance to incident

gonococcal, chlamydial and trichomonal genital infection. Journal of Infectious Diseases. 2010;**202**:1907-1915

[79] Wiesenfeld HC, Hiller SL, Krohn MA, Amortegui AJ, Heine RP, Landers DV, et al. Lower genital tract infection and endometritis: Insight into subclinical pelvic inflammatory disease. Obstetrics and Gynecology. 2002;**100**:456-463

[80] Ness RB, Kip KE, Hiller SL, Soper DE, Stamm CA, Sweet RL, et al. A cluster analysis of bacterial vaginosis-associated microflora and pelvic inflammatory disease. American Journal of Epidemiology. 2005;**162**:585-590

[81] Hebb JK, Cohen CR, Assete SG, Bukusi EA, Totten PA. Detection of novel organisms associated with salpingitis, by use of 16S rDNA polymerase chain reaction. Journal of Infectious Diseases. 2004;**190**:2109-2120

[82] Peipert JF, Lapane KL, Allsworth JE, Redding CA, Blume JD, Stein MD. Bacterial vaginosis, race and sexually transmitted infections: Does race modify the association? Journal of Sexually Transmitted Diseases. 2008;**35**(4):363-367

[83] Bacterial Vaginosis Centers For Disease Control and Prevention. CDC Publication No. 99-8825, updated June 4, 2015

[84] Al Ghazzewi FH, Teser RF. Biotherapeuticc agents and vaginal health. Journal of Applied Microbiology. 2016;**121**(1):18-27

[85] Sherrard J, Donders G, White D. 2011 European (IUSTI/WHO) Guideline on the Management of Vaginal Discharge. Lead Editor: JS Jensen; 2011

[86] Koumans EH, Kendrick JS, for the CDC Bacterial Vaginosis Working Group. A public health program and research agenda. CDC. Oct 2001;**28** N° 5:292-297

[87] Woodman Z. Can one size fit all? Approach to bacterial vaginosis in sub-Saharan Africa. Annals of Clinical Microbiology and Antimicrobials. 2016;**15**:16. DOI: 10.1186/s12941-016-0132-6

[88] Schellenberg JJ, Plummer FA. The microbiological context of HIV resistance: Vaginal microbiota and mucosal inflammation at the viral point of entry. International Journal of Inflammation. 2012;**2012**. article ID 131243:10 pages. DOI: 10.1155/2012/131243

[89] Royse KE, Kempf MC, McGwin Jr G, Wilson CM, Tang J, Shrestha S. Toll-like receptor gene variants associated with bacterial vaginosis among HIV-1 infected adolescents. Journal of Reproductive Immunology. 2012;**96**(1-2):84-89

[90] Doerfinger SY, Throop AL, Herbst-Kralovetz MM. Bacteria in the vaginal microbiome alter the innate immune response and barrier properties of the human vaginal epithelia in a species-specific manner. Journal of Infectious Diseases. 2014;**209**(12):1989-1999

[91] Alcaide ML, Strbo N, Romero L, Jones DL, Rodriguez VJ, Arheart K, Martinez O, Bolivar H, Podack ER, Fischi MA. Bacterial vaginosis is associated with loss of gamma delta T cells in the female reproductive tract in women in the Miami Women Interagency HIV Study (WIHS): A cross sectional study. PLOS One. 2016, Apr. 14;**11**(4):e0153045. DOI: 10.1371/journal.pone.0153045

[92] Briseden AM, Moncia BJ, Stevens CE, Hiller SL. Sialidases (neuraminidases) in bacterial vaginosis and bacterial vaginosis associated microflora. Journal of Clinical Microbiology. 1992;**30**(3):663-666

[93] Myziuk L, Romanowski B, Johnson SC, BVBlue test for diagnosis of bacterial vaginosis. Journal of Clinical Microbiology. 2003;**41**(5):1925-1928

[94] Wiggins R, Hicks SJ, Soothill PW, MIllar MR, Corfield AP. Mucinases and sialidases: Their role in the pathogenesis of sexually transmitted infections in the female genital tract. Sexually Transmitted Infections. 2001;**77**(6):402-408

[95] Lewis AL, Lewis WG. Host sialoglycans and bacterial sialidases: A mucosa perspective. Cellular Microbiology. 2012;**14**(8):1174-1182

[96] Stamatos NM, Gomatos PJ, Cox J, Fowler A, Dow N, Wohlhieter JA, et al. Desialylation of peripheral blood mononuclear cells promotes growth of HIV-1. Virology. 1997;**228**(2):123-131

[97] Stamatos NM, Curreli S, Zelia D, Cross AS. Desialylation of glycoconjugates on the surface of monocytes activates the extracellular signal-related kinases ERK ½ and results in enhanced production of specific cytokines. Journal of Leukocyte Biology. 2004;**75**(2):307-313

[98] Hu H, Shioda T, Moriya C, Xin X, Hasan MK, Miyake K, et al. Infectivities of human and other primate lentiviruses are activated by desialylation of the viron surface. Journal of Virology. 1996;**70**(11):7462-7470

[99] Scudder PR, Chantler EN. Control of human cervical mucin glycosylation by endogenous fucosyl and sialytransferases. Advances in Experimental Medicine and Biology. 1982;**144**:265-267

[100] Reid G, Milsap K, Bruce AW. Implantation of *Lactobacillus* case var rhamnosus into vagina. The Lancet. 1994;**344**(8931):1229

[101] Parma M, Stella Vanni V, Bertini M, Candiani M. Probiotics in the prevention of recurrences of bacterial vaginosis. Alternative Therapies in Health and Medicine. 2014;**20**:52-57

[102] Recine N, Musciola A, Moreira E. The benefits of topical vaginal therapy with Lactobacillus case sub-rhamnosus in preventing bacterial vaginosis relapses. In: Communication and Posters for the X National iBAT Conference Naples; 26-28 January 18(supll 1)

[103] Rossi A, Rossi T, Bertini M. The use of Lactobacillus rhamnosus in the therapy of bacterial vaginosis. Evaluation of clinical efficacy in a population of 40 women treated for 24 months. Archives of Gynecology and Obstetrics. 2010;**281**:1065-1069

[104] Bertini M. Is Lactobacillus rhamnosus BMX 54 vaginal application a strategy to counteract bacterial vaginosis recurrences? In: Ben-Rafael Z, editor, Proceedings of 18th World Congress on Controversies in Obstetrics, Gynecology & Infertility; October 24-27, 2013; Wien; 339-345. DOI: 10.12894/COGI/20131024

[105] Recine N, Palma E, Domenici L, Giorgini M, Imperiale L, Sassu C, Masella A, Marchetti C, Muzii L, Benedetti Panici PG. Restoring vaginal microbiota: Biological control of bacterial vaginosis. A prospective case-control study using Lactobacillus rhamnosus BMX 54 as adjuvant treatment against vacterial vaginosis. Archives of Gynecology and Obstetrics. January 2016;**23**(1):101-107. DOI: 10.1007/s00404-015-3810-2

[106] Marcone V, Calzolari E, Bertini M. Effectiveness of vaginal administration of *Lactobacillus rhamnosus* following conventional metronidazole therapy: How to lower the rate of recurrences. New Microbiologica. 2008;**31**(3):429-433

[107] Marcone V, Rocca B, Lichtner M, Calzolari E. Long-term vaginal administration of *Lactobacillus rhamnosus* as a complementary approach to management of bacterial vaginosis. International Journal of Gynecology & Obstetrics. 2010;**110**:223-226. DOI org/10.1016/I.ijgo.2010.04.026

[108] Stojanovic N, Plecas D, Plesinac S. Normal vaginal flora, disorders and application of probiotics in pregnancy. Archives of Gynecology and Obstetrics. 2012;**286**(2):325-332. DOI: 10.1007/S00404-012-2293-7

[109] Recine N, Palma E, Domenici L, Giorgini M, Pierangeli A, Benedetti Panici P. Long-term probiotic implementation to re-create a balanced vaginal ecosystem: A promising boost against HPV. In: Infection Communication and Poster of International Scientific Conference probiotics and prebiotics; 21st-23rd June 2016; Budapest Hungary

[110] EFSA Panel on Dietetic Products, Nutrition and Allergies (NDA). Scientific opinion on the substantiation of health claims related to a combination of *Lactobacillus fermentum* 57°, *Lactobacillus plantarum* 57B and *Lactobacillus gasseri* 57C and defence against vaginal pathogens (ID 934, further assessment) pursuant to Article 13(1) of Regulation (EC) no 1924/2006. EFSA Journal. 2012;**10**(6):2719

[111] Bradshaw CS, Morton AN, Hocking J, Garland SM, Morris MB, Moss LM, et al. High recurrence rates of bacterial vaginosis over the course of 12 months after oral metronidazole therapy and factors associated with recurrence. The Journal of Infectious Diseases. 2006;**193**(11):1478-1486

[112] Balkus JE, Manhart LE, Lee J, Anzala O, Kimani J, Schwebke J, Shafi J, Rivers C, Kabare E, McClelland S. Periodic presumptive treatment for vaginal infections may reduce the incidence of sexually transmitted bacterial infections. Journal of Infectious Diseases. 2016;**213**:1932-1937

[113] Schwebke Jr JR, Desmond RA. A randomized trial of metronidazole in asymptomatic bacterial vaginosis to prevent the acquisition of sexually transmitted diseases. American Journal of Obstetrics & Gynecology. 2007;**196**:S17.e1-S17.e6

[114] Allworth JE, Peipert JF. Severity of bacterial vaginosis and the risk of sexually trasmitted infection. American Journal of Obstetrics & Gynecology. 2011;**205**:113.e1-113.e6

[115] Allsworth JE, Peipert JF. Prevalence of bacterial vaginosis: 2001 – 2004 National Health and Nutrition Examination Survey data. Obstetrics and Gynecology. 2007;**109**:114-120

[116] Schwebke JR, Lee J, Lensig S, Philip SS, Wiesenfeld AC, Sena AC, Trainor N, Acevado N, Saylor L, Rompalo AM, et al. Home screening for bacterial vaginosis to prevent sexually transmitted diseases. Clinical Infectious Diseases. 2016;**62**(5):531-536. doi,org/10.1093/cid/civ975

[117] Workowski KA, Bolan GA. Sexually trasmitted diseases treatment guidelines, 2015. MMWR Recommendations and Reports. 2015;**64**:1-137

[118] Rajalaksmi R, Kalaivani S. Prevalence of asymptomatic infections in sexually transmitted diseases attendees diagnosed with bacterial vaginosis, vaginal candidiasis and trichomoniasis. Indian Journal of Sexually Transmitted Diseases. 2016;**37**(2):139-142

[119] Balkus JE, Richardson BA, Rabe LK, Taha TE, Mgodi N, Kasaro MP, Ramjee G, Hoffman IF, Abdol Karim SS. Bacterial vaginosis and the risk of *Trichomonas vaginalis* acquisition among HIV-1 negative women. Sexually Transmitted Infections. 2014;**41**(2):123-128. DOI: 10.1097/OLQ.00000000000075

[120] Sobel JD, Ferris D, Schwebke J, Nyirjesy P, Wiesenfeld HC, Peipert J, et al. Suppressive antibacterial therapy with 0.75% metronidazole vaginal gel to prevent recurrent bacterial vaginosis. American Journal of Obstetrics & Gynecology. 2006;**194**:1283-1289

[121] Balkus JE, Jahko W, Mandaliya K, Richardson BA, Mases L, Gitau R, et al. The posttrial effect of oral periodic presumptive treatment for vaginal infections on the incidence of bacterial vaginosis and *Lactobacillus* colonization. Sexually Transmitted Infections. 2012;**29**:361-365

[122] Serok AC, Verstraelen H, Temmerman M, Botta GA. Probiotics for the treatment of bacterial vaginosis. Cochrane Database of Systematic Reviews. 2009:CD006289

[123] Mitra A, Macinyre DA, Marchesi JR, Lee YS, Bennet PR, Kyrgiou M. The vaginal microbiota, human papillomavirus infection and cervical intraepithelial neoplasia: What do we know and where are we going next? Microbiome. 2016;**4**:58

11

The Advantages of Using Multiplex PCR for the Simultaneous Detection of Six Sexually Transmitted Diseases

Mihaela L. Vică, Horea V. Matei and
Costel V. Siserman

Abstract

Sexually transmitted diseases (STDs) are among the most common infections. Their clinical identification is difficult because STDs are often asymptomatic. Untreated infections with these pathogens can in time lead to serious consequences. It is documented that isolation of some of these bacteria from cultures is very difficult. Because there is a large number of STD pathogens which can generate coinfections, their simultaneous detection in a unique sample is very important. Multiplex polymerase chain reaction (PCR) is an advanced method of molecular biology which allows for simultaneous detection of multiple pathogens in the same sample. The advantages of the multiplex PCR method were assessed by various researchers by comparing the diagnosis results obtained with different other conventional methods. The sensitivity and specificity of these methods were analyzed on different specimens in comparison to traditional methods, such as culture media or direct microscopic examination. These studies demonstrated beyond any doubt that the multiplex PCR system is highly effective in the detection of each of multiple STD pathogens depicted from a single specimen and argued for multiplex PCR superiority in terms of sensitivity and rapidity.

Keywords: STD pathogens, DNA, simultaneous detection, multiplex PCR

1. Introduction

Sexually transmitted diseases (STDs) are an issue of great interest as they are among the most common of all infections. It is documented that STDs are more prevalent in economically underdeveloped populations. Only a few countries outside Western Europe and

North America have implemented monitoring systems for these infections. In the rest of the world, epidemiological studies are based on the results of samples provided by certain population segments (mainly symptomatic patients or prenatal controls) not necessarily representative for the majority of the population. Usually, persons presenting obvious signs (secretions, lesions or pain) interrupt their sexual activity and seek medical help. Ironically, most often those who actually transmit these infections are asymptomatic or present mild symptoms [1].

It is well-known that vaginal bacterial infections can induce human infertility, yet they are underestimated in infertility testing. Population screening and treatment of individuals presenting unexplained infertility that are detected as STD-infected persons seem appropriate in this context [2].

No STD can be regarded as an isolated problem since multiple infections are rather common and STD infections generally denote a high-risk sexual behavior that often can be associated with more serious infections. It is therefore important to acknowledge that STDs are often asymptomatic or cause nonspecific symptoms and that periodical STD testing is crucial in limiting the risk of human immunodeficiency virus (HIV) infection. STD control could significantly reduce HIV incidence worldwide, although the impact of interventions may vary depending on local epidemiological contexts. Analysis of data from several studies has suggested that a better management of STD cases is more likely to reduce HIV incidence in the early stages of an epidemic, when HIV infections are concentrated in population groups with a high prevalence of other curable STDs [3].

A correct STD diagnosis is needed to prevent further spreading of such infections in the healthy population. Several techniques and laboratory methods for highlighting these diseases were developed in the past decades. For instance, because of their high sensitivity, specificity and suitability for different types of samples, nucleic acid amplification tests (NAATs) are suitable for the diagnosis of urogenital infections. Lately, however, polymerase chain reaction (PCR) techniques are increasingly employed in such cases as they allow direct, sensitive, automated and usable detection of STD-causing pathogens on all sample types and even the simultaneous detection of several STDs.

2. The most frequent causative agent of STDs

Chlamydia trachomatis is an intracellular human pathogen. *C. trachomatis* infection is the most common STD reported in Western Europe developed countries [4]. About 75% of all cases involve young people aged 15–24 years, being more common in women than in men. It infects the epithelial cells of the endocervix in women and the urethra in men. Infection with *C. trachomatis* is often asymptomatic, especially in women, but presents a high risk for complications. The treatment is rather simple if early detected. Of note, the bacteria can be passed from mother to newborn during delivery [5].

Urogenital infection with *C. trachomatis* shows a broad spectrum of clinical manifestations, including urethritis, cervicitis and pelvic inflammatory disease (PID). Intense mucosal inflammation is characterized by erythema, swelling and mucous secretions caused by mucopurulent cervicitis in women and nongonococcal urehtritis (NGU) in men. It is very important to diagnose these bacteria in early stages of infection and beginning treatment as soon as possible to prevent long-term complications. It can persist in the genital tract for a long time, in a form that is resistant to immunodestruction; such symptoms are unnoticed in approximately 75–80% of women [6]. *C. trachomatis* genital infection significantly increases the risk of sequelae in the reproductive tract in women, including tubal deterioration, ectopic pregnancy and miscarriage [7]. The role of the *C. trachomatis* infection in decreasing male fertility is also well-known. Given the severity of the complications, several countries (e.g., France) made recommendations for screening these bacteria in asymptomatic young subjects [8].

Neisseria gonorrhoeae is the etiologic agent of gonorrhea, one of the most common sexually transmitted bacterial infections, producing more than 82 million new infections worldwide each year [9]. *N. gonorrhoeae* or gonorrhea is an aerobic Gram-negative bacterium presenting itself in the form of diplococci. Along with *C. trachomatis,* it is the most prevalent sexually transmitted bacterial infection. It causes urogenital mucosa infections in men and women, being a serious cause of morbidity. The disease is characterized by purulent inflammation of the urogenital system mucosa. It is also presumed that gonorrhea infection may increase susceptibility to HIV and its transmission [10].

Neisseria gonorrhoeae has developed mechanisms to alter the epithelial barriers in order to reach subepithelial tissues and colonize in the host organism. Emergence and spread of multiresistant *N. gonorrhoeae* strains and the absence of an effective vaccine are major problems worldwide. Gonococcal endocarditis is a rare (1–2%) but serious disease that occurs in patients with disseminated gonococcal infections, which are also rare (0.3–5%) [11].

Several data indicate the involvement of the gonococci in miscarriages. Screening and medical management of the *N. gonorrhoeae* infection, including screening of women visiting abortion centers, have been proposed in order to identify associated risk factors and to assess the benefits of systematic screening in avoiding complications [12].

Trichomonas vaginalis is the causative agent of trichomonosis, one of the nonviral STDs. This protozoan was first described in 1836 by Donné. Infection with this parasite can give birth to serious complications, especially in women. The spectrum of clinical presentation range from asymptomatic or slightly symptomatic, particularly in men, to severe vaginitis with abundant vaginal secretions in women [13]. Infections with this protozoan can lead to serious health problems such as infertility, preterm delivery, low birth weight [14, 15], susceptibility to cervical cancer [15] or increased prevalence of high risk human papillomavirus (HPV) infection [16]. Moreover, there is a strong association between *T. vaginalis* infection and acquisition of HIV [17]. Because it is sexually transmitted, trichomoniasis is common in populations at higher risk for other sexually transmitted infections. Its presence in an individual is a marker for high-risk behaviors and coincident STDs should be sought after. This infection is detected in approximately three quarters of the infected women's male sex partners [18]. For better cure rates, sexual partners should be treated simultaneously even if the infection is asymptomatic.

Trichomonas vaginalis infects squamous epithelial cells through direct contact, producing micro-ulcerations and microscopic bleedings in the vaginal walls and endocervix. In most cases, men are asymptomatic, but they transmit the infection to women. As the women's columnar epithelium is not affected, trichomonosis is manifest as vaginitis, but not endocervicitis. The simultaneous presence of an endocervicitis should alert the physician to check possible coinfections with *C. trachomatis* or *N. gonorrhoeae*. Severe infections are usually treated with nitroimidazole derivatives, but the number of resistant strains is constantly growing [19, 20].

The term mycoplasma is used to designate organisms in the Mollicutes class, the smallest free-living cell-wall-deficient microorganisms, the most simple life forms capable of replication outside a host cell. *Ureaplasma urealyticum, Ureaplasma parvum, Mycoplasma genitalium* and *Mycoplasma hominis* are the most common species of mycoplasmas in both men and women. Mycoplasma species (*U. urealiticum* and *M. hominis* in particular) are frequently detected in sexually active asymptomatic youngsters. However, they can induce a broad spectrum of pathological conditions in both women and men, including unexplained chronic symptoms of lower urinary tract, NGU, PID, pyelonephritis, chronic prostatitis, preterm labor and idiopathic abortion due to infection of the urogenital bodies [21].

Ureaplasma species are sometimes detected in the commensal bacteria of the lower genital tract, so their role among STD is still questioned. Some studies demonstrated that the association of *Ureaplasma* species with NGU depends on the detected species and that *U. urealiticum* is an etiologic agent of NGU, unlike *U. parvum*. In addition, it is reported that *U. urealyticum* can cause infections in the lower genital tract and is a pathogen agent of urethritis in males [22]. In assessing the role of these microorganisms in producing human diseases, their high prevalence among asymptomatic individuals should be taken into consideration.

M. genitalium is a microorganism associated with acute and chronic sexually transmitted non-gonococcal urethritis in men. Data regarding infections in women suggest that *M. genitalium* is associated with urethritis, cervicitis and PID. According to some authors, individuals with clinically-significant urethritis, persistent PID or cervicitis should be tested for *M. genitalium* [23]. As in the case of *C. trachomatis, M. genitalium* infection is often asymptomatic.

Several authors have reported that these organisms are engaged in women infertility, preterm delivery, premature rupture of membranes and chorioamnionitis [24, 25]. In addition, some studies present mycoplasma as causative agents of male infertility. It has been reported that these infections change various sperm characteristics, such as motility, density or morphology, and that antibiotic treatment improves the quality of the sperm [26]. A recent study found out that detection rates of *M. hominis* and *U. urealiticum* in infertile couples were about two times higher than in fertile couples [27].

3. STD detection methods

Chlamydia trachomatis was first isolated from the female genital tract in 1959 [28]. Culture techniques for the isolation of these bacteria were developed since 1965. Microimmunofluorescence tests for seroepidemiological studies and serotyping emerged later. Currently, detection of *C. trachomatis* is accomplished via bacteriological examination or enzyme-linked immunosorbent assay (ELISA) [29].

Due to technical difficulties resulting from the need to inoculate specimens immediately after sampling, culture assays present low sensitivity (50%) and are seldom used today in the microbiological detection of *C. trachomatis*.

It is thought that *Chlamydia* immunoglobulin (IgG) antibodies persist in the body for years and therefore are used as markers for *C. trachomatis* infections [30]. These markers can be useful if a previous infection could have produced changes in the reproductive tract, but the presence of antibodies is not indicative of an infection present in the body at the time of detection, so these markers cannot be used in diagnosis.

Today, there are numerous methods available for *C. trachomatis* diagnosis, but it should be underlined that the PCR direct approach is given great interest lately. Also, the quick and easy to use loop-mediated isothermal amplification (LAMP) is often employed in detecting *C. trachomatis* [31]. Molecular biology tests based on gene amplification improved diagnostic quality in terms of sensitivity and specificity and are gradually replacing all other techniques (cell cultures, antigen tests, molecular hybridization without amplification, etc.). These techniques confirmed the high frequency of asymptomatic infections, their prevalence in women and men and evaluation of the frequency of recurrent and/or persistent infections.

In detecting *N. gonorrhoeae* infections, bacteriological cultures are yet the gold standard for diagnosis as they allow further testing of antibiotic susceptibility. Culture assays using Thayer-Martin agar have long been seen as the standard method [32]. Due to difficulties in collecting, transferring and storing specimens, these tests exhibit low sensitivity and are unsuitable for screening. Although enriched agar cultivation is still widely used for the diagnosis of *N. gonorrhoeae* infections, recent years have seen extensive usage of NAATs, especially in detecting carriers. These genetic tests enable establishing a diagnosis in 2–3 days for gonococcal urethritis or cervicitis with a sensitivity of up to 99%. In contrast, cell cultures provide a sensitivity of 85–95% in acute urethral infections and below 50% in chronic forms in women. These figures largely depend on sampling conditions, as *N. gonorrhoeae* is a rather fragile organism [33].

Precise diagnosis of gonorrhea is needed to prevent severe complications and to control transmission, especially in the case of asymptomatic infections. Molecular approaches such as hybridization assays or nucleic acid amplification tests have revolutionized the diagnosis of gonococcal infection due to their increased accuracy compared to the culture media and their ability to simultaneously test multiple species. NAAT should be the technique of choice in the diagnosis of coinfections and screening. In addition to diagnostic, molecular approaches have been successfully applied for testing *N. gonorrhoeae* in tracking genetic diversity.

Suspicion of *T. vaginalis* is often considered by clinicians in symptomatic women presenting a combination of vaginal discharge, vulvar irritation and unpleasant smell. Unpleasant smell and low irritation is more likely to be correlated with bacterial vaginosis than with trichomonosis, the irritation being more prominent in the latter case. After completing the physical examination, it is useful to determine the pH of the vaginal secretion. Vaginal pH is higher than 4.7 in most women presenting trichomonosis, but high pH values are also seen in most women with bacterial vaginosis, therefore further investigations are required for an accurate diagnosis. A final diagnosis is based on the positive detection of this parasite. This can be determined microscopically in saline serum, using a magnification of 400×, but the sensitivity of this method is about 60%. A crucial step in the infection process involves a dramatic morphological change in the parasite. Free ovoid cells that resemble the familiar image of a flagellated protozoan take an amoeboid shape in contact with the urogenital tract [34], making microscopic detection more difficult. Pap smears can detect *Trichomonas* infections, but the Gram staining is useless here. Microscopic evaluation is time consuming and standardization in the interpretation of positive results is rather ambiguous [18]. Another disadvantage is that the microscopic examination should be performed within the first 10 min after sample collection [35].

Microscopic examination of the smear and/or culture is presently the most commonly used method in the detection of *T. vaginalis*. Because of its very slow growth rate, strict requirements for nutrients and specific culture embodiments that are not widely available, *T. vaginalis* is difficult to be grown in culture media [36]. Not only are such media very expensive, they also present a low sensitivity compared to the PCR methods recently introduced and require microscopic evaluation. Another disadvantage is that in women *T. vaginalis* is undetectable several months after metronidazole therapy [37]. Therefore, a precise diagnosis in women and men based on cell cultures is rather difficult to be made and the newer molecular techniques are more and more brought into action [38]. In the last decade, several PCR assays were developed and studies comparing the two methods in the detection of *T. vaginalis* demonstrated a higher sensitivity and specificity on behalf of the PCR.

The contribution of flow cytometry technology in investigating adhesion of the extracellular parasite to human host cells has been clearly demonstrated. This methodology can be optimized and the test can be used in a format in which several different strains may be analyzed simultaneously [39]. It is, however, a difficult method for the diagnosis of trichomooasis. A recent study [40] indicated the advantages of using DNA in the detection of *T. vaginalis*.

As mentioned above, *U. urealyticum, U. parvum, M. hominis* and *M. genitalium* are the most common mycoplasma species in both men and women. While the first three can be grown in culture media, the latter cannot. However, growing on culture embodiments is difficult and lasts longer, up to 4 days for *U. urealyticum* [36]. Also, the technique requires biochemical identification to determine the species of mycoplasma involved. Mycoplasmas are hard to grow in normal laboratory conditions, their simplistic genome demanding more complex environments. Difficulties in their cultivation and identification in clinical samples that often contain other bacteria or fungi have further complicated causal diagnosis and their association to disease. Mycoplasma infections are often associated with the presence of asymptomatic carriers that may or may not develop the disease [41]. Thus, identification of the virulence factors in mycoplasma has been complicated by the difficulties encountered in isolating the strains.

M. genitalium detection using culture cells is no longer employed in routine clinical practice because its growth takes several weeks and presents technical difficulties [42]. According to some authors, *M. genitalium* requires a special medium and incubating for up to 8 weeks to be successfully detected [43]. Although many researchers would rather turn to serological methods when documenting an infection caused by these bacteria [44], such diagnosis approach is not appropriate due to cross-reactivity with *M. pneumoniae*. For a precise diagnosis, a direct identification is therefore recommended.

The safe detection of *M. genitalium* and other bacteria was for a long time hampered by the absence of a commercially available diagnostic test. In recent years, however, NAATs revolutionized the detection and study of mycoplasma. These techniques contributed greatly to the DNA-based improvement of the detection, identification and serotyping methods [45]. In addition, the DNA-based method enabled the identification as separate species of *U. urealyticum* and *U. parvum*, previously considered as biovariants (biovar 1 and biovar 2) of *U. urealyticum* [46].

Over 50 mycoplasma genome sequences are now available in public databases, revealing a genetic diversity more complex than first predicted. This growing set of data is extremely valuable in the study of organisms otherwise difficult to cultivate, offering new means for testing and molecular diagnostics [47].

4. Multiplex PCR methods as diagnostic tools for STDs

Multiplex PCR methods for the simultaneous diagnosis of several STDs are more and more often employed in recent years. These methods place a number of primer pairs corresponding to specific DNA sequences of various STD pathogens all in one reaction tube, such commercial ready to use kits being available. While some kits can simultaneously detect two commonly associated STDs, such as *C. trachomatis* and *N. gonorrhoeae* infections, others can manage three pathogen detections. However, kits containing the primer pairs needed for the simultaneous detection of 6–12 STD pathogens are gaining momentum on the market. The most effective and widely used kits are presently those simultaneously detecting the top six most frequent STD agents, namely *C. trachomatis, N. gonorrhoeae, T. vaginalis, U. urealyticum, M. hominis* and *M. genitalium*, agents which play hard to get for other detection methods and often exhibit multiple associations.

Another asset is that easily collectable urine samples are adequate DNA sources for these PCR techniques along with the urethral/vaginal discharge swabs. About 30–50 mL of first void urine (FVU) samples collected in sterile polypropylene containers early in the morning, at least 4 h after the previous urination, are more than enough for a successful analysis. FVU is definitely less invasive compared to the harvesting of vaginal or urethral secretions, an aspect reported to have influenced a significant number of subjects to avoid STD identification tests previously [48]. As urine specimens can be self-collected in intimacy, an increased number of patients tend to favor such option that also enhances the applicability of the screening programs [49]. The fact that urethral secretions were found to present increased sensitivity and specificity compared to FVU in immunological analyzes for male subjects seems to hold lesser relevance, anyway differences have diminished since NAAT were first performed [46]. Concerning the female subjects, the use of urine specimens in STD identification produced similar results to vaginal or endocervical secretions [50]. It is known that assay sensitivity may decrease if samples are repeatedly frozen/thawed or stored for longer periods of time because nucleic acids can easily degrade. Urine samples hold another advantage as well: they can be stored at 4–8°C up to 7 days prior to the processing.

Thanks to this easy and noninvasive sampling, the multiplex PCR can be used to detect STDs in both symptomatic and asymptomatic individuals and could prove to be a useful screening tool for the general population.

A 15 min centrifugation at 15,000g and subsequent supernatant removal and pellet resuspension are needed as a successful DNA extraction requires concentrated pathogen suspensions. Both urethral/vaginal discharge swab specimens and urine samples should be brought to room temperature prior to the centrifugation. One can use up to 10 mL amounts of sample to increase the DNA extraction yield. Several commercially available kits for DNA extraction can be used according to the manufacturer's instructions, e.g., QIAamp® DNA Mini Kit (Qiagen, Hilden, Germany), AccuPrep Genomic DNA Extraction Kit (Bioneer, Seoul, Korea) or MasterPure™ Complete DNA and RNA Purification Kits (Epicentre Biotechnologies, USA).

In our marketing era, such new techniques and gadgets (kits) need to be accompanied by studies assessing their performance compared to other traditional methods.

One such study conducted in 2010 [36] compared the multiplex PCR assay for the simultaneous detection of *T. vaginalis, U. urealyticum* and *M. hominis* with data obtained using microscopic and culture techniques. Three cotton swabs were obtained from each of the 240 women enrolled in the study based on claims of lower genital tract infections. For the detection of *T. vaginalis,* swabs were inoculated in a modified Diamond's Trypticase-yeast medium including fetal bovine serum, streptomycin, penicillin G and amphotericin B and a wet mount was prepared for its detection by direct microscopic examination. The samples were incubated at 37°C in carbon dioxide atmosphere and observed for a week under a light microscope. The presence of *M. hominis* and *U. urealyticum* was assessed by culture detection using the Mycoplasma Duo kit (Sanofi Diagnostic). A number of different primer sets were synthesized, PCR amplifications and ethidium bromide detections in 1% agarose gels were performed for a multiplex PCR to be designed for the simultaneous detection of *T. vaginalis, M. hominis* and *U. urealyticum.* Results were then favorably compared to more conventional methods for the detection of *T. vaginalis, M. hominis* and *U. urealyticum.* When tested on vaginal swabs, the multiplex PCR correctly detected 14 out of 14 *T. vaginalis*-positives, 95 of 98 *U. urealyticum*-positives and 22 out of 22 *M. hominis*-positive samples. In contrast, the microscopic detection of *T. vaginalis* exhibited a 28.6% sensitivity, whereas culture methods identified 71.4% of the trichomonad infections documented with multiplex PCR. While the kit's sensitivity in the detection of *U. urealyticum* was 96.9%, a value comparable to culture test sensitivity (91.8%), identification of *M. hominis* was greatly improved (100 vs. 36.3% sensitivity). The study argued for multiplex PCR superiority in terms of sensitivity and rapidity (hours vs. days/weeks).

Another study [43] in 2011 compared the results of 113 STD patients tested for six sexually transmitted microorganisms (*C. trachomatis, M. hominis, M. genitalium, N. gonorrhoeae, T. vaginalis* and genital *Ureoplasma*) with an automated Seeplex® (Seegene, Korea) multiplex PCR-based STD6B autocapillary electrophoresis (ACE) system vs. culture and conventional PCR-based tests on genital and urinary specimens. *C. trachomatis* was cultured on cycloheximide-treated McCoy cells, while A7, arginine broth and agar media were used for *M. hominis* and *Ureaplasma*. Conventional culture media were employed for *N. gonorrhoeae. N. gonorrhoeae* and *C. trachomatis* was also tested with the PCR-based COBAS Amplicor. On the other hand, in-house validated PCR assays were performed for *T. vaginalis, N. gonorrhoeae* and *C. trachomatis*, while a Hy-Mycoplasma PCR Detection Kit (Hy-Labs, Israel) enabled the detection of *M. hominis, M. genitalium* and *Ureaplasma*. All six pathogens (*T. vaginalis, M. hominis, M. genitalium, C. trachomatis, N. gonorrhoeae* and *Ureaplasma*) were subjected to a multiplex PCR amplification and the products were separated and detected via automated capillary gel electrophoresis. The sensitivity of the STD6B ACE kit was 100% in case of *C. trachomatis, N. gonorrhoeae, M. genitalium, T. vaginalis* and *M. hominis*, and 98% for the *Ureaplasma*. Specificity was also 100% for *C. trachomatis, N. gonorrhoeae, M. genitalium* and *T. vaginalis*, while for *M. hominis* and *Ureaplasma* figures were 99 and 97%, respectively. These results prove beyond any doubt that the integrated STD6B ACE system is highly effective in the detection of each of the six STD pathogens depicted from a single specimen.

Seeplex® STD6 ACE Detection kit (Seegene, Korea) was evaluated in yet another Korean study, completed in 2012, which was conducted on 739 subjects [51]. Cervical swabs were collected from the women enrolled, while men were requested to provide 30–40 mL of FVU. The six pairs of dual priming oligonucleotide primers specifically targeting the *C. trachomatis, M. hominis, M. genitalium, N. gonorrhoeae, T. vaginalis* and *U. urealyticum* genes were tested against a combined monoplex PCR. All specimens were tested with the multiplex PCR for the six pathogens and amplification products were separated with a LabChip® DX Seeplex® assay system (Caliper, USA). All specimens were retested with six monoplex PCRs (one for each of the STD agents) and a duplex strand displacement amplification (SDA) for *C. trachomatis* and *N. gonorrhoeae* was accomplished with a BD ProbeTec™ (Becton–Dickinson Microbiology System, USA). An absolute correlation between the multiplex and monoplex PCRs was found in terms of both sensitivity and specificity. The results of the multiplex PCR and duplex SDA were 99.7% concordant in the case of *C. trachomatis* and 100% for *N. gonorrhoeae*. The results confirmed that the simultaneous detection of several species in one sample was feasible and that the clinical sensitivity provided by the multiplex PCR was on an equal footing with the monoplex PCR and duplex SDA, proving to be fully adequate for routine detection of several STDs while holding an upper hand in terms of cost-effectiveness and rapidity.

Anyplex™ II STI-7 Detection Kit (Seegene, Korea) was tested to the limit in a 2013 Korean study [46] aiming to investigate the accuracy and reliability of a real-time multiplex PCR assay employed for the detection of seven STD agents (*C. trachomatis, N. gonorrhoeae, T. vaginalis, M. genitalium, M. hominis, U. urealyticum* and *U. parvum*) in clinical samples. A total of 897 specimens (696 FVU and 201 endocervical swabs) were collected from 365 symptomatic patients and 532 asymptomatic volunteers and five diagnostic methods were employed as the specimens were subjected to parallel testing using four NAATs and one *Mycoplasma* detection kit. The RT-PCR amplification was performed for all seven microorganisms with Anyplex™ II STI-7 Detection Kit. PCR amplification was performed using the Seeplex® STD6 ACE Detection Kit, in accordance with the manufacturer's protocol. A battery of kits were deployed for detecting the pathogens: *C. trachomatis* and *N. gonorrhoeae*—SDA technology using BD ProbeTec™; *T. vaginalis* and *M. genitalium*—AmpliSens® (EPH PCR Kit-InterLabService Ltd, Russia); *M. hominis* and *U. urealyticum*—Mycoplasma IST 2 Kit (bioMérieux, France). Test sensitivity and specificity of each method for every STD agent were calculated in parallel and conclusions were that the multiplex real-time PCR (Anyplex™ II) demonstrated outstanding results compared with other diagnostic tools as it yielded 100% sensitivity and very high specificity in the detection of *C. trachomatis, N. gonorrhoeae, T. vaginalis, M. genitalium* and *M. hominis* and was also useful in discriminating between *U. urealyticum* and *U. parvum*. Despite the increased workload and higher costs due to the larger number of tests conducted, multiplex real-time PCR was found to be equivalent or superior to other assessment methods and in the future is expected to become a standard diagnostic tool.

We ourselves have used a Seeplex® STD6 ACE Detection kit in a study on 224 Romanian subjects including persons with STD symptoms and asymptomatic individuals involved in unprotected sex with multiple partners, couples experiencing unexplained infertility or others requesting STD screening for various reasons. Each individual contributed with 30–50 mL FVU samples and DNA extraction was accomplished with MasterPure™ Complete DNA and RNA Purification Kits (Epicentre Biotechnologies, USA). A 2% agarose gel containing ethidium bromide was used with 0.5× Tris-borate 0.1 mM EDTA (TBE) as running buffer. The PCR products were visualized using a UV transilluminator. An example of gel electrophoresis results can be visualized in **Figure 1**.

The accuracy of the method was demonstrated by the lack of contamination (no amplicons in the negative control band) and the presence of positive control bands corresponding to all six DNA fragments of known molecular weight included in the marker used to determine the size of the amplification products. Also, internal controls indicated proper PCR amplification in each microtube (see **Figure 1**).

About 74 (33.03%) of the 224 subjects, both symptomatic and asymptomatic, were positive for one or more STDs. All six pathogen agents were detected with the multiplex PCR kit, several double or triple infections demonstrating associative patterns. The following double associations were detected in the study: *C. trachomatis* and *N. gonorrhoeae*, *C. trachomatis* and *U. urealyticum*, *N. gonorrhoeae* and *U. urealyticum*, *C. trachomatis* and *M. hominis*. Several triple infections grouped *C. trachomatis*, *N. gonorrhoeae* and *U. urealyticum*.

The bacteria most frequently identified in the analyzed urine samples was *C. trachomatis*, found in 20.9% of the cases. Consequently, a number of associations between *C. trachomatis* and other STD agents (*N. gonorrhoeae*, *U. urealyticum* and *M. hominis*, respectively) were found. These results are consistent with studies conducted in other countries or international statistics indicating *C. trachomatis* as the most common STD agent [4, 52, 53]. Detection of *C. trachomatis* in several asymptomatic patients demonstrated again how easily this infection can pass unnoticed.

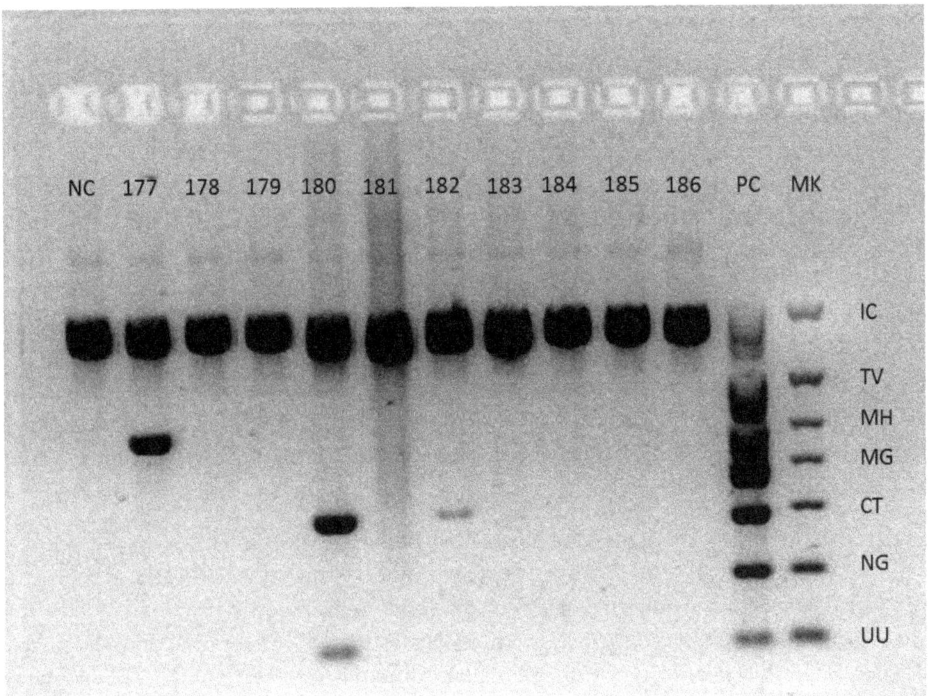

Figure 1. STD pathogens—agarose gel electrophoresis. NC: negative control, 177–186: samples, PC: positive control, MK: marker, TV: *T. vaginalis*, MH: *M. hominis*, MG: *M. genitalium*, CT: *C. trachomatis*, NG: *N. gonorrhoeae*, UU: *U. Urealyticum*.

Some studies recommended that all sexually active women should be tested, pregnant ones or those that have experienced miscarriages in particular, given the high prevalence of *C. trachomatis/N. gonorrhoeae* infections [54, 55]. In the US, concomitant empiric treatment of *C. trachomatis* and *N. gonorrhoeae* is recommended for all gonorrhea positives considering the frequent association between the two pathogens [56]. However, results indicate that several other associations (such as those between *C. trachomatis* and *U. urealyticum* or *M. hominis*) are often encountered, suggesting that a population screening for *C. trachomatis/N. gonorrhoeae* is not good enough and a multiplex method for the simultaneous detection of the most frequent six or more STD agents would be more appropriate, considering the different associations that may arise.

N. gonorrhoeae was detected in 7.1% of the cases, as was the case of *U. urealyticum*. These results are consistent with other studies indicating a high prevalence of both bacteria, the most frequent STD agents except for *C. trachomatis* [9, 57]. A notable finding is that we detected patients positive to *N. gonorrhoeae* that presented no or very atypical symptoms of gonococcal infection, which could have resulted in inadequate treatment without this DNA-based analysis that allowed us to identify the presence of the gonococcus. The *N. gonorrhoeae/U. urealyticum* coinfection we found was another confirmation that both *C. trachomatis* and *N. gonorrhoeae* can associate with other STD pathogens, an additional argument for the use of multiplex kits able to detect a large number of STDs in the same sample.

A recent study in Korea [58] found a 3.3% infection rate for *T. vaginalis* in the general population and argued that the rate was higher in women over 50 years of age. This followed a previous study documenting a 2.4% infection rate for *T. vaginalis* in the same area 15 years before and the significant increase lead researchers to recommend PCR-based testing of *T. vaginalis* in all women over 50 years old, irrespective of their symptomatology. Our study detected but one (0.44%) case of *T. vaginalis* infection, suggesting that in our area prevalence is much lower than the literature data based on other than NAAT determinations (e.g., physical and microscopy examinations or cell cultures) indicated. NAAT seems to be for now the only accurate method to diagnose this parasite. Our results are consistent with those conducted in other countries where *T. vaginalis* was detected in similarly low percentages compared to other STD [43, 51]. However, the incidence of trichomonosis has gradually decreased over the past 40 years. This may be due to the large amount of metronidazole and other imidazoles generally used in the treatment of bacterial vaginosis. Although the number of people infected with *T. vaginalis* is low, the analysis is justified considering its asymptomatic manifestation and the serious complications it produces.

In a study conducted in the United States, *M. hominis* and various *Ureaplasma* species were detected in 21–53% of the cases involving asymptomatic women and 40–80% of the sexually active women, respectively, their prevalence being slightly lower in men [59]. In our study, mycoplasma infections were detected in 25 individuals (a rate of 11.1%), the most commonly encountered being *U. urealyticum* (in 7.1% of the patients). Although *M. hominis* and *M. genitalium* were less represented (1.7 and 2.2% of the patients, respectively), these infections cannot be ignored. More so considering that *M. genitalium* was detected in an asymptomatic patient previously found negative for different STDs investigated on specific culture media (including ones for *M. genitalium*) in a number of different specimens (urine, urethral discharge). This last example reaffirmed the sensitivity of the multiplex PCR method over traditional alternatives.

5. Advantages of the multiplex PCR method

The advantages of the multiplex PCR method were assessed by various researchers comparing the diagnosis results obtained with different other conventional methods. The sensitivity and specificity of these methods were analyzed on different specimens in comparison to traditional methods, some of these considered to be the gold standard in diagnosis [36, 43, 46, 51]. Although this method can sometimes increase the workload, implying more protocol steps (DNA extraction, purification—if necessary, PCR amplification, electrophoresis), it still holds a huge advantage in terms of the exact diagnosis of STD. Except for special circumstances, such as when testing susceptibility to antibiotics of the various bacterial agents, NATTs have become the most sought after tests in STD detection. Regarding bacterial resistance to antibiotics, the DNA extracted and identified as belonging to such bacteria may be genetically tested to determine the genes that induce resistance to antibiotics or the different mutations that cause such resistance.

Although the symptoms are often similar, the treatment may differ depending on the STD agent detected. Without an accurate diagnosis, treatment is often ineffective. Clinicians often employ point-of-care (POC) tests to diagnose vaginal infections and STDs. For example, most clinicians rely on Amsel's clinical criteria in defining bacterial vaginosis: increased vaginal pH, the presence of amines, clue cells observed on wet mounts and homogeneous vaginal secretions [60]. Although bacterial cultures and other methods are still widely used in STD detection, PCR tests are relevant, reproducible, sensitive and specific enough tools implying low costs and simplicity. In addition, the availability of commercial NAATs that include several STD pathogens allows more detailed studies regarding the relationship between such organisms in the etiology of these diseases. As well documented, all STDs occur in populations at high risk for other sexually transmitted infections. Their presence in a given individual is a marker for high-risk behaviors and coincidental infections should be sought after, as well as other more serious sexually transmitted diseases such as HIV.

An advantage of this method is its great sensitivity consisting in the detection of STD pathogens in individuals who have previously been tested with conventional methods and came out with negative results.

The greatest advantage of this method is the detection of double or multiple coinfections. This is an important argument for promoting multiplex testing in the same sample. These results could have important implications in epidemiology and treatment by improvements in the accuracy of determining the possible synergies and interactions between such microorganisms.

STD screening for certain categories of population (e.g., patients attending sexual health clinics, infertile persons or women who had miscarriages) is necessary not only to identify symptomatic persons in order to diagnose and treat their infection but also to identify asymptomatic individuals who serve as possible infection carriers in order to reduce morbidity and help controlling these STDs. The multiplex PCR method provides a good opportunity to argue for STD screening.

Author details

Mihaela L. Vică[1]*, Horea V. Matei[1] and Costel V. Siserman[2]

*Address all correspondence to: mvica@umfcluj.ro

1 Department of Cell and Molecular Biology, "Iuliu Hatieganu" University of Medicine and Pharmacy, Cluj-Napoca, Romania

2 Department of Legal Medicine, "Iuliu Hatieganu" University of Medicine and Pharmacy Cluj-Napoca, Romania

References

[1] Holmes K.K., Handsfield H.H. Sexually transmitted diseases: overview and clinical approach. In: Harrison's Principles of Internal Medicine. 14th ed. Bucuresti: Teora; 2003. p. 881–893.

[2] Salah R.M., Allam A.M., Magdy A.M., Mohamed A.S. Bacterial vaginosis and infertility: cause or association?. Eur J Obstet Gynecol Reprod Biol. 2013;**167**(1):59–63. doi: 10.1016/j.ejogrb.2012.10.031

[3] Korenromp E.L., White R.G., Orroth K.K., Bakker R., Kamali A., Serwadda D., et al. Determinants of the impact of sexually transmitted infection treatment on prevention of HIV infection: a synthesis of evidence from the Mwanza, Rakai, and Masaka intervention trials. J Infect Dis. 2005;**191**(1):168–178. doi: 10.1086/425274

[4] ECDC.Annual epidemiological report on communicable diseases in Europe. Stockholm: European Centre for Disease Prevention and Control. 2010

[5] McGregor J.A., French J.I. *Chlamydia trachomatis* infection during pregnancy. Am J Obstet Gynecol. 1991;**164**(6):1782–1789. doi:10.1016/0002-9378(91)90560-E

[6] Witkin S.S., Linhares I.M. *Chlamydia trachomatis* in subfertile women undergoing uterine instrumentation. Hum Reprod. 2002;**17**(8):1938–1941

[7] Hafner L.M., McNeilly C. Vaccines for Chlamydia infections of the female genital tract. Future Microbiol. 2008;**3**(1):67–77. doi:10.2217/17460913.3.1.67

[8] Anaes. Evaluation of screening low urogenital *Chlamydia trachomatis* in France. Paris: National Accreditation and Health Evaluation Agency. 2003

[9] World Health Organization (WHO). Prevalence and incidence in 2005 of selected sexually transmitted infections. In: *Chlamydia trachomatis, Neisseria gonorrhoeae,* syphilis and *Trichomonas vaginalis*: methods and results used by WHO to generate 2005 estimates. WHO, Geneva. 2011

[10] Li S.Y. Global transmission of multiple-drug resistant *Neisseria gonorrhoeae* strains refractive to cephalosporin treatment. J Formos Med Assoc. 2012;**111**(9):463–464. doi:10.1016/j.jfma.2012.03.004

[11] Querci M., Rombini F., Spinola L., Boutureira M., Yetman M., Reyes D., et al. *Neisseria gonorrhoeae* infective endocarditis. A case report. Int J Antimicrob Ag 41S1. 2013;**S1–S34**:P53.

[12] Toyer A.L., Trignol-Viguier N., Mereghetti L., Joly B., Blin E., Body G., et al. Interest of simultaneous *Chlamydia trachomatis* and *Neisseria gonorrhoeae* screening at the time of preabortion consultation. Contraception. 2012;**86**:572–576. doi:10.1016/j.contraception.2012.04.012

[13] Gilbert R.O., Elia G., Beach D.H., Klaessig S., Singh B.N. Cytopathogenic effect of *Trichomonas vaginalis* on human vaginal epithelial cells cultured in vitro. Infect Immun. 2000;**68**(7):4200–4206.

[14] Cudmore S.L., Garber G.E. Prevention or treatment: the benefits of *Trichomonas vaginalis* vaccine. J Infect Public Health. 2010;**3**(2):47–53. doi:10.1016/j.jiph.2010.01.003

[15] Cotch M.F., Pastorek J.G., Nugent R.P., Hillier S.L., Gibbs R.S., Martin D.H., et al. *Trichomonas vaginalis* associated with low birth weight and preterm delivery. The Vaginal Infections and Prematurity Study Group. Sex Transm Dis. 1997;**24**(6):353–360.

[16] Noël J.C., Fayt I., Munoz M.R.R., Simon P., Engohan-Aloghe C. High prevalence of high-risk human papillomavirus infection among women with *Trichomonas vaginalis* infection on monolayer cytology. Arch Gynecol Obstet. 2010;**282**(5):503–505. doi:10.1007/s00404-009-1291-x

[17] Mayer K.H., Bush T., Henry K., Overton E.T., Hammer J., Richardson J., et al. Ongoing sexually transmitted disease acquisition and risk-taking behavior among US HIV-infected patients in primary care: implications for prevention interventions. Sex Transm Dis. 2012;**39**(1):1–7. doi:10.1097/OLQ.0b013e31823b1922

[18] Seña A.C., Miller W.C., Hobbs M.M., Schwebke J.R., Leone P.A., Swygard H., et al. *Trichomonas vaginalis* infection in male sexual partners: implications for diagnosis, treatment, and prevention. Clin Infect Dis. 2007;**44**(1):13–22. doi: 10.1086/511144

[19] Pal C., Bandyopadhyay U. Redox-active antiparasitic drugs. Antioxid Redox Signal. 2012;**17**(4):555–582. doi:10.1089/ars.2011.4436

[20] Sobel J.D., Nagappan V., Nyirjesy P. Metronidazole-resistant vaginal trichomoniasis—an emerging problem. N Engl J Med. 1999;**341**(4):292–293. doi:10.1056/NEJM199907223410417

[21] Baka S., Kouskouni E., Antonopoulou S., Sioutis D., Papakonstantinou M., Hassiakos D., et al. Prevalence of *Ureaplasma urealyticum* and *Mycoplasma hominis* in women with chronic urinary symptoms. Urology. 2009;**74**(1):62–66. doi: 10.1016/j.urology.2009.02.014

[22] Wetmore C.M., Manhart L.E., Lowens M.S., Golden M.R., Whittington W.L., Xet-Mull A.M., et al. Demographic, behavioral, and clinical characteristics of men with nongonococcal urethritis differ by etiology: a case-comparison study. Sex Transm Dis. 2011;**38**(3):180–186. doi:10.1097/OLQ.0b013e3182040de9

[23] Manhart L.E., Holmes K.K., Hughes J.P., Houston L.S., Totten P.A. *Mycoplasma genitalium* among young adults in the United States: an emerging sexually transmitted infection. Am J Public Health. 2007;**97**(6):1118–1125. doi: 10.2105/AJPH.2005.074062

[24] Gupta A., Gupta A., Gupta S., Mittal A., Chandra P., Gill A.K. Correlation of mycoplasma with unexplained infertility. Arch Gynecol Obstet. 2009;**280**(6):981–985. doi: 10.1007/s00404-009-1042-z

[25] Taylor-Robinson D. The role of mycoplasmas in pregnancy outcome. Best Pract Res Clin Obstet Gynaecol. 2007;**21**(3):425–438. doi:10.1016/j.bpobgyn.2007.01.011

[26] Reichart M., Kahane I., Bartoov B. In vivo and in vitro impairment of human and ram sperm nuclear chromatin integrity by sexually transmitted *Ureaplasma urealyticum* infection. Biol Reprod. 2000;**63**(4):1041–1048.

[27] Lee J.S., Kim K.T., Lee H.S., Yang K.M., Seo J.T., Choe J.H. Concordance of *Ureaplasma urealyticum* and *Mycoplasma hominis* in infertile couples: impact on semen parameters. Urology. 2013;**81**(6):1219–1224. doi: 10.1016/j.urology.2013.02.044

[28] Mirdh P.A., Paavonen J., Puolakkainen M, editors. Chlamydia. New York: Plenum Press Publishing Co; 1989.

[29] Bianchi A. *Chlamydia trachomatis et Chlamydia pneumoniae*: diagnostic problems. Med Mal Infect. 1999;**29**(Suppl. 1):38–50.

[30] Mol B.W., Dijkman B., Wertheim P., Lijmer J., van der Veen F., Bossuyt P.M. The accuracy of serum chlamydial antibodies in the diagnosis of tubal pathology: a meta-analysis. Fertil Steril. 1997;**67**(6):1031–1037.

[31] Dhama K., Karthik K., Chakraborty S., Tiwari R., Kapoor S., Kumar A., et al. Loop-mediated isothermal amplification of DNA (LAMP): a new diagnostic tool lights the world of diagnosis of animal and human pathogens: a review. Pak J Biol Sci. 2014;**17**(2):151–166.

[32] Van Dyck E., Ieven M., Pattyn S., Van Damme L., Laga M. Detection of *Chlamydia trachomatis* and *Neisseria gonorrhoeae* by enzyme immunoassay, culture, and three nucleic acid amplification tests. J Clin Microbiol. 2001;**39**(5):1751–1756. doi: 10.1128/JCM.39.5.1751-1756.2001

[33] Whiley D.M., Tapsall J.W., Sloots T.P. Nucleic acid amplification testing for *Neisseria gonorrhoeae*: an ongoing challenge. J Mol Diagn. 2006;**8**(1):3–15. doi: 10.2353/jmoldx.2006.050045

[34] Gould S:B., Woehle C., Kusdian G., Landan G., Tachezy J., Zimorski V., et al. Deep sequencing of *Trichomonas vaginalis* during the early infection of vaginal epithelial cells and amoeboid transition. Int J Parasitol. 2013;**43**(9):707–719. doi:10.1016/j.ijpara.2013.04.002

[35] Kissinger P. *Trichomonas vaginalis*: a review of epidemiologic, clinical and treatment issues. BMC Infect Dis. 2015;**15**(1):307. doi:10.1186/s12879-015-1055-0

[36] Diaz N., Dessì D., Dessole S., Fiori P.L., Rappelli P. Rapid detection of coinfections by *Trichomonas vaginalis, Mycoplasma hominis,* and *Ureaplasma urealyticum* by a new multiplex polymerase chain reaction. Diagn Microbiol Infect Dis. 2010;**67**(1):30–36. doi:10.1016/j.diagmicrobio.2009.12.022

[37] Gatski M., Mena L., Levison J., Clark R.A., Henderson H., Schmidt N., et al. Patient-delivered partner treatment and *Trichomonas vaginalis* repeat infection among human immunodeficiency virus-infected women. Sex Transm Dis. 2010;**37**(8):502–505. doi:10.1097/OLQ.0b013e3181d891fc

[38] Hobbs M.M., Lapple D.M., Lawing L.F., Schwebke J.R., Cohen M.S., Swygard H., et al. Methods for detection of *Trichomonas vaginalis* in the male partners of infected women: implications for control of trichomoniasis. J Clin Microbiol. 2006;**44**(11):3994–3999. doi:10.1128/JCM.00952-06

[39] Brooks A.E., Parsamand T., Kelly R.W., Simoes-Barbosa A. An improved quantitative method to assess adhesive properties of *Trichomonas vaginalis* to host vaginal ectocervical cells using flow cytometry. J Microbiol Methods. 2013;**92**(1):73–78. doi:10.1016/j.mimet.2012.10.011

[40] de Waaij D.J., Ouburg S., Dubbink J.H., Peters R.P.H., Morre S.A. Evaluation of Prestoplus assay and LightMix kit *Trichomonas vaginalis* assay for detection of *Trichomonas vaginalis* in dry vaginal swabs. J Microbiol Meth. 2016;**127**:102–104. doi:10.1016/j.mimet.2016.06.002

[41] Waites K.B., Talkington D. New developments of human diseases due to mycoplasmas. In: Blanchard A., Browning G., editors. Mycoplasmas: molecular biology, pathogenicity and strategies for control. Horizon bioscience; 2005. p. 289–354.

[42] Ross J.D., Jensen J.S. *Mycoplasma genitalium* as a sexually transmitted infection: implications for screening, testing, and treatment. Sex Transm Infect. 2006;**82**(4):269–271. doi:10.1136/sti.2005.017368

[43] Samra Z., Rosenberg S., Madar-Shapiro L. Direct simultaneous detection of 6 sexually transmitted pathogens from clinical specimens by multiplex polymerase chain reaction and auto-capillary electrophoresis. Diagn Microbiol Infect Dis. 2011;**70**(1):17–21. doi:10.1016/j.diagmicrobio.2010.12.001

[44] Baseman J.B., Cagle M., Korte J.E., Herrera C., Rasmussen W.G., Baseman J.G., et al. Diagnostic assessment of *Mycoplasma genitalium* in culture-positive women. J Clin Microbiol. 2004;**42**(1):203–211.

[45] Barré A., de Daruvar A., Blanchard A. MolliGen, a database dedicated to the comparative genomics of Mollicutes. Nucleic Acids Res. 2004;**32**:D307–D310. doi: 10.1093/nar/gkh114

[46] Choe H.S., Lee D.S., Lee S.J., Hong S.H., Park D.C., Lee M.K., et al. Performance of Anyplex™ II multiplex real-time PCR for the diagnosis of seven sexually transmitted infections: comparison with currently available methods. Int J Infect Dis. 2013;**17**(12):1134–1140. doi:10.1016/j.ijid.2013.07.011

[47] Citti C., Blanchard A. Mycoplasmas and their host: emerging and re-emerging minimal pathogens. Trends Microbiol. 2013;**21**(4):196–203. doi: 10.1016/j.tim.2013.01.003

[48] O'Byrne P. Self-directed sexually transmitted infection testing: providing noninvasive sexual health services. Appl Nurs Res. 2011;**24**(1):17–21. doi: 10.1016/j.apnr.2009.02.005

[49] Ostergaard L. Diagnosis of urogenital *Chlamydia trachomatis* infection by use of DNA amplification. APMIS Suppl. 1999;**89**:5–36.

[50] Fang J., Husman C., DeSilva L., Chang R., Peralta L. Evaluation of self-collected vaginal swab, first void urine, and endocervical swab specimens for the detection of *Chlamydia trachomatis* and *Neisseria gonorrhoeae* in adolescent females. J Pediatr Adolesc Gynecol. 2008;**21**(6):355–360. doi: 10.1016/j.jpag.2008.03.010

[51] Lee S.J., Park D.C., Lee D.S., Choe H.S., Cho Y.H. Evaluation of Seeplex® STD6 ACE detection kit for the diagnosis of six bacterial sexually transmitted infections. J Infect Chemother. 2012;**18**(4):494–500. doi:10.1007/s10156-011-0362-7

[52] Sturm-Ramirez K., Brumblay H., Diop K., Guèye-Ndiaye A., Sankalé J.L., Thior I., et al. Molecular epidemiology of genital *Chlamydia trachomatis* infection in high-risk women in Senegal, West Africa. J Clin Microbiol. 2000;**38**(1):138–145.

[53] Krõlov K., Frolova J., Tudoran O., Suhorutsenko J., Lehto T., Sibul H., et al. Sensitive and rapid detection of *Chlamydia trachomatis* by recombinase polymerase amplification directly from urine samples. J Mol Diagn. 2014;**16**(1):127–135. doi: 10.1016/j.jmoldx.2013.08.003

[54] U.S. Preventive Services Task Force. Screening for chlamydial infection: U.S. Preventive Services Task Force recommendation statement. Ann Intern Med. 2007;**147**(2):128–134.

[55] U.S. Preventive Services Task Force. Screening for Gonorrhea: recommendation statement. Ann Fam Med. 2005;**3**(3):263–267. doi:10.1370%2Fafm.337

[56] Stary A., Stary G. Sexually transmitted infection. In: Callen J.P., Cerroni L., Heymann W.R., Hruza G., Mancini A.J., Patterson J.W., et al, editors. Dermatology. 3rd ed. Elsevier; 2012. p. 1379–1383.

[57] Keane F.E., Thomas B.J., Gilroy C.B., Renton A., Taylor-Robinson D. The association of *Mycoplasma hominis, Ureaplasma urealyticum* and *Mycoplasma genitalium* with bacterial vaginosis: observations on heterosexual women and their male partners. Int J STD AIDS. 2000;**11**(6):356–360.

[58] Kim S.R., Kim J.H., Gu N.Y., Kim Y.S., Hong Y.C., Ryu J.S. Prevalence of trichomoniasis by PCR in women attending health screening in Korea. Korean J Parasitol. 2016;**54**(2):187–190. doi:10.3347/kjp.2016.54.2.187

[59] Waites K.B., Katz B., Schelonka R.L. Mycoplasmas and ureaplasmas as neonatal pathogens. Clin Microbiol Rev. 2005;**18**(4):757–789. doi:10.1128/CMR.18.4.757-789.2005

[60] Amsel R., Totten P.A., Spiegel C.A., Chen K.C., Eschenbach D., Holmes K.K. Nonspecific vaginitis. Diagnostic criteria and microbial and epidemiologic associations. Am J Med. 1983;**74**(1):14–22.

Permissions

All chapters in this book were first published in FSTI, by InTech Open; hereby published with permission under the Creative Commons Attribution License or equivalent. Every chapter published in this book has been scrutinized by our experts. Their significance has been extensively debated. The topics covered herein carry significant findings which will fuel the growth of the discipline. They may even be implemented as practical applications or may be referred to as a beginning point for another development.

The contributors of this book come from diverse backgrounds, making this book a truly international effort. This book will bring forth new frontiers with its revolutionizing research information and detailed analysis of the nascent developments around the world.

We would like to thank all the contributing authors for lending their expertise to make the book truly unique. They have played a crucial role in the development of this book. Without their invaluable contributions this book wouldn't have been possible. They have made vital efforts to compile up to date information on the varied aspects of this subject to make this book a valuable addition to the collection of many professionals and students.

This book was conceptualized with the vision of imparting up-to-date information and advanced data in this field. To ensure the same, a matchless editorial board was set up. Every individual on the board went through rigorous rounds of assessment to prove their worth. After which they invested a large part of their time researching and compiling the most relevant data for our readers.

The editorial board has been involved in producing this book since its inception. They have spent rigorous hours researching and exploring the diverse topics which have resulted in the successful publishing of this book. They have passed on their knowledge of decades through this book. To expedite this challenging task, the publisher supported the team at every step. A small team of assistant editors was also appointed to further simplify the editing procedure and attain best results for the readers.

Apart from the editorial board, the designing team has also invested a significant amount of their time in understanding the subject and creating the most relevant covers. They scrutinized every image to scout for the most suitable representation of the subject and create an appropriate cover for the book.

The publishing team has been an ardent support to the editorial, designing and production team. Their endless efforts to recruit the best for this project, has resulted in the accomplishment of this book. They are a veteran in the field of academics and their pool of knowledge is as vast as their experience in printing. Their expertise and guidance has proved useful at every step. Their uncompromising quality standards have made this book an exceptional effort. Their encouragement from time to time has been an inspiration for everyone.

The publisher and the editorial board hope that this book will prove to be a valuable piece of knowledge for researchers, students, practitioners and scholars across the globe.

List of Contributors

Agustín Luján, Silvina Fili and María Teresa Damiani
Laboratory of Phagocytosis and Intracellular Transport, IHEM-CONICET, School of Medicine, University of Cuyo, Mendoza, Argentina

Selma Emre
Department of Dermatology, Medical School, Yildirim Beyazit University, Ankara, Turkey

Ayse Akkus
Dermatology Clinic, Tunceli State Hospital, Tunceli, Turkey

Adriana Ancer-Arellano, Jesus Ancer-Rodríguez, Alberto Niderhauser-Garcia and Alvarez-Cuevas Salomón
Faculty of Medicine, Department of Pathology, Autonomous University of Nuevo León, México

David Hardisson
Department of Pathology, Hospital Universitario La Paz, Faculty of Medicine, Universidad Autonoma de Madrid, Madrid, Spain

Jose Sanchez-Hernández and Guadalupe Gallegos-Avila
Sertoli Lab Asociados, Civil Association, Monterrey, Nuevo León, México

Özge Aşkın
Department of Dermatology, Memorial Atasehir Hospital, Istanbul, Turkey

Naveed Shahzad
School of Biological Sciences, University of the Punjab, Lahore, Pakistan

Roman Farooq and Bilal Aslam
Department of Microbiology, Government College University Faisalabad, Pakistan

Muhammad Umer
National Institute for Biotechnology and Genetic Engineering, Faisalabad, Pakistan

Thana Khawcharoenporn
Division of Infectious Diseases, Faculty of Medicine, Thammasat University, Pathumthani, Thailand

Beverly E. Sha
Division of Infectious Diseases, Rush University Medical Center, Chicago, IL, USA

Inaya Hajj Hussein
Oakland University William Beaumont School of Medicine, Rochester, MI, The United States of America

Ibrahim Mortada
Faculty of Medicine, American University of Beirut Medical Center, Beirut, Lebanon

Alice Gerges Geagea
Department of Experimental Biomedicine and Clinical Neuroscience, Section of Human Anatomy, (BIONEC), University of Palermo, Italy

Abdo Jurjus
Department of Anatomy, Cell Biology and Physiological Sciences, Faculty of Medicine, American University of Beirut, Beirut, Lebanon

Marco Vella, Alberto Abrate and Alchiede Simonato
Urological Section, Department of Surgical, Oncological and Stomatological Science, University of Palermo, Palermo, Italy

Antonina Argo
Medico-Legal Section, Department for Health Promotion, Maternal and Child Care, University of Palermo, Palermo, Italy

Tamunomie K Nyengidiki, Goddy Bassey and Ikechukwu Durugbo
Gynaecological Oncology Unit, Department of Obstetrics and Gynaecology, University of Port Harcourt Teaching Hospital, Port Harcourt, Rivers State, Nigeria

Marco Bertini
R&D Department, Laboratori Baldacci SpA, Pisa, Italy

Mihaela L. Vică and Horea V. Matei
Department of Cell and Molecular Biology, "Iuliu Hatieganu" University of Medicine and Pharmacy, Cluj-Napoca, Romania

Costel V. Siserman
Department of Legal Medicine, "Iuliu Hatieganu" University of Medicine and Pharmacy Cluj-Napoca, Romania

Index

www.ingramcontent.com/pod-product-compliance
Lightning Source LLC
LaVergne TN
LVHW080623210926
848485LV00003B/202
9781639894819